Special Care Baby Unit; 3-50

AIDS/HIV INFECTION

A

REFERENCE GUIDE

FOR

NURSING PROFESSIONALS

Jacquelyn Haak Flaskerud, RN, PhD, FAAN

Associate Professor, School of Nursing
Center for Interdisciplinary Research in Immunology and Diseases
University of California, Los Angeles
Los Angeles, California

In cooperation with
The National Institute of Allergy and Infectious Diseases
American Nurses' Association

1989
W.B. SAUNDERS COMPANY
Harcourt Brace Jovanovich, Inc.

Philadelphia · London · Toronto · Montreal · Sydney · Tokyo

W. B. SAUNDERS COMPANY
Harcourt Brace Jovanovich, Inc.

The Curtis Center
Independence Square West
Philadelphia, PA 19106

Library of Congress Cataloging-in-Publication Data

AIDS/HIV infection.

 1. AIDS (Disease)—Nursing. I. Flaskerud,
Jacquelyn Haak. [DNLM: 1. Acquired Immunodeficiency
Syndrome—nurses' instruction. WD 308 A28832]
RC607.A26A3473   1989   610.73'699   88-6645
ISBN 0-7216-2756-0

Editor: Thomas Eoyang
Designer: Joanne Carroll
Production Manager: Carolyn Naylor
Manuscript Editor: Cathy Fix
Indexer: Angela Holt

Aids Reference Guide for Nursing Professionals   ISBN 0-7216-2756-0

Last digit is the print number: 9   8   7   6   5   4   3   2

Dedicated to
the nurses engaged in the
prevention of HIV infection and
the care of persons with HIV infection

and

In Memory Of
those who are gone too soon

Contributors

Jacquelyn Haak Flaskerud R.N., Ph.D., F.A.A.N.
Associate Professor
School of Nursing, UCLA
Center for Interdisciplinary Research in Immunology and
  Diseases (CIRID), UCLA
Los Angeles, California

Elizabeth A. Chaney R.N., M.S.N., J.D.
Attorney-at-Law
Lecturer in Nursing Law
Los Angeles, California

Marsha D. M. Fowler R.N., Ph.D.
Associate Professor, School of Nursing
Graduate School of Theology
Azusa Pacific University
Los Angeles, California

Christine Grady R.N., M.S.N., C.S.
Clinical Nurse Specialist
National Institutes of Health
Bethesda, Maryland

Rose Haque R.N., M.S.N., C.S.
Coordinator, Psychiatric Day Hospital
Hinsdale Hospital
Hinsdale, Illinois

Michael Hedderman R.N., B.S.N.
Nurse Manager, AIDS Services
Los Angeles County/USC Medical Center
Los Angeles, California

Ronnie E. Leibowitz   R.N., M.A., C.I.C.
Nurse Epidemiologist
Veterans Administration Medical Center
New York, New York

Keeta De Stefano Lewis   R.N., B.S.N., P.H.N.
Special Education School Nurse
Napa County Office of Education
Napa, California

Adeline M. Nyamathi   R.N., Ph.D.
Assistant Professor
School of Nursing, UCLA
Los Angeles, California

Nancy B. Parris   R.N., M.P.H.
Nurse Epidemiologist
Department of Hospital Infection Control
UCLA Medical Center
Los Angeles, California

Helen Bosson Thomson   R.N., B.S.N., P.H.N.
Special Education School Nurse
Napa County Office of Education
Napa, California

Peter J. Ungvarski   R.N.C., M.S.N. Candidate
Clinical Nurse Specialist, HIV Infection
Visiting Nurse Service of New York
New York, New York

Peter Wolfe   M.D.
Assistant Clinical Professor
School of Medicine, UCLA
Los Angeles, California

Preface

AIDS/HIV infection is an individual and public health problem in which nurses and nursing care play a vital role. This text grew out of a need among nurses for information about AIDS and HIV infection. The content of the book is based on a national survey of nurses in which they identified: (1) their needs for information about AIDS/HIV infection, (2) the groups to which they were providing counseling, education, and referrals for HIV infection, and (3) the resources they used or preferred to use to gain knowledge of AIDS/HIV infection. The book provides a comprehensive view of the spectrum of HIV infection to assist the nurse in clinical practice, whether that practice be in primary, secondary or tertiary prevention of HIV infection. It serves, as well, as an in-depth text for students learning the practice of nursing or specializing in a nursing clinical area.

Chapters 1 through 3 provide a context into which the AIDS epidemic and the consequent demands on nursing care can be placed:
- The history of the AIDS epidemic and nurses' identified needs for information about AIDS/HIV infection.
- An overview of the sociodemographic distribution of AIDS in the United States, including geographic distribution and transmission groups.
- A description of immunity and how HIV infection affects the immune system.

Nurses' needs for information, as identified in the survey, about the care of persons infected with HIV are addressed in Chapters 4 through 8 and in Chapter 11. These chapters provide guidelines for nursing care that can be applied in the hospital or the community:
- Common infections and neoplasms associated with AIDS and their medical treatment.
- A comprehensive nursing care plan for managing the adult client with HIV infection through primary, secondary, and tertiary prevention measures; the plan is based on symptom assessment and organized by nursing diagnosis.
- A multifaceted look at the nursing care of children with HIV infection and AIDS and the opportunity for prevention of HIV infection through education programs in the schools.
- Infection control guidelines applicable to both the hospital and the community; information on risk to health care workers and household contacts.
- The psychosocial needs of persons with HIV infection, their families, lovers, spouses, and friends, and the nurses caring for them; guidelines for neuropsychiatric assessment and nursing care.

- The ethical and legal concerns of nurses regarding HIV infection: obligation to treat, withholding and withdrawing treatment, mandatory testing, and rights of the nurse with HIV infection.

Information that will assist nurses in counseling, education and referrals is provided in the next two chapters (Chapters 9 and 10) and the final chapter (Chapter 13).

- A detailed account of risk factors and how they provide exposure to HIV and trigger the expression of disease with special attention to transmission groups, minority groups, women and children; information central to health education programs.
- The various community activities that occur surrounding HIV infection: education, counseling, referrals, home care, and hospice care.
- A comprehensive national list of education, health, and community resources, including AIDS service agencies.

Finally, bringing together and giving meaning to much of the information presented in other chapters, a nurse shares her personal experience of living with and caring for a brother with AIDS (Chapter 12).

Readers of this text should be aware of two phenomena associated with the burgeoning literature on HIV infection and AIDS. First, information on HIV infection is constantly developing. Knowledge of infection and the disease may change on a day-by-day basis. Two examples: (1) the sociodemographic distribution of the disease changes daily; and (2) during the editing of this book, it was reported that HIV infects cells of the bowel and rectum directly. This information and other information like it will affect the care and teaching that nurses provide. Nurses should be cognizant of this constant change and keep themselves up-to-date through continuing education courses and by reading the voluminous literature on HIV infection.

Second, because of the vast amount of literature available, there is a diversity of opinion on risk of infection, transmission, and disease expression. This diversity is common to all areas of knowledge that are developing and constantly changing but is exaggerated in the case of AIDS because of the high rate of mortality associated with the disease and because of the social stigma and moral disapproval associated with the largest transmission groups. There are currently many unknowns regarding HIV infection and AIDS. This is partially due to the constant and consistent change in information and partially to the differences in human nature. Opinion on what current information means can reflect attempts to exploit public fear for personal or political gain, competition in the scientific community, public policy and political expediency, professional vs. lay opinion, individual pessimism vs. optimism, and the focus of one discipline as opposed to another. It is important that nurses stay well-informed and abreast of information on HIV infection so that they can sift through the diversity of opinion, give informed care to their clients, and allay their own fears and those of the public. It is in this spirit and with confidence in the intelligence, sensitivity, intentions, and motivation of nurses that the book was written.

Several persons and organizations made important contributions to the development of this text. The survey of nurses' information needs and staff support for the project was funded by the National Institute of Allergy and Infectious Diseases. Special appreciation goes to John Fahey, Director of the Center for Interdisciplinary Research in Immunology and Diseases (CIRID) at UCLA for his belief in and support of the value of the project and his constant encouragement, interest, and ideas. CIRID staff members Diana Shin and Joanne Avers provided valuable assistance and support. The American Nurses' Association (ANA) cooperated with the project by providing sampling lists, position papers, and resource materials. Margaret Fisher analyzed the data. The contributing authors were spirited, cooperative, and inspiring, an intelligent and knowledgeable group with whom it was an honor to work. Peter Ungvarski deserves special recognition for his contributions to several chapters in addition to his own, review of the manuscript, and promotion of the entire project from beginning to end. James Welch, Chair of the ANA Coordinating Committee on AIDS, reviewed the manuscript and provided valuable suggestions. Cecilia Rush and Sean Clark deserve special appreciation. No one put in longer hours on the book than they did. They are commended for their special skills, talents, perseverance, and attention to detail that went into producing this text. Our editor, Tom Eoyang, facilitated this project through his constant belief in it and his unflagging attention, assistance, and string-pulling. Thanks to John Murray for being a source of joy and pride in my life. And finally, a special thank you to my best friend, John Flaskerud, who gave me encouragement, valued critiques and suggestions, good cheer, love, and dinners out.

Contents

APPENDIX B

APPENDIX C

APPENDIX D

Chapter 1

Overview: AIDS/HIV Infection and Nurses' Needs for Information

Jacquelyn Haak Flaskerud

As of this writing, there are over 50,000 cases of AIDS documented in the United States and between 1.5 to 2 million people are believed to be infected by the causative virus. There is no known cure and predictions are that AIDS will be with us until the 21st century (Coolfont Report, 1986).

What Is HIV Infection?

In order to speak knowledgeably and to understand the disease known as AIDS, it is necessary to define the problem in all of its complexity. Acquired immunodeficiency syndrome (AIDS) is the most severe disease state observed to date of a continuum of illnesses related to infection by human immunodeficiency virus (HIV). The virus has also been known as HTLV-III or human T-cell lymphotropic virus type III and LAV or lymphadenopathy-associated virus. HIV infection and AIDS are not synonymous. HIV infection can give rise to a spectrum of outcomes. The spectrum can range from asymptomatic infection to full-blown AIDS. The clinical presentation of HIV infection varies (Fig. 1–1). (Abrams, 1986, 1987; Bennett, 1986; Lang et al., 1985; Schietinger, 1986).

Primary HIV Infection

In many people, the primary HIV infection is subclinical; that is, they experience no symptoms but become seropositive for antibodies to HIV. In some

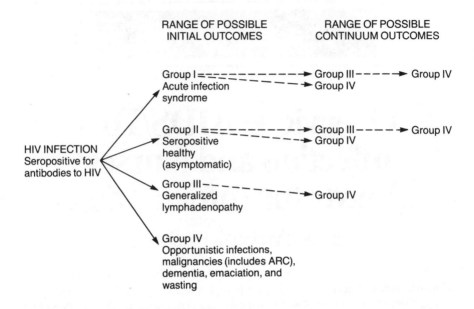

Figure 1–1. Outcomes of HIV infection based on Centers for Disease Control classifications. Dashed lines indicate that some infections in Groups I to III can progress to Groups III and IV.

cases, however, the HIV infection is manifested as an acute illness that occurs two to six weeks after infection. Signs and symptoms may include fever, rigors, arthralgias, and myalgias lasting two to three weeks. Rashes, abdominal cramps, diarrhea, and acute meningitis may also occur. Immunologic abnormalities during primary illness may include mild leukopenia, lymphopenia, thrombocytopenia, elevated erythrocyte sedimentation rate, and relative monocytosis (Abrams, 1987; Bennett, 1986).

HIV Seropositivity

Persons who have had a primary HIV infection will test seropositive on a blood test for antibodies to HIV. Tests commonly in use are the enzyme-linked immunosorbent assay (ELISA), and the Western blot assay and immunofluorescent assay (IFA) techniques for confirming positive results. Used correctly and repeatedly, these tests together have the capability of identifying previous exposure to the virus and avoiding false positive results. A number of situations exist where error might occur but, in general, these tests are over 99% accurate (Abrams, 1986; Ascher & Francis, 1987). An antigen test which is currently being developed will permit early and accurate detection of infection by the virus.

Lymphadenopathy Syndrome (LAS) or Persistent Generalized Lymphadenopathy (PGL)

LAS is a chronic, diffuse, non-cancerous lymph node enlargement. When accompanied by fever, it may be called lymphadenopathy fever syndrome. These terms are used when lymph nodes in at least two extrainguinal sites are swollen to a size of more than 1 cm and remain swollen for three months or longer. Symptoms consist of swollen, sometimes painful nodes, sometimes accompanied by fever, night sweats, weight loss, and enlarged spleen. Prospective studies of persons with LAS project that 20–25% of persons with LAS go on to develop AIDS (Abrams, 1987).

AIDS-Related Complex (ARC)

This term is used when a person who has been infected by HIV has at least two well-developed symptoms of immunodeficiency with at least two laboratory abnormalities. Symptoms such as fever, drenching night sweats, weight loss, fatigue, and lymphadenopathy in the absence of an opportunistic infection or Kaposi's sarcoma have come to be known as ARC. ARC may be a prodrome (precursor) to AIDS or it may be a mild form and the dominant pattern of HIV disease. Whether ARC reflects chronic active infection or is due only to immune abnormalities is not known. As yet there is no way to predict whether a person with ARC will go on to develop full-blown AIDS. Also, patients have developed AIDS without any preceding symptoms (Abrams, 1987).

Acquired Immunodeficiency Syndrome (AIDS)

AIDS is the life-threatening complications of HIV infection, defined as (1) the presence of reliably diagnosed disease at least moderately indicative of underlying cellular immunodeficiency (Kaposi's sarcoma in a patient under 60 years of age, *Pneumocystis carinii* pneumonia or other opportunistic infection, dementia, emaciation, or wasting), and (2) the absence of known causes of underlying immunodeficiency and of any other reduced resistance reported to be associated with the disease (CDC, 1986). These classifications and the diseases associated with HIV infection are discussed in depth in Chapters 3 and 4.

History of AIDS

The history of the AIDS epidemic in the United States is very recent

(Abrams, 1986, 1987; Beckham & Rudy, 1986; CDC, 1981a,b, 1985; Lang et al., 1985; *Time*, Feb. 16, 1987, April 13, 1987).

The name AIDS dates back only to 1982. In June 1981, the first description of what would soon be referred to as AIDS appeared in the Centers for Disease Control's (CDC) *Morbidity and Mortality Weekly Report*. This report described the occurrence of *Pneumocystis carinii* pneumonia (PCP) in five previously healthy, sexually active young homosexual men from Los Angeles, California. This was quickly followed by case reports in New York City of an unusual and extremely rare tumor, Kaposi's sarcoma (KS), also in a male homosexual population.

Both of these conditions occur infrequently. PCP is seen almost exclusively in immunosuppressed individuals. It is a protozoan infection that produces an atypical pneumonia. KS in its classic form was a relatively rare, systemic, multi-centric, neoplastic, angiomatous growth of unknown origin composed of proliferating vascular and fibroelastic elements. It occurred in an indolent form in predominantly elderly males, of black, Italian, and Jewish origin. A more aggressive form of the disease has been seen in young African males. Both the indolent and aggressive forms have been seen in persons, who are immunosuppressed (Abrams, 1986; Ungvarski, 1983).

Throughout the summer of 1981, similar cases were reported to the CDC in increasing numbers. The numbers of cases initially were doubling every six months. In addition to PCP and KS, other types of unusual viral, fungal, and parasitic infections were being diagnosed in young homosexual men. Again, these diseases were previously seen only in severely immunosuppressed individuals. Laboratory studies done on patients with these opportunistic infections and cancers revealed that all of them had severe immunologic deficiencies; clinically they succumbed quickly to these unusual infections.

At first it was thought that only homosexual and bisexual men were affected, and it was hypothesized that some aspect of the gay lifestyle was the probable cause of the immune deficiency. The disease was named gay-related immune deficiency at that stage.

However, as the complex of diseases became more widely known and recognized, other cases were reported to the CDC that made it obvious that AIDS was not a homosexual disease. The same infections and tumors were reported in heterosexual intravenous (IV) drug abusers, Haitian immigrants, persons with hemophilia A, spouses, sexual partners, and children of persons with AIDS or at risk for AIDS, and recipients of blood or blood components from persons infected with AIDS. With the exception of those Haitian immigrants who were found to belong to one of the other risk behavior groups, these others became and currently are the groups at highest risk for AIDS. It soon became apparent that AIDS was transmitted through an exchange of body fluids and principally through blood and semen. Persons who are at increased risk of contracting AIDS were identified as those who were sexually promiscuous, shared needles, received blood or blood products from AIDS-infected individuals, or were the sexual partners or children of these persons. Although sexual transmission occurs both heterosexually and homosexually, currently the largest risk behavior groups in the United States are bisexual and homosexual males followed by IV drug abusers, although the proportion of newly diagnosed IV drug abusers appears to be increasing (Joseph, 1987). These two groups currently account for 90% of persons with AIDS, and males account for 93% (CDC, 1988).

While the number of cases was mounting in the United States, AIDS started appearing in Europe and an interesting phenomenon was observed. Many of the cases were occurring in immigrants from central Africa or in Europeans who plied the major trade routes in central and east Africa. When investigators turned their attention to Africa, they discovered an already existing epidemic, which could be traced to the mid-1970's. A quite different aspect of the epidemic in Africa was that it was affecting men and women equally and cases were widespread in the heterosexual population. The disease has spread to 47 countries in Africa and has been transmitted principally through sexual contact with multiple partners (Lang et al., 1985; WHO, 1988).

There is speculation that AIDS may have existed in Africa for a long time but that it was isolated and not widespread. Either because of a mutation that made it more virulent or transmissible or because of increased travel in a rapidly developing region, AIDS spread to new populations quickly (Lang et al., 1985).

Not until early 1983 in France was there any indication that a virus first discovered in 1980, human T-cell leukemia/lymphotropic virus (HTLV), might be the causative agent. In 1984, in the United States, investigators reported the isolation of a group of cytopathic retroviruses and antibodies against these viruses in AIDS patients. Researchers from the National Institutes of Health reported these findings and termed their virus discovery "human T-lymphotropic virus III (HTLV-III)." Scientists at the Institute Pasteur in France had termed theirs "lymphadenopathy-associated virus (LAV)." For the sake of standardization and communication, the virus is now known worldwide as human immunodeficiency virus (HIV). With the identification of the virus, a test to determine the presence of HIV antibody in the blood was developed. This test made it possible to determine which persons had been infected by HIV and also made possible the screening of blood and blood products to prevent transmission by blood transfusion (Abrams, 1986).

Since 1981, the AIDS epidemic has assumed major proportions; projections indicate that if progress is not made against it, it will rank with history's greatest killers. According to the World Health Organization (1988), cases of AIDS have been reported in over 160 countries. WHO officials estimate that between 5 and 10 million people in the world carry the virus and project that as many as 100 million will become infected in the next 10 years. By 1991, WHO estimates that between 500,000 and 3 million infected people will develop AIDS.

· In the United States, over 50,000 cases have been reported and between 1.5

and 2 million people are estimated to carry the virus. If the epidemic had continued at its current rate, the CDC had expected 270,000 cases by 1991 with a death toll of 179,000. With the new case definitions of AIDS released by the CDC in the summer of 1987, projections are higher.

In Africa, the WHO estimates that 2 to 5 million people are infected, that at least 50,000 people have already died of the disease, and that if a vaccine is not found, another 1.5 million more may succumb. In some African countries 15–25% of the adult population is affected. In Nairobi, Kenya, a study of prostitutes showed that 88% carried the AIDS virus. Epidemiologists have predicted that some countries in Africa could lose 25% of their populations if a cure is not found (*Time*, Feb. 16, 1987).

However, progress has been made against the disease. To summarize that progress since 1981: The probable causative agent of AIDS has been discovered, the virus has been cloned, a bloodscreening program has been implemented, work has begun on the development of a vaccine, and various therapies that extend life have been identified.

Research is going forward on many fronts but currently there is no cure for AIDS and there is no vaccine against it. Prevention is the only effective measure against the disease. Many drugs, chemotherapy, and radiation therapy are used to combat the opportunistic infections and cancers and to enhance the immune system, but so far these have had limited success. The most that can be expected of them thus far is that they will extend life. In the meantime, the number of cases of AIDS has grown to the point where in some cities it is taxing medical resources and is posing an economic threat. It has been predicted that by 1991 most people in certain cities will know someone who has AIDS. It is virtually impossible to provide health care services in those cities without knowledge of AIDS.

The explosion of knowledge about AIDS has been phenomenal. Nurses and other health care workers have a need for in-depth and up-to-date knowledge of AIDS in order to practice. Nurses have close and constant contact with AIDS patients in a variety of settings, and nursing is also one of the principal professions involved in AIDS education and prevention.

Why Nurses Need Knowledge of AIDS/HIV Infection

With few exceptions the care and management of persons with AIDS (PWAs) becomes the responsibility of nurses in secondary and tertiary care centers. In acute care hospitals, nurses provide constant, direct care to AIDS patients who are experiencing exacerbations of their disease. To do so, they need knowledge regarding nursing management of the alterations in health status caused by the disease and precautions to prevent transmission in the workplace.

In home health settings, and in intermediate and long-term care settings, nurses are often the only professionals involved with patients in the remission or chronic phase of their disease on a daily basis. Knowledge regarding prevention, precautions, infection control in the home, nutrition, transmission among household contacts, and safer sexual practices is necessary.

In the younger school population both children and their parents, as well as teachers, might request information from nurses on how HIV infection is spread to allay their fears of having a child with AIDS in the classroom. In addition, the teenage population needs information on safer sexual practices to reduce the likelihood of transmission.

In primary care settings, nurses are in positions to screen and counsel populations at risk for HIV infection and AIDS and to assist in the identification of cases. Nurses have contact with AIDS patients and families in a variety of nursing care and occupational settings and may assume one or more roles in the prevention or care of actual or potential AIDS patients. Nurses working in occupational health settings and nurses working as independent practitioners need assessment skills in determining whether a client might need to be referred for a possible diagnosis of AIDS.

Knowledge of the psychosocial aspects of AIDS and HIV infection is needed by nurses in acute care settings and those working in mental health centers who might be dealing with the depression that accompanies terminal illness, in addition to the dementia associated with AIDS. Knowledge of HIV infection is necessary for counseling persons who have tested positive for HIV antibodies, for those with lymphadenopathy and ARC, and for the "worried well."

Knowledge of supportive therapies to deal with death and dying is needed by mental health nurses, hospital nurses, and community health nurses, as well as by nurses working in hospice settings.

In community settings, nurses need information on prevention, transmission, HIV antibody testing, and psychosocial support to be of service to their clients. In addition they need knowledge of the sexual and lifestyle practices of various subcultures within the United States in order to work effectively and educate. Nurses are also commonly the source of referrals for many of the problems associated with AIDS. Nurses in all settings provide referrals for PWAs, families and friends and are a source of information regarding AIDS to the general public.

Nurses need knowledge about HIV infection and AIDS and the care of PWAs because they have a greater range of contact with AIDS patients and their families than any other single health care professional group. Nurses are also contacted frequently by the public, whether individually or in groups to provide information on AIDS. Finally, in order to give safe and sensitive care to PWAs, nurses must understand the disease and its effects on patients, transmission, and precautions for avoiding infection, and the supportive care needs of patients. Questions have been raised about whether nurses have adequate knowledge of AIDS and the care of PWAs and whether their attitudes interfere with sensitive, supportive, and safe care.

Nurses' Knowledge and Attitudes
and Effect on Practice

Often knowledge and attitudes are interrelated in the care of PWAs. Anxiety, fear, discomfort, embarrassment, and negative social attitudes usually decrease with increased knowledge of the disease and its transmission and experience working with PWAs (Battan & Tabor, 1983; Christ & Wiener, 1985; Frank, 1986; Staff, *Hospitals*, 1984; Nelson et al., 1984; Van Servellen et al., 1988). Fear of the disease and its transmissibility has been probably the most overriding concern of both nurses and physicians. This fear has been translated into nurses leaving their jobs, refusing to care for PWAs, giving only minimal care to these patients, and isolating them inappropriately. In other instances nurses have been observed to use inappropriate precautions and isolation techniques with patients with AIDS (e.g., double gloves, masks and gowns, surgical boots).

The American Nurses' Association in February 1986 released a survey of state nurses' associations' (SNAs') responses to a questionnaire on AIDS that addressed a variety of issues. Twenty-eight SNAs and eight state affiliates of the Emergency Nurses Association responded. Instances of registered nurses refusing to care for AIDS patients were reported by 14 SNAs or affiliates. These were isolated cases that occurred early in the AIDS epidemic; fears were alleviated by education and information on transmission. Employees were being permitted to request reassignment to avoid caring for AIDS patients in nine states; this was not allowed in eight states. If allowed to request reassignment, the employee had to meet certain requirements such as pregnancy or immunosuppressed condition. Only two states reported having to take disciplinary action. In most cases nurses backed down on threats to resign when told that refusal to care for patients with AIDS would result in termination of employment. At the time of the survey, all hospitals and health care facilities in one state were adopting specific guidelines regarding care of PWAs and employee protection from exposure; most hospitals and facilities in seven states were doing so and some hospitals and facilities were doing so in fifteen states.

Nurses' knowledge of AIDS and its transmission as well as clear institutional policies regarding obligation to treat appear to influence attitudes toward caring for PWAs. Knowledge, however, might be inaccurate and inadequate. In January 1986, the Veterans Administration Medical Center in Washington, D.C., and the National Institutes of Health surveyed knowledge of AIDS in 1194 hospital employees (including nurses) of a large urban hospital in Washington, D.C. Significant findings included the following inaccurate beliefs and information regarding AIDS and the consequent effect on the care of patients with AIDS:

1. 50% believed that AIDS could be spread through casual contact
2. 20% believed AIDS could be spread through coughing and sneezing

3. Over 50% said they would wear a gown and mask when caring for an AIDS patient

4. 49% said they spent less time with AIDS patients than with other patients

5. 35% reported actively avoiding involvement with patients with AIDS (Macks, 1986).

A survey of nurses in California (N = 1019) demonstrated other areas of knowledge deficit of AIDS and consequent behavior toward persons with AIDS (Van Servellen et al., 1988). About half of these nurses had cared for a patient with AIDS in the last six months and two-thirds cared for patients at risk for or concerned about contracting AIDS; 62% of the sample were general staff nurses. Knowledge and practice deficits occurred in correctly distinguishing the symptoms of AIDS (88% could not) and in taking a sexual history (91% did not). However, 69% were able to identify the groups at risk for AIDS, and 82% could identify the correct infection control procedures. The effect on patient care could be inferred from the findings: 23% said they absolutely would not care for patients with AIDS and 54% said that nurses should be allowed to refuse care for patients having or suspected of having AIDS. Nurses who had recently cared for AIDS patients and those at risk and who had attended lectures and education forums on AIDS were more likely to have knowledge of AIDS symptoms, groups at risk and necessary precautions. They were also more willing to care for PWAs.

Other studies have shown that accurate knowledge about AIDS has been significantly correlated with low anxiety, willingness to work with PWAs, and appropriate professional behavior toward PWAs (Christ & Wiener, 1985; Macks, 1986). In general, accurate and regular in-service education on transmission and infection control, clear and consistent institutional policies on precautions for health care workers, and clear and consistent institutional guidelines on the obligation to treat have decreased the fear and inappropriate behaviors of nurses working with patients with AIDS (Malik-Nitto & Plantemoli, 1986). These fears and behaviors have decreased as accurate knowledge of AIDS and its transmission has become available to health care workers.

For some time now, available evidence has indicated that the risk to health care workers is small and that the recommendations for precautions for health care personnel in the workplace are adequate. In addition, the Centers for Disease Control's prospective study of percutaneous injuries to health care workers caring for patients with AIDS has further quieted fears about the risk of acquiring AIDS to nurses in the workplace (1987). There remains, however, evidence of some paranoia among nurses and physicians that the government, their hospital, researchers, or the Centers for Disease Control are withholding information on the transmission of AIDS (Ostrow & Gayle, 1986; Simmons-Alling, 1984). This attitude appears to be most prevalent among health care workers who have had less contact with PWAs and less knowledge of AIDS. In the study by Van Servellen et al. (1988) about 25% of nurses surveyed believed they were at high to moderate risk for contracting AIDS because of occupational or environmental exposure in their current work role. These nurses were also less knowledgeable of the correct precautions to take when caring for patients with AIDS and were uncomfortable caring for male homosexual patients.

This finding focuses attention on a second area of difficulty, which has arisen because nurses have made moral and social judgments about the worth and value of persons with AIDS. Nurses have refused to care for clients because of negative attitudes toward the sexual behaviors and lifestyles of some groups, such as homosexuals, IV drug abusers, and prostitutes. In several studies of health care workers' attitudes toward homosexuals, homophobia among physicians and nurses was assessed. The first study done at Cornell University surveyed 37 medical staff and 91 registered nurses in the New York area, and the second study surveyed 250 registered nurses living in San Francisco. Physicians in San Diego were also surveyed. Using the Index of Homophobia scale these studies reported low-grade homophobia among the nurses and physicians surveyed in New York, San Diego, and San Francisco. Having a gay friend or relative was significantly correlated with more positive attitudes and feelings toward homosexuals. About 10% believed that persons with AIDS were getting what they deserved (Douglas et al., 1985; Macks, 1986; Matthews et al., 1986).

In the study by Van Servellen et al. (1988) about half the nurses surveyed felt that the average nurse was uncomfortable discussing sexual matters with male homosexual patients and 38% indicated moderate to great discomfort compared to their colleagues when caring for these patients. These nurses were more likely to believe that they should be allowed to refuse to care for AIDS patients and that they were at high risk for contracting AIDS, and to use overly cautious isolation techniques. They were also less knowledgeable about AIDS symptoms, risk groups, and correct precautions.

Nurses' Needs for AIDS Information

Nurses have responded to the AIDS epidemic by identifying their specific informational needs and by identifying which resources can best meet their needs for information and education.

An American Nurses' Association Survey (February, 1986) asked SNAs to identify their needs for assistance in dealing with AIDS. The states identified the following areas of concern to nurses:

1. education on AIDS, nursing care of AIDS patients and transmission in the workplace through workshops, featured articles in nursing journals and newspapers, pamphlets for nurses and a speaker's bureau.

2. legislative updates; and

3. a professional position statement or policy statement and guidelines for nurses and nursing care in legal and ethical areas.

The American Nurses' Association (ANA) has responded to these requests from nurses through its Cabinet on Human Rights, Committee on AIDS (ANA,

1986b,c). The ANA has developed a strategic plan regarding AIDS that addresses the following broad issues:

1. Education for health care workers and the public
2. Prevention and risk reduction
3. Protection of civil and human rights of affected persons and care givers
4. Funding for care, research, and dissemination of information.

To implement these goals, the ANA has developed policy statements, established linkages and coordinated with other organizations to share information and resources, encouraged registered nurse representation on local and state AIDS task forces, and distributed AIDS educational materials to SNAs. In this last regard, ANA has developed and distributed an annotated AIDS bibliography (1986), participated in an AIDS teleconference sponsored by the Bureau of National Affairs and the Public Broadcasting Services, and assisted in distributing booklets on AIDS produced by the Surgeon General's Office, the National Institute of Mental Health, and the Centers for Disease Control. The most recent publication of the ANA defines nursing's role and ethical perspectives in the prevention and treatment of HIV infection as these affect nursing care, coordination of services, education, advocacy, and research. Materials referred to here can be obtained from the ANA in Kansas City to assist nurses in meeting their educational needs. The ANA has also served as a cooperating agency in the production of this text.

In addition to the ANA survey of its SNAs to determine nurses' needs for AIDS information, other surveys of nurses themselves have been conducted. Nurses have reaffirmed the same areas of needs in these other surveys and have indicated an eagerness for information and education. In 1985, the Center for Interdisciplinary Research in Immunology and Diseases (CIRID) at UCLA surveyed a sample of health professionals ($N = 163$) who had purchased their publication, *AIDS Reference Guide for Medical Professionals.* The purpose of the survey was to determine whether the Guide was meeting consumers' needs for information and education on AIDS. Of those responding to the survey, 35% were nurses who were using this educational resource. Nurse respondents were using the Guide for general professional interest (100%), for patient information (57%), and for patient's family information (93%); 56% indicated that they used the Guide frequently. Nurse respondents shared information with colleagues (75%), the public (23%), and students (2%). In addition to presenting a picture of health professionals who were interested in information on AIDS, nurse respondents identified specific areas in which they needed more information.

Nurses as a group used the section of the Guide on psychosocial aspects of AIDS more than other health professionals. They indicated that they needed even more information in this area (psychosocial needs of patients), as well as information on legal and ethical aspects of the care of PWAs, and on prevention of, precautions against, and transmission of the disease.

Furthermore, nurses identified their preferred sources for education: 83%

used continuing education courses to learn more about AIDS; 96.3% used professional journals; 94% used newspapers and magazines, and 77% used television as a source of information on AIDS. Despite these sources, nurse respondents asked for more information: 100% wanted information on AIDS research; 85% wanted more continuing education courses; and 74.3% wanted more frequent updates on AIDS information. About a third (31.7%) wanted to be updated every one to two months and 42.6%, every three to four months. These data suggested a picture of nurses as interested consumers of AIDS education who could specify their educational needs and identify their preferred sources of information.

Because the sample for the above data was small and located mostly in California, the CIRID conducted an extensive national survey of nurses, asking them to identify their needs for information about AIDS and their preferred sources of information. The purpose of this survey was to provide the data needed to produce a comprehensive reference guide for nurses on AIDS. This text is the result of that survey.

Data were collected from August 1986 through March 1987 from 832 nurses in 48 states and the District of Columbia. Respondents represented four groups: medical-surgical nurses (N=194), community health nurses (N=194), psychiatric-mental health nurses (N=233), and school nurses (N=211). The sample was well educated: 93.7% had a bachelor's degree in nursing or higher degree. Their primary occupational settings were schools (23.4%), hospitals (24.3%), community health facilities (17.6%), schools of nursing (21.7%), and mental health facilities (10.7%). They had practiced their present occupation from 1–47 years with a mean of 12 years. They ranged in age from 22–72 years with a mean of 44.3 years, and 97% were female.

Just over 50% of respondents considered it very likely that they would see a patient with AIDS in the next six months (Table 1–1). Respondents were asked to indicate their needs for a variety of information on AIDS. In general, need for information was high in every category queried despite a substantial nursing and related medical literature on the topic of AIDS and the care of AIDS patients, and frequent attention to AIDS in nursing continuing education courses, programs and conferences. Results of the survey accompany each of the chapters in this text. A general summary of the results is provided here.

Nurses were asked to indicate their needs for information on:
1. case definition,
2. case reporting,
3. groups at risk,
4. transmission in the workplace,
5. precautions,
6. AIDS symptom assessment,
7. neuropsychiatric syndromes,
8. psychosocial care,
9. prevention,

Table 1-1. Nurses' Contact With AIDS Patients

	MS	CH	PMH	SCH
Likelihood of seeing a patient with AIDS in the next six months	N=194 %	N=194 %	N=233 %	N=211 %
Very likely	69	61	60	19
Not likely	31	39	40	81

10. safer sexual practices,
11. legal and ethical aspects, and
12. resources and services available to patients and families.

Over 50% of the sample indicated need for information in all of the categories queried. In some categories over 70% of the sample indicated need for information (Table 1-2). As in previous surveys of nurses, information needs on psychosocial issues, legal and ethical issues, transmission, and precautions remained paramount. In addition nurses identified need for information on case definitions of AIDS, ARC, and HIV infection, AIDS symptom assessment and neuropsychiatric syndromes, prevention, and safer sexual practices. They were particularly interested in resources or services provided by community medical centers and referral centers.

These informational needs were fairly consistent across the four groups of nurses surveyed. However, school nurses' needs for information in the various categories, while high, were consistently lower than the other groups, except when the issue was pediatric AIDS. In all four groups, large percentages of respondents indicated needs for information in the areas of prevention and precautions for nurses and other health care workers (HCWs). Medical-surgical nurse respondents indicated the greatest number of categories of need; community health nurses were next, followed by psychiatric-mental health nurses and then school nurses.

In addition to the direct care they provide to patients, nurses also provide information or assistance through education, counseling, and referrals to a wide range of persons interested in AIDS. Nurses surveyed were asked to identify the groups to whom they provide such assistance. They were asked to indicate their likelihood of providing AIDS-related education, counseling, or referrals to:

1. the groups at risk,
2. community groups, and
3. other health care workers.

One quarter to three quarters of the nurses surveyed assist all of these groups by providing information, counseling, or referrals. They are most likely to assist other health care workers, especially those in in-patient settings who give direct care to patients (Table 1-3).

Differences in giving assistance occurred according to clinical specialty

Table 1–2. Nurses' Needs for AIDS Information

Needs for Information	MS N=194 %	CH N=194 %	PMH N=233 %	SCH N=211 %
Case definition				
AIDS	81	75	69	74
ARC	78	75	64	73
Pediatric AIDS	43	69	44	84
HIV infection	82	77	68	77
Case reporting				
Adult AIDS	72	73	58	45
Pediatric AIDS	43	65	36	68
HIV positive	74	76	58	55
Groups at risk				
Homosexually-bisexually active males	59	69	68	42
IV drug users	64	64	58	41
Blood recipients	69	64	47	60
Prostitutes	50	63	51	25
Sexual partners of above	66	70	71	39
Transmission in the workplace	85	79	76	78
Precautions				
For nurses/health professionals	91	90	82	86
For persons living with AIDS patients	86	85	73	69
For minimizing infection	85	81	72	67
Assessment of symptoms	93	80	73	76
Neuropsychiatric syndromes	83	75	86	60
Psychosocial care				
Of patients	89	83	82	65
Of families	88	84	82	68
Of HCWs	87	84	86	66
Prevention	88	87	84	86
Safer sexual practices	73	80	83	66
Legal-ethical aspects				
Rights of HCWs	89	87	78	78
Rights of patients	85	87	76	73
Ethical issues	93	86	82	73
Confidentiality/privacy	76	81	81	73
Resources/services available				
Home health nursing	80	75	67	57
Community medical	79	75	68	70
University medical	63	65	58	61
Referral centers	79	78	71	72
AIDS hotlines	66	70	63	63
Financial assistance	66	72	61	56
HIV testing sites	69	67	62	56

group, but probably more importantly according to work setting. All four groups of nurses appeared to provide assistance to their fellow workers as well as to persons with whom they would be expected to come in contact in their respective settings (e.g., schools, community, hospitals, mental health facilities). Of the groups at risk, homosexuals/bisexuals and IV drug abusers were assisted most often by

Table 1–3. Groups Nurses Assist Through Education, Counseling, and Referrals

Groups Assisted	MS	CH	PMH	SCH
	N=194	N=194	N=233	N=211
	%	%	%	%
Groups at risk				
Homosexually-bisexually active males	44	50	65	20
-Families of	56	63	62	40
-Sexual partners of	44	56	61	20
IV drug abusers	44	46	53	18
-Families of	48	55	54	34
-Sexual partners of	37	49	53	17
Prostitutes	18	34	33	5
-Families of	25	32	31	16
-Sexual partners of	22	37	36	10
Blood recipients/hemophiliacs	74	58	32	66
-Families of	70	61	34	69
-Sexual partners of	52	48	32	22
Community groups				
School-age children	26	47	22	84
-Parents of	36	62	36	89
Teenagers	35	59	44	80
-Parents of	45	58	49	79
Teachers, principals	32	57	31	94
Teaching assistants	29	48	24	91
Police	37	42	24	17
Firefighters	33	38	22	15
Health care workers (HCWs)				
Other nurses	87	82	79	62
Nursing assistants	86	81	77	62
Social workers/psychologists	59	71	70	74
Hospice workers	46	61	36	15
Home health aides	40	70	35	16
Clerical workers	56	63	50	66
Food service workers	48	42	34	68
Maintenance workers	48	36	33	70

community health and psychiatric-mental health nurses. Blood recipients and hemophiliacs were assisted by medical-surgical and school nurses. School and community nurses were assisting children, teenagers, and their parents. Groups receiving the least assistance from any of the nurse specialty groups were prostitutes, police, and firefighters. Groups receiving assistance from all the nurse specialty groups were other nurses, nursing assistants, and social workers/psychologists. These differences indicate which groups of nurses have contact with which population groups and provide direction for supplying appropriate information to nurses according to their specialty that will enhance their practice.

Finally, the nurses surveyed were asked to identify their preferred sources of information on AIDS and the care of patients with AIDS. Respondents overwhelmingly preferred continuing education courses; professional journals, newspapers, magazines; and TV/radio as sources of information about AIDS

Table 1–4. Nurses' Preferred Resources for Information

Educational Resources	MS	CH	PMH	SCH
	N=194	N=194	N=233	N=211
	%	%	%	%
CE conferences & workshops	89	83	81	95
General nursing journals	87	86	77	72
Specialty nursing journals	83	74	86	89
CDC Reports	32	60	32	49
Local public health newsletters	16	19	14	58
Newspapers/magazines	83	84	89	91
TV/radio	81	80	86	81
AIDS nursing update newsletter	39	41	43	50

(Table 1–4). Respondents were offered the choice of other sources of information such as interdisciplinary journals as well as newsletters, computer networks, and periodic reports. In addition to general sources of information preferred by all groups of respondents, each clinical specialty group had favorite sources such as clinical specialty journals and newsletters or reports.

The data gathered from the survey demonstrated that the scope of nurses' needs for AIDS education and information is quite comprehensive. This information is needed for direct care of AIDS patients (51% expect to give direct care) and to provide indirect care through counseling, public education and referral. The scope of nurses' indirect care giving is wide ranging. From the data it can be ascertained that the information nurses need should address:

1. physical care and emotional support of patients and their families in institutions, the home, and the community;

2. prevention of the spread of infectious agents in the environment;

3. protection of the patient, the public, and nurses; and

4. guidelines for care within individual settings that address legal and ethical issues, protect both the needs and rights of patients and the rights of workers, and allow professional judgment in the delivery of care.

Nurses' identified needs for information guided the development and content of the chapters in this book. In addition, information that provided a context for the identified educational information needed was included also.

These data can be used by nurses using the text to guide them in designing continuing education offerings or in-service education workshops. They can be used to give direction to the content or emphasis of educational publications on AIDS or audiovisual presentations on the topic. They can be used also to select the sources preferred by nurses for presenting information to specific groups of nurses.

The data will be used by the Editor of this text as a baseline for comparing nurses' needs for information before and after use of the text. In addition, these data will serve as a foundation for updating the text through an AIDS nursing update periodical publication. This periodical will be based on nurses' follow-up evaluations and on identification of future needs for AIDS information.

In this regard it is important to note that information about AIDS is changing so rapidly that it is impossible to publish anything that is completely up to date. For this reason, it is especially important for nurses to remain aware of new developments and changes in information about AIDS. Close attention to AIDS-related research, conferences, and information in the popular media can assist nurses in keeping up with the various issues and information surrounding AIDS.

Survey results are reported in raw form so that other nurses can also use them as a baseline for identifying changes in nurses' needs for information regarding AIDS. By using these data in this fashion, it would be possible to create a network of AIDS information for nurses that would increase their knowledge, influence their attitudes, and provide the basis for safe and sensitive care of persons with HIV infection and AIDS. Such a network could also lay the ground work for cooperative nursing research on AIDS. Nurses interested in pursuing any of the ideas suggested here should contact the Principal Investigator/Editor of this text.

References

Abrams, D.I. (1986). AIDS: Battling a retroviral enemy. *California Nursing Review, 8*(6), 10–16, 36–37, 44.

Abrams, D.I. (1987). AIDS: A search for hope. *California Nursing Review, 9*(1), 4–7, 11–13, 38–40.

American Nurses' Association (February 1986a). Survey of state nurses' associations. Questionnaire on AIDS. Kansas City, MO.

American Nurses' Association (July 1986b). Informational Report of Cabinet on Human Rights. Acquired immune deficiency syndrome (AIDS). Kansas City, MO.

American Nurses' Association (November 1986c). Cabinet of Economic and General Welfare. Statement on serologic testing of health care workers for human immunodeficiency virus antibody. Kansas City, MO.

American Nurses Association (1986d). Task Force on AIDS. Annotated bibliography on AIDS. Kansas City, MO.

American Nurses Association (1988). Nursing and the Human Responses to AIDS/HIV Infection, Kansas City, MO

Ascher, M.S. & Francis, D.P. (1987). Is the blood supply safe from AIDS? *California Physician, 4*(7), 18–19.

Battan, C. & Tabor, R. (1983). Nursing the patient with AIDS. *Cancer Nursing, 79* (10), 19–22.

Beckman, M.M. & Rudy, E.B. (1986). Acquired immunodeficiency syndrome. *Journal of Neuroscience Nursing, 18*(1), 5–10.

Bennett, J.A. (1986). AIDS: what we know. *American Journal of Nursing, 86*, 1016–1020.

Centers for Disease Control (1981). Pneumocystis pneumonia–Los Angeles. *Morbidity & Mortality Weekly Report, 30*, 250–253.

Centers for Disease Control (1981). Kaposi's sarcoma and pneumocystis pneumonia among homosexual men–New York City and California. *Morbidity & Mortality Weekly Report,* 30, 305–309.

Centers for Disease Control (1985). WHO workshop: Conclusions and Recommendations on AIDS. *Morbidity & Mortality Weekly Report, 34*, 275.

Centers for Disease Control (1986). Classification system for human T–lymphotropic virus III/lymphadenopathy–associated virus infections. *Morbidity & Mortality Weekly Report, 35*, 335.

Centers for Disease Control (1987). Update: Human immunodeficiency virus infections in health care workers exposed to blood of infected persons. *Morbidity & Mortality Weekly Report, 36*(19), 285–289.

Centers for Disease Control (February, 1988) *AIDS Weekly Surveillance Report.* United States AIDS Program, Atlanta, GA.

Christ, G.H. & Wiener, L.S. (1985). Psychosocial issues in AIDS. In V.T. DeVita Jr., Editor. *AIDS Etiology, Diagnosis, Treatment and Prevention*. Philadelphia: J.B. Lippincott, pp. 275–297.

Coolfont Report (1986). A PHS plan for prevention and control of AIDS and the AIDS virus. *Public Health Report, 101*, 341–348.

Douglas, C.J., Kalman, C.M., & Kalman, T.P. (1985). Homophobia among physicians and nurses: An empirical study. *Hospital and Community Psychiatry, 36*(12), 1309 1311.

Frank, H. (1986). AIDS – The responsibility of health workers to assume some degree of personal risk. *Western Journal of Medicine, 144*(3), 363–364.

Joseph, S.C. (1987). AIDS in New York City: Moving ahead on effective public health approaches. *New York State Journal of Medicine, 87*(5), 257–258.

Lang, J.M., Spiegel, J., & Strigle, S.M. (eds). (1985). *Living with AIDS*. AIDS Project Los Angeles, Los Angeles, CA.

Macks, J. (1986). The Paris AIDS conference: psychosocial research. *Focus. 1*(10), 1–2.

Malik–Nitto, S. & Plantemoli, L. (1986). A strategic plan for the management of patients with AIDS. *Nursing Management, 17*(6), 46–48.

Matthews, W.C., Booth, M.W., Turney, J.D., et al. (1986). Physicians' attitudes toward homosexuality: survey of a California medical society. *Western Journal of Medicine, 144*, 106–110.

Nelson, W.J., Maxey, L., & Keith, S. (July 1984). Are we abandoning the AIDS patient? *RN, 47*, 18–19.

Ostrow, D.G., & Gayle, T.C. (August 1986). Psychosocial and ethical issues of AIDS health care programs. *Quality Review Bulletin, 12*, 284–294.

Schietinger, H. (1986). A home care plan for AIDS. *American Journal of Nursing, 86*, 1021–1028.

Simmons–Alling, S. (1984). AIDS: psychosocial needs of the health care worker. *Topics in Clinical Nursing, 6*, 31– 37.

Staff (Feb. 1, 1984). Educating staff about AIDS eases hysteria. *Hospitals, 58*, 40–43.

Time (Feb. 16, 1987). The big chill, fear of AIDS; "You haven't heard anything yet;" In the grip of the scourge. pp. 56–59.

Time (April 13, 1987). Yalta of AIDS. p. 60.

Ungvarski, P. (1983). Acquired immune deficiency syndrome. *Nursing Mirror, 157*, 17–20.

Van Servellen, G.M., Lewis, C.E., & Leake, B. (1988). Nurses' knowledge, attitudes, and fears about AIDS. *Nursing Management*, (in press).

World Health Organization data, February 1988.

Chapter 2

Sociodemographic Distribution of AIDS

Ronnie E. Leibowitz

Epidemics have often been more influential than statesmen and soldiers in shaping the course of political history, and diseases may also color the moods of civilizations.

René and Jean Dubos, *in* The White Plague.

Based on World Health Organization (WHO) data, AIDS must be considered a worldwide epidemic, necessitating a global effort to control its transmission. Since a vaccine or any curative therapy for AIDS is currently not available, this disease must be considered the most serious epidemic of the past 50 years (Quinn et al., 1986). Cultural differences, endemic diseases, and other unidentified risk factors may affect the epidemiologic and clinical features of HIV infection in different countries. However, the immunopathogenesis of HIV infection for the most part is similar in most persons with AIDS (Quinn et al., 1986). Because the number of cases of AIDS worldwide and in the United States is constantly increasing, numbers in this chapter will be out of date at the time of publication. Numbers and percentages do, however, reflect trends in the distribution of AIDS and the magnitude of the problem. They should be viewed from that perspective.

As of February 1988, over 75,392 cases of AIDS were reported to the WHO from 161 countries representing all continents (Table 2–1). However, official reports grossly understate the true magnitude of the AIDS epidemic, particularly in Africa and the Caribbean, where many cases are neither diagnosed nor counted according to WHO. The largest percentage (79.1%) of the cases have been reported from the Americas. Europe has reported 11% of the total; Africa 8.6% of the total;

Table 2–1. Worldwide Reported Cases of AIDS
WHO Data as of February 1988
Total Cases = 75,392

Continent	% of Total	# of Countries Reporting Cases
Americas	79.1	44
Europe	11.0	28
Africa	8.6	47
Oceania	1.0	14
Asia	0.3	28
Total	100.0	161

Oceania 1% of the total; and Asia 0.3% of the total. Slightly over 90% of the cases have been reported to the WHO from 12 countries, with the United States leading the list with 69.7% (Table 2–2).

Africa

Although the fact is often denied, this region of the world is the most affected by HIV infection and AIDS. The African continent probably has the highest proportion of HIV infection in the healthy population and the highest incidence of clinical AIDS (Assad & Mann, 1987). Denial of disease in Africa may be the result of national pride, fear of stigmatization, economic repercussions of admitting the existence of AIDS (e.g., decreased tourism), and concerns about the local, social, and political consequences of a disease for which prevention and treatment resources are unavailable (Imperato, 1987).

HIV infection has been detected in increasing numbers in areas of Africa thought to be free of infection (Quinn et al., 1986). It is difficult to determine,

Table 2–2. Reported Cases of AIDS in Selected Countries
WHO Data as of February 1988
Total Cases = 75,392

Country	Continent	% of Total
United States	America	69.7
Brazil	America	3.2
France	Europe	3.1
Uganda	Africa	2.1
Tanzania	Africa	2.1
Federal Republic of Germany	Europe	2.0
Canada	America	1.9
Haiti	America	1.6
United Kingdom	Europe	1.5
Rwanda	Africa	1.3
Italy	Europe	1.2
Australia	Oceania	0.9

Table 2–3. Factors in Heterosexual Transmission of HIV Infection in Africa*

1. Ratio of male to female cases is 1:1.
2. Female cases = younger age and single marital status.
3. Case-control studies have shown:
   a. Cases have a significantly higher number of heterosexual partners than controls (mean = 32 vs. 3).
   b. Male patients have had sex significantly more often with female prostitutes (81 vs. 34%).
   c. Risk of seropositivity increases significantly with the number of different sexual partners per year and with a history of other sexually transmitted diseases.
   d. Risk of seropositivity increases significantly in individuals who are sexual partners of infected persons.
4. Prostitutes have the highest infection rate (27 to 88%).

* Adapted from Quinn et al. (1986) and Quinn (1987).

however, if the virus has been introduced to these areas recently or if the virus has been recognized only recently (i.e., increasing awareness of the virus more recently). The areas most severely affected appear to be the countries in central and eastern Africa. Risk factors for transmission of HIV infection in Africa include, but are not limited to, heterosexual activity, blood transfusions, transmission from mother to infant, and frequent exposure to unsterilized needles or other invasive equipment (Imperato, 1986; Quinn, 1987). It must be noted that both national and international experts in sexually transmitted diseases have failed to verify homosexuality and/or intravenous drug abuse as risk factors in Africa (Quinn et al., 1986). Additionally, amplification of HIV transmission has been attributed to urbanization, major population shifts from rural villages to urban centers, and increased numbers of (and visitations to) prostitutes in cities (Francis & Chin, 1987). There is a low prevalence rate of HIV infection in 2 to 14 year olds, an indication that this is not an arthropod-transmitted disease, for which one would expect a high infection rate in this age group (Quinn, 1987; Zuckerman, 1986).

Heterosexual Transmission. Evidence for heterosexual transmission of HIV infection in Africa can be seen in Table 2–3. Bidirectional transmission (from female-to-male as well as male-to-female) of HIV may occur among heterosexual contacts since the virus has been isolated from cervical-vaginal secretions as well as semen. African males with AIDS, as well as males with AIDS who previously lived in Africa, frequently report a history of sexual contact with prostitutes. An increasing number of heterosexual males presenting for treatment at sexually transmitted disease clinics are HIV seropositive, thus suggesting female-to-male transmission (Fauci, 1986; Quinn et al., 1986). Furthermore, 90 to 100% of heterosexual males in Zaire had serologic evidence of infection with cytomegalovirus, Epstein-Barr virus and hepatitis B virus, which is comparable to the incidence in homosexual males in the United States (Fauci, 1986).

Blood Transfusions. The seroprevalence rate of HIV among blood donors in Uganda, Rwanda, and Zaire range from 8% to 18% and therefore the risk of transmission of HIV infection to transfusion recipients in these African countries and in countries to which blood from Africa is exported is high (Quinn et al.,

1986). Additional information which supports blood transfusion as a risk factor for transmission of HIV in Africa includes the following:

1. screening of donors for hepatitis B and HIV is not done in many areas;

2. storage and processing facilities are rudimentary in many areas of the continent; and

3. efforts to identify and exclude high-risk donors based on epidemiologic or clinical grounds have been largely unsuccessful thus far.

The potential spread of HIV infection in Africa may actually be a result of the medical overuse of transfusions as well as patient expectations of blood transfusions in treatment of disease (Quinn et al., 1986).

Perinatal Transmission. A large number of African women of childbearing age are exposed to HIV as a result of heterosexual transmission. A strong association appears to be present between maternal HIV infection and infant seropositivity in Africa, as it is in the United States. However, it is unclear whether these children acquired maternal HIV antibody passively or acquired the virus perinatally (Quinn et al., 1986).

Injections. There are several regional practices in Africa related to needles that should be mentioned:

1. there is often a preference for parenteral rather than oral therapy—it is felt to be more effective;

2. personnel inadequately trained in aseptic techniques may be administering injections and/or causing scarifications with needles; and

3. disposable equipment is often reused and therefore may be contaminated or inadequately sterilized (Quinn et al., 1986).

United States

As of February 1988, over 52,256 cases of AIDS in the United States were reported to the Centers for Disease Control (CDC) with a total of 29,206 (55.9%) deaths (CDC, 1988). Table 2–4 displays a cumulative total of AIDS cases and deaths reported to the CDC by transmission categories. Based on the number of cases reported to the CDC, New York State led the list with 26.5% of the total, California was second with 22.0%, Florida was third with 7.3%, Texas was fourth with 7.0%, and New Jersey was fifth with 6.3% (CDC, 1988). Ninety-three percent of the cases reported to the CDC have occurred in males and 7% have occurred in females. Forty-seven percent of the cases have been in the 30–39 age group, and 21% each have been in the 20–29 and 40–49 age groups (CDC, 1988). AIDS is now the leading cause of death in New York City among men aged 25–44 and women aged 25–29 (Joseph, 1987a). The age distribution of cases of AIDS by racial/ethnic group is displayed in Table 2–5. See Table 2–6 for a display of the transmission categories of cases of AIDS by racial/ethnic group.

Homosexual/Bisexual Males. Sixty-six percent of the cases of AIDS reported

Table 2–4. Distribution of AIDS Cases and Deaths by Transmission Categories
as Reported to the CDC by February 1988

Transmission Categories[1]	Cumulative Cases and Deaths Since June 1981			
	# Cases	%	# Deaths	%
Adults/Adolescents				
Homosexual/Bisexual Male	33,369	(64.8)	18,248	(63.5)
Intravenous Drug Abuser (IVDA)	8,877	(17.2)	5,091	(17.7)
Homosexual Male and IVDA	3,858	(7.5)	2,248	(7.8)
Hemophilia/Coagulation Disorder	519	(1.0)	305	(1.1)
Heterosexual Cases	2,058	(4.0)	1,139	(4.0)
Transfusion, Blood/Components	1,206	(2.3)	813	(2.8)
Undetermined	1,580	(3.1)	888	(3.1)
SUBTOTAL	51,467	(100.0)	28,732	(100.0)
Children[2]				
Hemophilia/Coagulation Disorder	43	(5.4)	27	(5.7)
Parent with/at risk of AIDS[3]	603	(76.4)	360	(75.9)
Transfusion, Blood/Components	108	(13.7)	69	(14.6)
Undetermined	35	(4.4)	18	(3.8)
SUBTOTAL	789	(100.0)	474	(100.0)
TOTAL	52,256		29,206	

[1] Cases with more than one risk factor other than the combinations listed in the table are tabulated only in the category listed first.
[2] Includes all patients under 13 years of age at time of diagnosis.
[3] Epidemiologic data suggest transmission from an infected mother to her fetus or infant during the perinatal period.
Source: CDC, 1988.

to the CDC are in the homosexual/bisexual male transmission category. An additional 8% of cases reported occurred in the homosexual male and intravenous drug abusers (IVDA) category (CDC, 1988). It is interesting to note that, proportionately, the numbers of cases in each of the major risk categories have remained fairly constant since surveillance began in 1981 in the United States, with the

Table 2-5. Cumulative Age Distribution of AIDS Cases by Racial/Ethnic Group
as Reported to the CDC by February 1988

Age Group	White[1]		Black[1]		Hispanic		Other[2]/ Unknown		Total	
	#	(%)	#	(%)	#	(%)	#	(%)	#	(%)
Under 5	124	(0)	384	(3)	164	(2)	4	(1)	676	(1)
5 – 12	53	(0)	39	(0)	19	(0)	2	(0)	113	(0)
13 – 19	103	(0)	70	(1)	39	(1)	5	(1)	217	(0)
20 – 29	6,005	(19)	3,139	(24)	1,609	(23)	87	(18)	10,840	(21)
30 – 39	14,298	(45)	6,328	(48)	3,372	(47)	212	(44)	24,210	(46)
40 – 49	7,131	(23)	2,270	(17)	1,375	(19)	120	(25)	10,896	(21)
Over 50	3,746	(12)	947	(7)	557	(8)	54	(11)	5,304	(10)
Total [% of all cases]	31,460	[60]	13,177	[25]	7,135	[14]	484	[1]	52,256	[100]

[1] Does not include Hispanic cases.
[2] Includes patients whose race/ethnicity is Asian/Pacific Islander (305 persons) and American Indian/Alaskan Native (53 persons).
Source: CDC, 1988.

Table 2–6. Distribution of AIDS Cases by Transmission Categories[1] and Racial/Ethnic Groups as Reported to the CDC by February 1988

	White[2]		Black[2]		Hispanic		Other[3] Unknown		Total	
	#	(%)	#	(%)	#	(%)	#	(%)	#	(%)
Adults/Adolescents										
Homosexual/Bisexual Male	24,740	(79)	4,981	(39)	3,321	(48)	327	(68)	33,369	(65)
Intravenous Drug Abuser (IVDA)	1,773	(6)	4,573	(36)	2,484	(36)	47	(10)	8,877	(17)
Homosexual Male and IVDA	2,463	(8)	913	(7)	459	(7)	23	(5)	3,858	(7)
Hemophilia/Coagulation Disorder	441	(1)	33	(0)	33	(0)	12	(3)	519	(1)
Heterosexual Cases	344	(1)	1,446	(11)	259	(4)	9	(2)	2,058	(4)
Transfusion, Blood/Components	913	(3)	178	(1)	84	(1)	31	(6)	1,206	(2)
Undetermined	609	(2)	630	(5)	312	(4)	29	(6)	1,580	(3)
SUBTOTAL [% of all cases]	31,283	[61]	12,754	[25]	6,952	[14]	478	[1]	51,467	[100]
Children										
Hemophilia/Coagulation Disorder	29	(16)	6	(1)	6	(3)	2	(33)	43	(5)
Parent with/at risk of AIDS[4]	78	(44)	373	(88)	148	(81)	4	(67)	603	(76)
Transfusion, Blood/Components	59	(33)	27	(6)	22	(12)	–		108	(14)
Undetermined	11	(6)	17	(4)	7	(4)	–		35	(4)
SUBTOTAL [% of all cases]	177	[22]	423	[54]	183	[23]	6	[1]	789	[100]
TOTAL [% of all cases]	31,460	[60]	13,177	[25]	7,135	[14]	484	[1]	52,256	[100]

[1] Cases with more than one risk factor other than the combinations listed in the table are tabulated only in the category listed first.

[2] Does not include Hispanic cases.

[3] Includes patients whose race/ethnicity is Asian/Pacific Islander (305 persons) and American Indian/Alaskan Native (53 persons).

[4] Epidemiologic data suggest transmission from an infected mother to her fetus or infant during the perinatal period.

Source: CDC, 1988.

majority of cases occurring in homosexual or bisexual males. In this group, anal receptive intercourse appears to be a more effective method of HIV transmission than anal insertive intercourse or any type of genital-oral intercourse (Darrow et al., 1987; Francis & Chin, 1987; Moss et al., 1987).

Closer analysis of New York City data indicates that 73% of cases reported in 1981 were in the homosexual/bisexual male transmission category, whereas the incidence in that transmission category declined to 66% in 1986 (Joseph, 1987b). This reduction in incidence is attributed to the effect of educational efforts and counseling on reducing high-risk behaviors. In an effort to determine the impact of AIDS on gay males in New York City, Martin (1987) found that the number of different sexual partners and sexual activity declined by approximately 78%, the frequency of sexual episodes involving the exchange of body fluids and mucous membrane contact declined by an average of 70%, and the frequency of condom use during anal intercourse increased from 1.5 to 20% after respondents heard about AIDS.

Studies have documented the fact that there are both homosexual and heterosexual individuals who have had repeated sexual intercourse with persons known to be infected with HIV who have not become infected. Other studies have reported seroconversion following only one sexual encounter. The risk, therefore, of HIV infection for a susceptible person following one sexual encounter with an infected person is unknown (Francis & Chin, 1987). Case-control studies in homosexual men have indicated that certain co-factors (e.g., prior history of other sexually transmitted diseases, use of nitrites) may predispose to HIV infection or to the development of clinical AIDS following HIV infection (Francis & Chin, 1987; Osborn, 1986).

Kaposi's sarcoma has a greater prevalence among homosexual men with AIDS than in other risk categories (Cohen, 1987; Moss et al., 1987). An association has been made between nitrite use and transient immunosuppression, which may be a risk factor for Kaposi's sarcoma rather than for opportunistic infections (Moss et al., 1987). In case-control studies of risk factors for AIDS and HIV infection in homosexual men in San Francisco, Moss et al. (1987) found only nitrites (poppers) possibly associated with risk. Infection may be facilitated as a result of the vasodilator effect of nitrites or their possible effect of increasing tolerance to rectal abrasions.

Intravenous Drug Abusers. Seventeen percent of cases of AIDS were reported to the CDC in the intravenous drug abuser (IVDA) transmission category (CDC, 1988). Of these, 79.3% were males and 20.7% were females. Of the women with AIDS in the United States, 49% have been IVDAs. Additionally, 8% of cases of AIDS have been reported in the homosexual male and IVDA transmission category (CDC, 1988). Eighty percent of the cases of AIDS in the IVDA transmission category have occurred in Black and Hispanic individuals (50% and 30%, respectively) whereas only 19% have occurred in Caucasian individuals. In contrast, 74% of the cases of AIDS in the homosexual/bisexual male transmission category have occurred in Caucasian individuals with only 25% in Black and Hispanic individuals (15% and 10%, respectively) (CDC, 1988). Although the nationwide data have remained fairly constant since 1981, the proportion of AIDS cases among IVDAs in New York City has increased from 22% in 1981 to 36% in 1986 (Joseph, 1987b). It is estimated that 50% to 60% of the approximately 200,000 IVDAs in New York City are infected with HIV.

Viral transmission in IVDAs can be attributed primarily to the sharing of drug injecting equipment (needles and syringes, called "works" by IVDAs) as well as by homosexual and heterosexual contact (Des Jarlais et al., 1987). Little is known about the effect on the incidence of HIV infection in IVDAs of sharing equipment used to dissolve heroin or cocaine (called the "cooker" by IVDAs), utilization of services at "shooting galleries" (i.e., buying drugs, being injected by someone else, renting of previously used needles and syringes) or cleaning unsterile works before use (Marmor et al., 1987). Pathogenesis of HIV may be influenced by the immunologic status of the IVDA but there is limited information available in this area. Brown et al. (1986) demonstrated that the duration of drug use and the route of administration were the factors most significantly associated with a greater prevalence of immunologic abnormalities in 97 patients (71 males and 26 females) applying for admission or currently enrolled in clinics of the Addiction Research and Treatment Corporation in New York City. Additionally, findings indicated that abnormal liver function may have contributed to altered immune status. Yet to be studied are some other factors that might contribute to the IVDA's immunologic changes: asepsis in administration techniques, the type of diluents or contaminants gaining entry in the course of drug use, the frequency of infection and neoplastic disorders, and nutritional impairment (Brown et al., 1986).

A high prevalence of HIV infection in IVDAs affects the increasing number of women and children with AIDS. According to CDC data, most IVDAs are heterosexual men who presumably are transmitting HIV to their female sexual partners who are not IVDAs. Seventy-eight percent of children with AIDS have been born to mothers with or at risk for AIDS, presumably women who are IVDAs or who have been infected by sexual contact with IVDAs (CDC, 1988). In contrast to the national data, 62% of the women in New York City who have developed AIDS have been IVDAs (versus 49% nationally). Estimates indicate that the number of HIV-infected children who will be born in New York City each year will be between 300 and 800 (Joseph, 1987a). Obviously, studies focusing on the use of intravenous drugs in the pathogenesis of HIV would have significant public health implications beyond the actual risk group.

Heterosexual Cases. As of February 1988, a total of 2,058 (4%) cases of AIDS were reported to the CDC in the heterosexual cases transmission category. Of these, 47.4% have been males and 52.6% have been females. This is the only transmission category in which women outnumber men. This category includes persons who have had heterosexual contact with a person with AIDS or at risk for AIDS as well as persons without other identified risks who were born in countries in which heterosexual transmission is believed to play a major role, although precise means of transmission have not yet been fully identified (CDC, 1988).

Heterosexual transmission of HIV has become a major focus of concern in the United States, largely based on evidence of heterosexual transmission reported in Africa. It is currently unclear whether or not there is a difference in transmission efficiency between anal and vaginal intercourse and further studies are needed in this area (Francis & Chin, 1987; Joseph, 1987a). In a study of 45 heterosexual partners (spouses) of index cases with AIDS, Fischl et al. (1987)

reported an incidence rate of HIV seropositivity of 58%. When spouses with other heterosexual partners were eliminated from the data analysis, the incidence of HIV infection was 50%. At enrollment in the study, 13 spouses were seropositive and of the remaining 32 spouses, 13 (41%) seroconverted during the study. In more than half of the couples, vaginal intercourse was the only type of sexual activity practiced; anal intercourse was not a common practice (Fischl et al., 1987). In surveys of heterosexual males with AIDS in Kenya, Zaire, and Rwanda, specific sexual activities, including anal intercourse reported by 4–8% of the respondents, were not associated with HIV infection (Quinn et al., 1986).

Based on what is currently known about the epidemiology of HIV infection, it is likely that the incidence of infection will increase among heterosexuals who are closest to the high-risk behavior groups. The strongest bridge to heterosexual transmission currently exists in the sexual partners of IVDAs and other infected persons. In comparing the relative risk of developing AIDS among females who inject drugs versus females who do not inject drugs but are the heterosexual partners of male IVDAs, Des Jarlais et al. (1987) reported that the risk of heterosexual transmission is relatively small compared with the risk of transmission from IV drug use. In New York City, over 90% of the heterosexually transmitted HIV infection is from sexual contact with IVDAs (Joseph, 1987a).

The degree to which HIV infection will spread outside the high-risk transmission categories will be directly related to the prevalence of HIV infection, the number of sexual partners, the frequency of sexual contacts, and the role of co-factors in infection susceptibility (Fauci, 1986; Imperato, 1987). The prevalence of HIV seropositivity among prescreened blood donors in the United States is reported to be less than 0.03% (Fauci, 1986). In contrast, seroprevalence rates of HIV infection in blood donors range from 0.7% in Zaire to 18% in Kigali, Rwanda (Quinn et al., 1986). In certain central African countries where there is increased incidence of AIDS, studies have determined that 10% of the population is infected (Fauci, 1986).

A review of the data generated from serologic screening of 789,578 civilian applicants for military service between October 1985 and December 1986 indicated an overall rate of seropositivity of 1.5 per 1,000 individuals tested (CDC, 1987a). The population volunteering for military service may not be representative of the U.S. population at large because of the exclusion of hemophiliacs, IVDAs and admittedly homosexual men. Additionally, applicants do not equally represent all socioeconomic and demographic groups in the general population. Seroprevalence of HIV per 1,000 applicants by age was 0.6 for 17–20 year olds, 2.5 for 21–25 year olds and 4.1 for those 26 years of age and older. By sex, seroprevalence was 1.6 for males and 0.6 for females (CDC, 1987a). In contrast, age at diagnosis of total reported cases of AIDS in the U.S. is older, with 0.7% between 13 and 20 years of age, 6.5% between 21 and 25 years and 92.8% diagnosed at or after 26 years of age (CDC, 1988). The ratio of seroprevalence between male and female military recruit applicants was 3:1, the same as for total persons with AIDS in the U.S. if homosexual and hemophilia-associated cases are excluded. The male-to-female ratio among all persons with AIDS is 13:1 (CDC, 1986a).

The number of sexual partners and the frequency of sexual contacts are closely associated with the prevalence factor in relation to transmission of HIV outside the high-risk transmission categories. There are likely to be more sexual contacts by the male partners of a bisexual husband than by his suburban housewife whom he has infected (Imperato, 1987). Adolescents between the ages of 13 and 19 may be a high-risk behavior group for heterosexual transmission of HIV infection because of their early age of first intercourse, the number and choice of sexual partners, rates of sexually transmitted diseases, and current contraceptive practices (Hein, 1987).

In central Africa, prevalence of AIDS among males was associated with a history of frequent sex with prostitutes and an increased prevalence of HIV infection in male heterosexuals who were patients in sexually transmitted disease clinics (Fauci, 1986). In a study of 295 males without homosexual or IVDA risk factors attending a sexually transmitted disease clinic in New York City, Rabkin et al. (1987) found that HIV seropositivity was significantly associated with a history of sexually transmitted diseases. However, in contrast, exposure to prostitutes was not associated with increased odds of HIV seropositivity in these sexually transmitted disease clinic patrons. Des Jarlais et al. (1987) reported that HIV-infected prostitutes in New York City apparently rarely transmitted HIV to their clients, primarily as a result of safer sexual practices (i.e., use of condoms).

The presence of co-factors may enhance an individual's susceptibility to HIV infection and the subsequent development of AIDS. Prior or ongoing infection with cytomegalovirus (CMV), Epstein-Barr virus (EBV), or hepatitis B virus (HBV) and the resultant immunosuppression may increase the chances of HIV progressing to infection in an exposed individual (Osborn, 1986). Ninety to 100% of heterosexual men in Zaire and homosexual men in the United States had comparable serologic evidence of CMV, EBV and HBV. In contrast, a significantly lower prevalence of infection with these viral agents was detected in heterosexuals in the United States (Fauci, 1986). Immunosuppression may occur as a result of exposure to semen as well as opiates, nitrites (poppers), and marijuana (Osborn, 1986).

Activation of the immune system may enhance the efficiency and pathogenesis of HIV infection (Fauci, 1986). Sexually active homosexual males with multiple sexual partners often have a history of parasitic, bacterial, and viral illnesses and a resultant antigenic stimulation and overload. In the process of needle-sharing, IVDAs are exposed to multiple infections, such as viral hepatitis and bacterial endocarditis. Haitians, who at one time were listed as a separate transmission category by the CDC, often have a history of parasitic infections and endemic tubercular infections resulting in antigenic overstimulation (Osborn, 1986). Suboptimal nutritional status, especially of the IVDA, may also contribute to disease progression.

Transfusion-Associated Cases. A total of 1,206 (2%) cases of AIDS were reported to the CDC in the transfusion, blood/components transmission category (CDC, 1988). Of these, 64.6% were males and 35.4% were females. Twelve percent of the children with AIDS have been in this transmission category (CDC, 1988). Although infants are estimated to receive less than 2% of the red blood cells or whole blood transfusions, they make up a higher proportion of transfusion-associated cases of AIDS than would be expected (Peterman, 1987; Peterman et al., 1985). It is postulated that:

1. infants may be more susceptible to the development of AIDS as a result of their immature immune systems;

2. infants have a larger exposure to the virus via one transfusion relative to their body size and weight;

3. there is a shorter incubation period for infants (mean, 21 months versus 31 months in adults), resulting in a higher incidence rate of AIDS; and

4. there may be an increased incidence of unrecognized co-factors in infants (Fisher, 1987; Peterman et al., 1985).

Adults over 70 years of age have accounted for a relatively small number of transfusion-associated cases of AIDS, perhaps because individuals in that age group do not live long enough to develop AIDS after becoming infected with HIV (Peterman et al., 1985).

In studying the 194 cases of transfusion-associated cases of AIDS that had been reported to the CDC by August 1985, Peterman and colleagues (1985) determined that HIV was transmitted equally well by transfusion of red cells, platelets, plasma, and whole blood. There was no indication that HIV was more likely to be transmitted by any of the components. Blood transfusion is an apparently extremely efficient mechanism for transmission of HIV infection; studies have not been able to identify a transfusion recipient who did not acquire HIV infection from a transfusion from an infected donor (Peterman, 1987).

In March 1983, the Public Health Service recommended that potential blood donors from groups at high risk for AIDS voluntarily refrain from donating blood or plasma (Fisher, 1987; Peterman et al., 1985). Between 1983 and 1985 (when enzyme-linked immunosorbent assay [ELISA] and Western blot assay tests for determination of antibody to HIV were approved by the Food and Drug Administration) the rate of donation from individuals at high risk for AIDS declined greatly. Use of the screening tests (ELISA and Western blot assay) on all donated blood virtually eliminated transfusion with HIV-infected blood.

An additional comment must be made about the importance of voluntary deferment of high-risk donors along with screening of all donated blood. In June 1986, the CDC (1986b) reported HIV seropositivity in two individuals who had received blood from a donor who was seronegative at the time of blood donation in August 1985. The donor, a 31 year old man, had donated blood at the same center in April, August, and November 1985. He was seronegative in April and August and seropositive in November. The donor stated that he had had sexual contact with one male partner since May 15, 1985, and therefore did not believe that he was at risk for AIDS. He gave no history of acute viral illness and was asymptomatic for AIDS or AIDS-related complex (ARC) in 1985 and 1986.

Hemophilia/Coagulation Disorder. One percent of cases of AIDS reported to the CDC were in the hemophilia/coagulation disorder transmission category by February 1988. Of these, 97.8% were males and 2.2% were females. Five percent of the children with AIDS were in this transmission category (CDC, 1988). The majority of cases had hemophilia A or factor VIII deficiency, whereas the rest had hemophilia B or factor IX deficiency, von Willebrand's disease (a genetic coagulation disorder), or other blood coagulation defects. Patients with hemophilia A receive more clotting factor concentration, probably because their disease is more severe than the others (Cohen, 1987).

In 1984, heat-treated factor concentrates were introduced for use in treating hemophiliacs because unheated concentrates had been linked epidemiologically to the high incidence of HIV infection in that population in the United States (CDC, 1987b). Since that time there have been a few reports of patients who seroconverted after receipt of unscreened, heat-treated factor concentrates. Although it has been reported that seroconversion in other risk categories occurs within 8 to 12 weeks after HIV exposure, it is unclear whether this can be applied to hemophiliac patients (CDC, 1987b). It may take up to 26 months for seroconversion to occur following HIV exposure in this population. Between February and July 1986, most hemophilia treatment centers converted to using donor-screened, heat-treated factor concentrate products and since that time no cases of seroconversion have been reported (CDC, 1987b).

Undetermined. Three percent of cases of AIDS reported to the CDC were in the undetermined transmission category. Of these, 77.4% were males and 22.6% were females. Four percent of children with AIDS fall into this transmission category (CDC, 1988). This category includes patients on whom risk information is incomplete (due to death, refusal to be interviewed, or loss to follow-up), patients still under investigation (and who may be placed in another category at a later date), men reported only to have heterosexual contact with a prostitute, and interviewed patients for whom no specific risk was identified.

Organ and Semen Donation. HIV transmission has been reported by organ transplantation from a donor screened for HIV antibody (CDC, 1987c). A blood sample taken two days after the donor received a large number of blood transfusions was negative for HIV antibody. A later sample taken when the donor's kidneys, heart and liver were removed was found to be HIV antibody positive when tested at one of the transplantation centers and after the organs had been transplanted. Two persons who survived the transplant procedures were subsequently found to be HIV antibody positive. A blood sample from the organ donor taken on admission (prior to any transfusions) was found to be positive for HIV antibody when tested. The large number of transfusions the organ donor received before his serum was tested for HIV probably caused the false-negative HIV antibody result (CDC, 1987c).

HIV as well as other microorganisms has been transmitted via donor semen to artificially inseminated women. Four of eight women in Australia were HIV antibody positive after insemination with cryopreserved semen from an infected donor (Francis & Chin, 1987; Mascola & Guinan, 1987). Agreement is lacking, however, on when semen donors should be screened. A negative antibody test on the day of semen donation will not guarantee that the donor is not infected with HIV (just as it also does not guarantee absence of HIV infection in blood donors) since in most cases seroconversion may not occur for 6 to 12 weeks following exposure.

Health Care Workers

Although the risk of acquisition of HIV infection purely as a consequence of health care employment is extremely low, it seems prudent to discuss the epidemiologic data on HIV infection and AIDS in this risk group. The relative absence of HIV transmission in health care settings, even following needlestick injuries from infected persons, is in direct contrast to the high infection rate with hepatitis B virus after such accidents (Francis & Chin, 1987). As a result of the increasing prevalence of HIV infection, health care workers are at an increasing risk of exposure to the blood of HIV-infected persons (CDC, 1987d). McCray and the Cooperative Needlestick Surveillance Group (1986) have prospectively followed 883 health care workers with documented parenteral or mucous membrane exposure for the development of antibody to HIV. A total of four health care workers developed antibody to HIV, one for whom heterosexual transmission could not be ruled out and three without any other documented risk factors for infection. There are two other prospective studies of health care workers currently ongoing in the United States and both studies have failed to document any seroconversions (CDC, 1987d).

Additionally, eight persons who denied other risk factors and who provided care to HIV-infected persons have been reported to have acquired HIV infection (CDC, 1987d). Three individuals reported needlestick exposure to blood of infected persons and two others reported extensive contact with blood or other body fluids without needlestick injuries. The remaining three health care workers reported skin or mucous membrane exposures to blood from infected persons (CDC, 1987e). These three health care workers did not identify any other risk factors for acquisition of HIV infection, although this does not completely rule out the unrecognized or forgotten exposure. All three had direct contact of their skin with blood from infected patients, all had skin lesions which may have been contaminated by blood, and one also had a mucous membrane exposure (CDC, 1987e).

Out of a total of 1,231 dentists and hygienists who participated in a study to determine the prevalence of HIV antibody, only one dentist (0.1%) had antibody to HIV. No other risk factors for HIV infection were identified, although the dentist did not have an exposure to a known HIV-infected person. He did give a history of needlestick injuries, trauma to his hands, and not routinely wearing gloves during dental procedures (CDC, 1987e).

Household Contacts

It is important to note that prospective studies of transmission of HIV infection in household (non-sexual) contacts of persons with AIDS have failed to demonstrate any seroconversion. This has been true in spite of practices such as sharing household items and facilities and close personal interactions with the person with AIDS (Fischl et al., 1987; Friedland et al., 1986).

Women

By February 1988, 51,467 adult cases of AIDS had been reported to the CDC. Of those, 7% have been in women. The most common route of transmission in women is intravenous drug use (49% of the adult female cases) with shared injection equipment being the mode of spread. The only transmission category in which women outnumber men is in heterosexual transmission (52.6% of the female cases versus 47.4% of the male cases), which is the second most common route of transmission in women (30% of the adult female causes of AIDS) (CDC, 1988). The heterosexual transmission category includes persons who have had heterosexual contact with a person with AIDS or at risk for AIDS, or with a person without other identified risks who was born in a country in which heterosexual transmission is believed to play a major role, although precise means of transmission have not yet been fully defined. AIDS is the leading cause of death in women 25–29 years of age in New York City (Joseph, 1987a). Since the majority of women with AIDS are within their childbearing years, this affects the children with AIDS: 78% of the pediatric cases of AIDS are a consequence of infected mothers (CDC, 1988; Wofsy, 1987).

Certain factors probably account for the number of heterosexually acquired cases of AIDS in women:

1. a woman is more likely than a man to encounter an infected partner since there are more men with AIDS (and presumably HIV infection) than women;

2. female-to-male transmission of HIV is probably less efficient than male-to-female transmission (similar to the spread of gonococcal infections) although bidirectional transmission has been documented; and

3. some women may have been unaware of their exposure to a male in a high-risk category for HIV infection (i.e., recent IVDA or bisexual male with

multiple sexual partners) (Evans, 1987; Fauci, 1986; Guinan & Hardy, 1987; Joseph, 1987a; Quinn et al., 1986).

Apparent female-to-female sexual transmission of HIV was reported by Marmor and colleagues (1986). The second person, who apparently acquired HIV infection through sexual contact with the first person (the index case), reported having oral-vaginal and oral-anal contact during the index case's menses. Both women reported vaginal bleeding as a result of traumatic sexual activities.

Children

As of February 1988, 789 children less than 13 years of age with AIDS had been reported to the CDC, representing 1.4% of the total number reported. The majority (78%) were children with a parent with AIDS or at risk for AIDS, most likely an infected mother who transmitted HIV to her fetus or infant during the perinatal period. The other transmission categories include: transfusion, blood/components (12%), hemophilia/coagulation disorder (5%), and undetermined (4%). Fifty-four percent were Black, 24% were Hispanic and 21% were Caucasian. Two-thirds of the pediatric cases of AIDS have been reported from four states: New York, New Jersey, Florida, and California (CDC, 1988).

As a result of the routine screening of blood and blood products for the presence of HIV antibody, as well as the continuation of voluntary deferment of high-risk donors, the category of children infected by transfusions should be eliminated in the near future (Novick & Rubinstein, 1987; Rogers et al., 1987). However, this will not result in a decrease in the incidence of HIV infection in children because it is anticipated that the number of perinatally transmitted cases of AIDS will increase, based on the projected increase in HIV infection in women of childbearing age secondary to heterosexual transmission.

HIV transmission from infected mothers to their infants during the perinatal period is the most common mode of HIV transmission. There have been reports of transmission of HIV via breastfeeding (the mother was infused post-partum with HIV-infected blood) and the isolation of HIV in breast milk (Rogers et al., 1987).

One case has been reported to CDC (1986c) of transmission of HIV from a child to his mother. The child most likely acquired HIV infection from a blood transfusion (one of many transfusions required by the child's presenting illness) from a donor in 1984, later found to be seropositive. The child's mother provided extensive nursing care to the child at home, which included extensive contact with his blood and other body substances. She did not follow recommended precautions, often did not wear gloves, and frequently did not wash her hands immediately following exposure.

Summary

The AIDS virus, the epidemic and our understanding of it are constantly evolving and changing. Historically, epidemiologic data contributed to the identification of the etiologic agent and its mode of transmission. The data are currently assisting in understanding the pathogenesis (and the differences in the pathogenesis) of HIV in different individuals with varying infection risks. As the number of cases increases and the epidemiologic data change, new information about infection and transmission might become apparent. As various aspects are researched and published, more is learned about the sociodemographic distribution of AIDS that may be able to be extrapolated to HIV infection. For the present, the only means to control the epidemic are education, health promotion, and risk reduction.

References

Assad, F., & Mann, J.M. (1987). AIDS—An international perspective. *Ethiopian Medical Journal*, 25(2), 97–100.

Brown, L.S., Evans, R., Murphy, D., et al. (1986). Drug use patterns: Implications for the acquired immunodeficiency syndrome. *Journal of the American Medical Association*, 78(12), 1145–1151.

Centers for Disease Control. (1983). Prevention of acquired immune deficiency syndrome (AIDS): Report of inter-agency recommendation. *Morbidity and Mortality Weekly Report*, 32, 101–103.

Centers for Disease Control. (1986a). Human T-lymphotropic virus type III/lymphadenopathy-associated virus antibody prevalence in U.S. military recruit applicants. *Morbidity and Mortality Weekly Report*, 35(26), 421–424.

Centers for Disease Control. (1986b). Transfusion-associated human T-lymphotropic virus type III/lymphadenopathy-associated virus infection from a seronegative donor—Colorado. *Morbidity and Mortality Weekly Report*, 35(24), 389–391.

Centers for Disease Control. (1986c). Apparent transmission of human T-lymphotropic virus type III/lymphadenopathy-associated virus from a child to a mother providing health care. *Morbidity and Mortality Weekly Report*, 35(5), 76–79.

Centers for Disease Control. (1987a). Trends in human immunodeficiency virus infection among civilian applicants for military service—United States, October, 1985–December, 1986. *Morbidity and Mortality Weekly Report*, 36(18), 273–276.

Centers for Disease Control. (1987b). Survey on non-US hemophilia treatment centers for HIV seroconversions following therapy with heat-treated factor concentrates. *Morbidity and Mortality Weekly Report*, 36(9), 121–124.

Centers for Disease Control. (1987c). Human immunodeficiency virus infection transmitted from an organ donor screened for HIV antibody. *Morbidity and Mortality Weekly Report*, 36(20), 306–308.

Centers for Disease Control. (1987d). Recommendations for prevention of HIV transmission in health care settings. *Morbidity and Mortality Weekly Report*, Supplement, 36(2S), 1–18.

Centers for Disease Control. (1987e). Update: Human immunodeficiency virus infections in health care workers exposed to blood of infected persons. *Morbidity and Mortality Weekly Report*, 36(19), 285–289.

Centers for Disease Control. (1988, February). AIDS Weekly Surveillance Report. United States AIDS Program, Atlanta, GA.

Cohen, F.L. (1987). The epidemiology and etiology of AIDS. In J.D. Durham & F.L. Cohen (Eds.), *The Person with AIDS: Nursing Perspectives* (pp. 9–51). New York: Springer Publishing Company.

Darrow, W.W., Echenberg, D.F., Jaffe, H.W., et al. (1987). Risk factors for human immuno-deficiency virus (HIV) infections in homosexual men. *American Journal of Public Health*, 77(4), 479–483.

Des Jarlais, D.C., Wish, E., Friedman, S.R., et al. (1987). Intravenous drug use and the heterosexual transmission of the human immunodeficiency virus. *New York State Journal of Medicine*, 87(5), 283–286.

Evans, K.M. (1987). The female AIDS patient. *Health Care for Women International*, 8, 1–7.

Fauci, A.S. (1986). Current issues in developing a strategy for dealing with the acquired immunodeficiency syndrome. *Proceedings of the National Academy of Science*, 83, 9278–9283.

Fischl, M.A., Dickinson, G.M., Scott, G.B., et al. (1987). Evaluation of heterosexual partners, children and household contacts of adults with AIDS. *Journal of the American Medical Association*, 257(5), 640–644.

Fisher, M.C. (1987). Transfusion-associated acquired immunodeficiency syndrome—What is the risk? *Pediatrics*, 79(1), 157–159.

Francis, D.P., & Chin, J. (1987). The prevention of acquired immuno-deficiency syndrome in the United States. *Journal of the American Medical Association*, 257(10), 1357–1366.

Friedland, G.H., Saltzman, B.R., Rogers, M.F., et al. (1986). Lack of transmission of HTLV-III/LAV infection to household contacts of patients with AIDS or AIDS-related complex with oral candidiasis. *New England Journal of Medicine*, 314(6), 344–349.

Guinan, M.E., & Hardy, A. (1987). Epidemiology of AIDS in women in the United States—1981 through 1986. *Journal of the American Medical Association*, 257(15), 2039–2042.

Hein, K. (1987). AIDS in adolescents: A rationale for concern. *New York State Journal of Medicine*, 87(5), 290–295.

Hilgartner, M.W. (1987). AIDS in the transfused patient. *American Journal of Diseases in Children*, 141(2), 194–198.

Imperato, P.J. (1986). The epidemiology of the acquired immunodeficiency syndrome in Africa. *New York State Journal of Medicine*, 86, 118–121.

Imperato, P.J. (1987). Acquired immunodeficiency syndrome—1987. *New York State Journal of Medicine*, 87(5), 251–255.

Joseph, S.C. (1987a). Remarks presented to the New York State Assembly Standing Committee on Health, Hearing on AIDS.

Joseph, S.C. (1987b). AIDS in New York City: Moving ahead on effective public health approaches. *New York State Journal of Medicine*, 87(5), 257–258.

Marmor, M., Des Jarlais, D.C., Cohen, H., et al. (1987). Risk factors for infection with human immuno-deficiency virus among intravenous drug abusers in New York City. *AIDS*, 1(1), 39–44.

Marmor, M., Weiss, L.R., Lyden, M., et al. (1986). Possible female-to-female transmission of human immunodeficiency virus [letter]. *Annals of Internal Medicine*, 105(6), 969.

Martin, J.L. (1987). The impact of AIDS on gay male sexual behavior patterns in New York City. *American Journal of Public Health*, 77(5), 578–581.

Mascola, L., & Guinan, M.E. (1987). Semen donors as the source of sexually transmitted diseases in artifically inseminated women: The saga unfolds. *Journal of the American Medical Association*, 257(8), 1093–1094.

McCray, E., & The Cooperative Needlestick Surveillance Group. (1986). Occupational risk of the acquired immunodeficiency syndrome among health care workers. *New England Journal of Medicine*, 314, 1127–1132.

McGrady, G.A., Jason, J.M., & Evatt, B.L. (1987). The course of the epidemic of acquired immunodeficiency syndrome in the United States hemophilia population. *American Journal of Epidemiology*, 126(1), 25–30.

Moss, A.R., Osmond, D., Bacchatti, P., et al. (1987). Risk factors for AIDS and HIV seropositivity in homosexual men. *American Journal of Epidemiology*, 125(2), 1035–1047.

Novick, B.E., & Rubinstein, A. (1987). AIDS—the pediatric perspective. *AIDS*, 1(1), 3–7.

Osborn, J.E. (1986). Co-factors and HIV: What determines the pathogenesis of AIDS? *BioEssays*, 5(6), 287–289.

Peterman, T.A. (1987). Transfusion-associated acquired immunodeficiency syndrome. *World Journal of Surgery*, 11(1), 36–40.

Peterman, T.A., Jaffee, H.W., Feorino, P.M., et al. (1985). Transfusion-associated acquired immunodeficiency syndrome in the United States. *Journal of the American Medical Association*, 254(20), 2913–2917.

Quinn, T.C. (1987). AIDS in Africa: Evidence for heterosexual transmission of the human im-munodeficiency virus. *New York State Journal of Medicine*, 87(5), 286–289.

Quinn, T.C., Mann, J.M., Curran, J.W., et al. (1986). AIDS in Africa: An epidemiologic paradigm. *Science*, 234, 955–963.

Rabkin, C.S., Thomas, P.A., Jaffe, H.W., et al. (1987). Prevalence of antibody to HTLV-III/LAV in a population attending a sexually transmitted diseases clinic. *Sexually Transmitted Diseases*, 14(1), 48–51.

Rogers, M.F., Thomas, P.A., Starcher, E.T., et al. (1987). Acquired immunodeficiency syndrome in children: Report of the Centers for Disease Control national surveillance, 1982–1985. *Pediatrics*, 79(6), 1008–1014.

Wofsy, C.B. (1987). Human immunodeficiency virus infection in women. *Journal of the American Medical Association*, 257(15), 2074–2076.

Zuckerman, A.J. (1986). AIDS and insects. *British Medical Journal*, 292, 1094–1095.

Chapter 3

The Immune System and AIDS/HIV Infection

Christine Grady

The immune system, part of the body's host defense mechanisms, is a highly sophisticated, integrative system designed to help protect the host against the ravages of infectious microorganisms, environmental toxins, and cell mutations.

Structure of the Immune System. The immune system comprises organs and cells located throughout the body that carry out this protective function. The organs of the immune system include the bone marrow, thymus gland, spleen, lymphatic system, and peripheral blood. It is in these organs that the cells of the immune system develop, mature, and are stored, poised for action whenever necessary. The cells of the immune system are the lymphocytes and the monocytes/macrophages. They are the mononuclear portion of the white blood cells (as opposed to the polymorphonuclear granulocytes). There are two main types of lymphocytes: T cells and B cells (Table 3–1). Another lymphocyte, the large granular lymphocyte (LGL), also known as the natural killer cell (NK), makes up a small portion of the lymphocyte pool. The NK cell is believed to function nonspecifically to destroy mutated cells and virally infected cells (Bellanti, 1985; Roitt et al., 1985; Stites et al., 1984).

T cells are lymphocytes derived from the bone marrow stem cell, which develop and mature in the thymus gland (T = thymus derived lymphocyte or thymocyte). Most of our circulating lymphocytes are T cells (approximately 80%) (Roitt et al., 1985). T cells are further subdivided into at least two subsets with distinct functions and surface proteins. One subset is the T4 cell subset, so called because the cells have a surface protein (T4 or CD4) recognized by the OKT4 monoclonal antibody (Fauci, 1987; Roitt et al., 1985; Stites et al., 1984). T4 cells are inducer cells and helper cells and are the key cells in cell mediated immunity. The other subset is the T8 cell. T8 cells function as cytotoxic cells and as suppres-

Table 3–1. Differences Between T and B Lymphocytes

	T cells	B cells
Responsible for	Cell-mediated immunity	Humoral immunity
% in peripheral blood	80%	15–20%
Products elaborated	Lymphokines	Antibody
Provide protection against	Intracellular organisms (virus, fungi, parasites), malignant cells, allografts	Bacteria, virus, soluble antigens
Subsets	T4 inducer, helper T8 suppressor, cytotoxic cell	

sor cells. Normally T4 cells outnumber T8 cells in the peripheral blood by approximately 2:1 (Lane, 1987; Roitt et al., 1985).

The other major lymphocyte is the B cell. B cells are also derived from the bone marrow stem cell. They make up approximately 10–20% of the circulating pool of lymphocytes but are more abundant in the bone marrow, spleen, and certain other lymphoid tissues such as the GALT (gut associated lymphoid tissue) in the intestine (Bellanti, 1985; Roitt et al., 1985; Stites et al., 1984). When stimulated and activated, B cells make antibody. B cells are responsible for humoral immunity.

Monocytes are white blood cells that have several functions. Monocytes develop into tissue macrophages, which are essentially big scavenger cells (literally big eaters). They are critical cells in phagocytosis and in killing certain microorganisms, in killing certain tumor cells, in clearing antigens bound to antibody, and in presenting antigen to lymphocytes (Bellanti, 1985; Roitt et al., 1985; Stites et al., 1984).

The Immune Response. There are two main arms to the immune response: cell mediated immunity (CMI) and humoral immunity (Figure 3–1). Although distinguished by the cells involved and their specific function, there is extensive collaboration and cooperation between them.

Humoral immunity is provided by the B cell and its product, antibody. Activated B cells proliferate and differentiate into plasma cells. Plasma cells are antibody factories producing large amounts of specific antibody (Bellanti, 1985; Roitt et al., 1985; Stites et al., 1984). Although specific to the inciting antigen, antibody in humans is always one of five classes: IgG, IgA, IgM, IgD, or IgE (Stites et al., 1984) (Table 3–2). Antibody binds to the antigen, forming an antibody-antigen complex or immune complex. Some antibodies are capable of neutralizing an antigen simply by preventing its attachment to and subsequent infection of a host target cell. Antibodies usually function like adaptors. After binding with the antigen, the antibody binds at the other end to another cell or substance which can help to destroy or eliminate the antigen and the whole complex. Sometimes this destruction is carried out by a macrophage, sometimes by other phagocytic cells, and sometimes with the aid of complement (Bellanti, 1985; Stites et al., 1984).

HUMORAL IMMUNITY

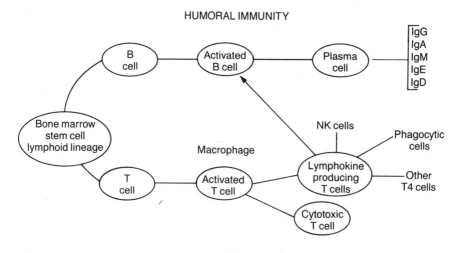

CELL-MEDIATED IMMUNITY

Figure 3–1. The Immune Response.

Humoral immunity generally protects against bacteria, some viruses, and the potentially deleterious effects of certain soluble antigens (Bellanti, 1985; Stites et al., 1984). Most of the time a B cell will not become activated unless it receives a signal from the T cell. The helper T cell (T4), itself stimulated by recognizing an antigen, sends a message to the B cell to join in the effort and make antibody. When there seems to have been a sufficient response to the antigen, the suppressor T cell (T8) signals to cease the production of antibody. It is clear that the T cell has a crucial role in regulating humoral or B cell immunity (Bellanti, 1985; Roitt et al., 1985; Stites et al., 1984).

Cell mediated immunity (CMI) or T cell immunity is different from humoral immunity. Activated T4 cells do not produce antibody, but produce mediator substances known as lymphokines. Activated T8 cells function as cytotoxic cells and

Table 3–2. Classes of Human Immunoglobulins

Class	Characteristics
IgG	Most abundant antibody, important in the secondary response, only Ig that crosses the placenta
IgA	Secretory antibody, important in virus and toxin neutralization, found in breast milk
IgM	Intravascular, important in the primary response, the largest molecule
IgE	Found bound to mast cells and basophils, important in the type 1 immediate hypersensitivity reaction (allergenic antibody)
IgD	Function unknown, found on the surface of B lymphocytes

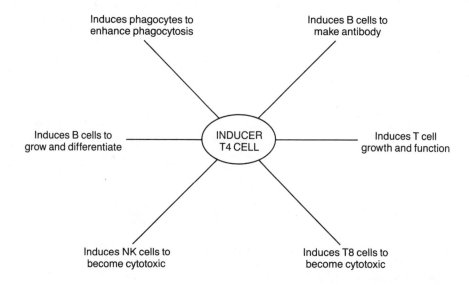

Figure 3–2. Functions of the Inducer T4 Cell.

destroy infected or mutated target cells. CMI primarily protects against intracellular organisms such as viruses, parasites, and fungi, and also against malignancy (Bellanti, 1985; Roitt et al., 1985; Stites et al., 1984). The T4 lymphokine producer is known as the inducer cell (Figure 3–2). When stimulated, it induces (via lymphokines) all of the other cells of the immune system (i.e., T8 cells, B cells, NK cells, macrophages) to carry out their programmed function (Fauci, 1987). The T4 cell is sometimes thought of as the conductor of the immune orchestra; without it the symphony becomes discordant and malfunctions. Lymphokines produced by the T4 cell include:

- substances that enhance phagocytosis, such as: macrophage chemotactic factor (MCF), macrophage inhibition factor (MIF), macrophage activation factor (MAF), and others.
- substances that enhance T cell growth and function, such as: interleukin-2 (IL-2), and gamma interferon (IFN-γ).
- substances that enhance B cell growth and function, such as: B cell growth factor (BCGF) and B cell differentiation factor (BCDF).
- substances that enhance cytotoxicity, such as: gamma interferon and IL-2 (Stites et al., 1984).

A typical immune response to an invading microorganism is as follows: the microorganism enters the body and gets past the nonspecific defenses. It is picked up by a macrophage, enzymatically chewed up, and degraded. Then a piece of it is presented, almost like a flag, on the macrophage surface. The macrophage then waves its flag at the T4 cell which recognizes the antigen in association with the self HLA class II protein (DR molecule) on the macrophage surface (Roitt et al., 1985; Stites et al., 1984). Once the T4 cell recognizes the antigen in this way, it becomes activated, proliferates, and differentiates into lymphokine-producing cells and memory cells. The T4 cell, depending upon which responses would be most efficient against this invader, secretes lymphokines to induce B cells, NK cells, T8 cells, other T4 cells or phagocytes. The virus is then eliminated by antibody, T8 cytotoxicity, NK cytotoxicity, phagocytosis, or a combination of these (Bellanti, 1985; Halliburton, 1986; Laurence, 1985; Roitt et al., 1985; Stites et al., 1984).

Clinical Immunology. Basic knowledge of the immune system and its functions has increased rapidly over recent years. Clinical immunology is the application of this basic knowledge about the immune system to clinical conditions and situations. Applying this knowledge allows:

1. enhancement of immunity by certain therapeutic techniques, for example, immunizations and immunotherapy;

2. prevention of problems that may occur with certain therapeutic modalities used for other purposes, for example, preventing transfusion reactions, transplant rejection, and excessive immunosuppression; and

3. understanding and treating or controlling malfunctions of the immune system, i.e., hypersensitivities, immunodeficiencies, and autoimmune diseases.

Human Immunodeficiency Virus. The acquired immunodeficiency syndrome (AIDS) is, as the name implies, a syndrome of clinical events that occur because of an acquired immunodeficiency. We know that this immunodeficiency is due to an infection with a virus. The virus that causes AIDS is known as the human immunodeficiency virus (HIV), previously also called HTLV III (human T cell lymphotropic virus-III), LAV (lymphadenopathy associated virus), ARV (AIDS-related virus), and other names (Coffin et al., 1986; Durham & Cohen, 1987; Gallo, 1987; Margolick et al., 1987).

The human immunodeficiency virus is an RNA virus; i.e., it is essentially a piece of RNA (genetic material) surrounded by a coat or envelope. HIV is also a retrovirus that has a unique method of propagating itself (Gallo, 1987; Laurence, 1985; Urba & Longo, 1985). Once inside the host, HIV attaches itself to the target cell membrane via a receptor or surface molecule. The viral coat opens up and the RNA enters the cell (Figure 3–3). Retroviral RNA has an enzyme with it known as reverse transcriptase. This enzyme enables the RNA to make a DNA copy of itself. The newly created DNA then finds its way to the nucleus and the DNA of the cell. Viral DNA integrates itself into the cellular DNA or genome of the cell, creating a provirus (Gallo, 1987; Laurence, 1985; Margolick et al., 1987; Margolick & Fauci, 1987). Once the provirus is in place, the cell is confused. Its genetic machinery is no longer pure cell but part virus, and so the cell may function abnormally. In addition, when cell products are made, one of the products (coded

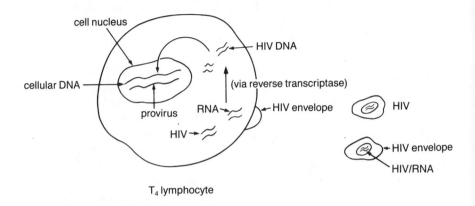

Figure 3–3. HIV Infecting a T lymphocyte.

by the viral DNA), is new virus (Bennett, 1986; Gallo, 1987; Laurence, 1985). Thus, there is an infected cell capable of producing virus. It is known that this virus can remain latent inside of a cell for a variable length of time. Only when the cell becomes activated, does active infection occur (Bowen et al., 1985; Margolick et al., 1987; Margolick & Fauci, 1987).

Human Immunodeficiency Virus Type 2 (HIV-2). HIV-2 was first reported in 1986 in West Africa, where the virus is believed to be endemic. HIV-2 is closely related to, but distinct from, HIV-1. A majority of persons with documented HIV-2 infection in Africa have a clinical syndrome indistinguishable from AIDS, others have HIV-1 type symptoms (similar to ARC) and some are asymptomatic (Clavel, 1987). In addition, the modes of transmission of HIV-2 are similar to those of HIV-1, the major mechanism of spread being sexual intercourse (CDC, 1988).

Several well documented cases of HIV-2 infection and disease have been reported among Europeans and especially West Africans living in Europe. In January, 1987, the Centers for Disease Control (CDC) and the Food and Drug Administration (FDA) initiated surveillance for HIV-2 in the United States. As of January 1988 approximately 22,699 serum samples have been screened, and no case of HIV-2 infection has been found (CDC, 1988). In December, 1987, a case of AIDS caused by HIV-2 was reported from New Jersey. The patient was a West African woman with cerebral toxoplasmosis (CDC, 1988). She tested negative on ELISA (enzyme-linked immunosorbent assay) for HIV-1 and positive on both ELISA and Western blot for HIV-2. The CDC states that occasional cases of infection with HIV-2 should be anticipated in the United States. The CDC estimates that between 40 and 90% of HIV-2 infections will be detected by HIV-1 ELISA; however, surveillance for HIV-2 will also continue. Education and prevention measures for HIV-1 and HIV-2 are the same.

HIV and the Immune System. HIV selectively infects the T4 (or CD4+) cell (Bowen et al., 1985; Gallo, 1987; Lane & Fauci, 1985; Margolick et al., 1987). In fact, some studies have shown that the cellular receptor for the virus is actually the CD4 molecule itself (Bowen et al., 1985; Fauci, 1987; Margolick et al., 1987; Margolick & Fauci, 1987). HIV is cytopathic for infected cells, eventually leading to their destruction. The result is a quantitative defect in T4 cells (Bowen et al., 1985; Lane & Fauci, 1985; Lane, 1987; Laurence, 1985; Margolick et al., 1987). Persons who are immunologically normal have between 600 and 1200 T4 cells/mm^3. Persons with AIDS generally have from 0–500 T4 cells, and even asymptomatic HIV-infected individuals often have a lower than normal number of T4 lymphocytes (Lane, 1987). The number of T4 cells seems to correlate with clinical course. Persons with very low T4 cell numbers tend to have more clinical problems, especially infection, than those with a higher T4 cell number (Lane & Fauci, 1987). Due to a low number of T4 cells, the individual is also usually lymphopenic (low total lymphocyte count), and his or her ratio of T4/T8 cells (normally 2:1) is low (Bowen et al., 1985; Lane & Fauci, 1985; Laurence, 1985; Margolick et al., 1987). The number of T8 cells in AIDS is generally normal, but may be slightly increased or decreased.

Besides an abnormal number of T4 cells, the function of infected T4 cells is also defective (Bowen et al., 1985; Lane & Fauci, 1985; Laurence, 1985; Margolick et al., 1987; Margolick & Fauci, 1987). In persons with AIDS (PWAs), all of the normal functions of the T4 cell are either absent or depressed (Bowen et al., 1985; Lane & Fauci, 1985; Margolick et al., 1987; Margolick & Fauci, 1987). This includes:

1. decreased ability of T4 cells to release lymphokines,
2. decreased cytotoxicity,
3. decreased T cell help to B cells for Ig synthesis, and
4. decreased ability of T cells to proliferate in mixed lymphocyte cultures.

Possibly the most significant finding is that T4 cells are unresponsive or less responsive to specific antigen (as demonstrated by in vitro and in vivo tests with tetanus toxoid), and therefore lack all of the antigen induced T4 cell functions (Lane, 1987; Margolick et al., 1987; Margolick & Fauci, 1987). The result is abnormal function in almost every part of the immune system. In other words, without the conductor, the symphony does not play well together. Some players don't play at all, others play feverishly and don't know when to stop, and still others are playing the wrong music. Clinically what is seen are the results of a defective CMI manifested by opportunistic infections and tumors.

As mentioned earlier, research has demonstrated that activated T4 lymphocytes are more easily infected and more productive of virus than resting T4 cells (Fauci, 1987; Lane & Fauci, 1985; Margolick et al., 1987; Margolick & Fauci, 1987). There are several immune stimulators that activate lymphocytes and therefore could be co-factors necessary for active infection and disease. Theoretical possibilities include: other infectious agents (such as cytomegalovirus [CMV],

Epstein-Barr virus [EBV], parasitic infections), environmental antigens, drugs, toxic substances, and genetic factors (Fauci, 1987; Margolick et al., 1987). In the clinical situation this means educating PWAs to prevent infection and to avoid drugs and other toxic substances that may serve as immune activators.

Humoral immunity or B cell abnormalities seen in AIDS may be due to the aforementioned lack of induction and regulation by the T cell; to direct activation of the B cell by HIV, EBV, or CMV; or possibly to an excess secretion of lymphokines that stimulate B cells (Bowen et al., 1985; Lane & Fauci, 1985; Margolick et al., 1987; Margolick & Fauci, 1987). Whatever the cause, B cells in AIDS are polyclonally activated, which results in a hypergammaglobulinemia (high level of circulating IgG, IgA, IgM) and increased levels of circulating immune complexes and autoantibodies (Lane & Fauci, 1985; Margolick & Fauci, 1987). At the same time, B cells will not mount an antibody response to a new antigen. Some individuals with AIDS experience clinical problems related to circulating immune complexes or autoantibodies, for example thrombocytopenia, Reiter's disease, and others (Fauci, 1987; Lane & Fauci, 1985). The lack of ability to mount an antibody response has clinical significance in that serologic criteria for diagnosing certain infections are unreliable (Bowen et al., 1985; Lane & Fauci, 1985; Margolick et al., 1987). In addition, a PWA will probably not respond to immunization (e.g., pneumococcal vaccine or influenza vaccine) with appropriate production of antibody (Lane & Fauci, 1985; Lane, 1987). PWAs should never be vaccinated with any vaccine made with live virus (Stites et al., 1984).

Monocytes/macrophages in HIV infection have also been shown to be abnormal. In vitro tests show: (1) decreased intracellular killing following phagocytosis; (2) decreased chemotaxis; and (3) decreased expression of class II HLA antigens (Lane & Fauci, 1985; Margolick & Fauci, 1987). These defects may be due to a lack of gamma interferon and other monocyte stimulating lymphokines from the T4 cell, as well as direct infection of monocytes/macrophages with HIV (Bowen et al., 1985; Margolick et al., 1987; Margolick & Fauci, 1987). The monocyte defect is important clinically because it contributes to the frequent occurrence of diseases due to parasites and intracellular organisms (Bowen et al., 1985).

Clinically, a PWA is usually lymphopenic with a low number of T4 cells, a low T4/T8 ratio, and anergy. In addition the PWA shows manifestations of opportunistic diseases which normally would be handled by T cell immunity, hypergammaglobulinemia, an inability to make new antibody, and an inability to kill intracellular organisms efficiently (Table 3–3).

HIV Antibody. When an individual is adequately exposed to HIV, he or she will begin to make antibody to the virus. This antibody is usually detectable by current measures within three months of exposure. Antibody to HIV is measured by a test known as the ELISA (enzyme-linked immunosorbent assay) (Durham &

Table 3–3. Immunologic Abnormalities in AIDS

T cell number	low T4 cell number—lymphopenia
T cell function	decreased ability to release lymphokines decreased cytotoxicity decreased B cell help decreased proliferation in mixed lymphocyte culture decreased responsiveness to specific antigen
B cell number	normal

B cell function	polyclonal activation with increased Ig levels and
	    increased circulating immune complexes
	inability to respond to new antigen by
	    antibody production

Macrophage number	normal
Macrophage function	decreased intracellular killing during phagocytosis decreased chemotaxis decreased expression of class II HLA antigens

Cohen, 1987). After the virus was discovered and isolated in spring of 1984, work began on the development of a test to detect antibody. By the spring of 1985 this test was in place for the purpose of screening donated blood. Screening of blood by the ELISA is done at all blood banks and blood collection centers in the United States and in many places around the world. If a sample of donated blood tests positive, the blood is not used. A second ELISA is always run on another sample of the blood, and a confirmatory test (Western blot analysis) is done before the person is determined to be positive for antibody to HIV. The ELISA test has also been used to test individuals who want to know whether or not they have been infected with HIV. The test is available through private physicians, health departments and clinics, and at alternative testing sites. It is important to remember that the HIV antibody test is not a test for AIDS. Having a positive test for antibody does not mean the person has AIDS or will necessarily develop AIDS. Preliminary studies show that approximately 30% of persons who test positive for antibody to HIV will develop AIDS within 5–10 years (Fauci, 1987).

The ELISA test uses beads or microtiter wells coated with inactivated HIV antigen to which is added goat anti-human immunoglobulin linked to an enzyme. The blood to be tested is placed in the antigen-coated wells; if antibody is present it will bind to antigen. This antibody is then detected by the antihuman antibodies conjugated to enzyme, which when bound produce a color. Because the ELISA is very sensitive, it is always confirmed by repeating it several times to look for repeated reactivity and by using the Western blot analysis (which is more specific). The Western blot is able to identify antibodies to HIV proteins of specific molecular weights. Therefore, besides being more specific, it gives information about the particular antibodies that HIV antigens may elicit, specifically antibodies against gp120, gp41, and p24 (parts of the virus). A person who is both ELISA positive and Western blot positive has antibody to HIV and is believed to be infected and also considered infectious. It is probable that persons who are antibody positive will be so for the rest of their lives. Some of them will develop AIDS.

p24 Antigen Capture Assay. A test that has received a great deal of attention recently is a test for HIV antigen, specifically the part of the antigen known as p24. This is not a test for antibody. It is a test that measures the amount of p24 antigen. p24 is a piece of the HIV referred to as core antigen. In the p24 antigen assay, a monoclonal antibody to p24 is reacted with the patient's serum. If p24 antigen is present, the monoclonal antibody will attach to it. Then, a second labeled antibody is added to detect captured antigen. As it binds, a color is enzymatically produced. The amount of color measures the amount of p24 antigen present (Lane, 1987). The p24 antigen capture assay is a test used primarily by researchers involved in basic research and clinical trials. It is not a licensed or commercially available test. The detection of p24 antigen is an indication of the presence of active HIV infection and is, therefore, a useful indicator to monitor the effectiveness of experimental antiviral therapy. Some studies have attempted to correlate higher levels of p24 antigen with an increase in symptoms and a declining clinical course. Two studies presented at the Third International Conference on AIDS (Pedersen et al., 1987 and Phair et al., 1987) suggest that HIV antigenemia (as measured by p24 antigen) precedes the development of clinical symptoms or opportunistic infections and is associated with a depletion of T4 cells. Exactly if and how the p24 antigen capture assay can be used as an indicator of clinical course is yet to be determined.

Clinical Manifestations in HIV Infection

There is a broad spectrum of consequences of infection with HIV; full-blown AIDS represents only a relatively small part. Most HIV-infected individuals are asymptomatic and physically feel fine. The Centers for Disease Control (CDC) in May 1986 devised a classification scheme which is helpful in understanding the spectrum of HIV infection (Table 3–4). The classification is intended for use with future case reporting and in disease coding and recording systems. In the classification, each group is distinct, i.e., a person can only be classified in one group at a time although classifications can change. The classification is also hierarchical, i.e., from Group I a person can only move to Group II and then to Group III, etc., but not back from a higher group to Group I (Durham & Cohen, 1987; CDC, 1986).

An acute HIV infection (CDC Group I) has been described in which a person experiences fever, malaise, rash, lymphadenopathy, and muscle aches, in essence a mononucleosis-like illness approximately two to three weeks after exposure to HIV. The syndrome resolves within a week or so. In persons in whom this type of

Table 3–4. Summary of Classification System for Human Immunodeficiency Virus (HIV) Infection

Group I.	Acute infection
Group II.	Asymptomatic infection*
Group III.	Persistent generalized lymphadenopathy*
Group IV.	Other disease

    Subgroup A. Constitutional
    Subgroup B. Neurologic disease
    Subgroup C. Secondary infectious diseases
        Category C-1. Specified secondary infectious diseases listed in the CDC surveillance definitions for AIDS†
        Category C-2. Other specified secondary infectious diseases
    Subgroup D. Secondary cancers†
    Subgroup E. Other conditions

---

*Patients in Groups II and III may be subclassified on the basis of a laboratory evaluation.
†Includes those patients whose clinical presentation fulfills the definitions of AIDS used by the CDC for national reporting.

From: Classification system for human T-lymphotropic virus III/lymphadenopathy associated virus infections (1986). *Morbidity and Mortality Weekly Report*, 35, 335.

illness has been documented, seroconversion to HIV antibody positive occurs shortly thereafter, usually within three months of initial exposure (Durham & Cohen, 1987).

There are an estimated 1.5 to 2 million individuals in the United States who are HIV-infected and asymptomatic; they are classified by the CDC as Group II.

CDC Group III are persons with persistent generalized lymphadenopathy (PGL). This group consists of HIV-infected individuals who essentially feel well but have persistent (longer than three months), palpable lymphadenopathy with lymph node enlargement of greater than 1 cm, at more than one extra-inguinal site, and the absence of a concurrent illness other than HIV infection which would explain the lymphadenopathy.

Group IV includes patients with clinical symptoms and diseases other than or in addition to lymphadenopathy. Group IV is divided into four subgroups and each group may include people who are mildly symptomatic or severely ill. A patient may fall into more than one of the subgroups at any given time. It is important to note that only those who fall into subgroup C, category C-1, and subgroup D are by definition diagnosed as having AIDS (CDC, 1986). In-depth information on the most recent CDC case definitions for diagnosing AIDS can be found in Appendix B.

Subgroup A: Constitutional Disease. This group includes persons with one or more of the following: fever persisting for more than one month, involuntary weight loss of more than 10% of body weight, or diarrhea for more than one month, and the absence of a concurrent illness other than HIV infection to explain these symptoms (CDC, 1986). Most of the persons that are referred to as having AIDS-related complex (ARC) fit into this subgroup.

Subgroup B: Neurologic Disease. Patients fall into this group if they have dementia, myelopathy, or peripheral neuropathy in the absence of concurrent illness other than HIV infection to explain these symptoms. Besides the several opportunistic infections that affect the central nervous system, it is now known that between 30% (Ho, 1985) and 60% (McArthur & McArthur, 1986) of persons with AIDS (PWAs) have some signs or symptoms of AIDS dementia or subacute encephalitis. It is believed to be caused by direct HIV infection of the brain. Typical symptoms include apathy, depression, and withdrawal (Beckham & Rudy, 1986; Lane & Fauci, 1987). Dementia is usually progressive and over time a person may develop memory loss, confusion, deterioration in intellectual functioning, and inability to care for self. This differential diagnosis between AIDS dementia, the opportunistic infections or neoplasms that affect the central nervous system, and depression or psychosis is critical for appropriate management and care. Central nervous system complications and neurologic dysfunctions are discussed in greater depth in Chapters 5 and 8.

Subgroup C: Secondary Infectious Diseases. This subgroup is further divided into two categories. Category C-1 includes persons diagnosed with one of the opportunistic infections listed in the CDC surveillance definition of AIDS. These include: *Pneumocystis carinii* pneumonia, chronic cryptosporidiosis, toxoplasmosis, candidiasis (esophageal, bronchial, or pulmonary), cryptococcosis, histoplasmosis, isosporiasis, mycobacterial infection with *Mycobacterium avium* or *Mycobacterium kansasii*, cytomegalovirus infection, chronic mucocutaneous or disseminated herpes simplex infection, and progressive multifocal encephalopathy. Category C-2 includes patients with invasive disease with one of the following: oral hairy leukoplakia, multidermatomal herpes zoster, recurrent Salmonella bacteremia, nocardiasis, tuberculosis, or oral candida (Durham & Cohen, 1987).

Subgroup D: Secondary Cancers. This group includes those individuals who have one of the types of cancer that is known to be associated with HIV infection and is listed in the CDC surveillance definition. This includes: Kaposi's sarcoma, non-Hodgkin's lymphoma, or primary lymphoma of the brain.

Subgroup E: Other. This is a catch-all group for any clinical findings or diseases that are not classifiable in the other groups, yet may be attributed to HIV infection and/or may be indicative of a cell-mediated immunodeficiency. Examples might include patients with chronic interstitial pneumonitis or with thrombocytopenia. It is probable that as new information and diagnostic techniques are available, more clinical symptoms will be defined that may not be classifiable except in this subgroup. Periodic revision of the classification scheme may have to be made.

Specific Diseases in AIDS

The clinical presentation of AIDS is the secondary opportunistic infection or neoplasm that occurs because of the immune defect. PWAs suffer from infections caused by protozoa, viruses, fungi, and atypical bacteria, as well as from specific forms of cancer. Following is a brief description of the signs and symptoms of common clinical manifestations, as well as some information about diagnostic tests (Tables 3–5 and 3–6). For an in-depth discussion of medical treatment and nursing care, see Chapters 4 and 5, respectively.

Opportunistic Infections. *Pneumocystis carinii* pneumonia (PCP), caused by the protozoal pneumocyst, is the most common opportunistic infection in AIDS, occurring in at least 60% of PWAs, and recurring in many (Durham & Cohen, 1987; Kaplan et al., 1987; Kovacs & Masur, 1985; Volberding, 1985). PCP in AIDS is a diffuse pneumonia manifested by cough, fever, and shortness of breath. Unlike other cell-mediated immunodeficient conditions, the onset of symptoms in AIDS is generally insidious, with many patients having symptoms for two to three weeks or longer before being diagnosed (Kovacs & Masur, 1985). In PWAs the cough and dyspnea are often not as severe as in non-AIDS patients, but without timely treatment PCP in AIDS can progress to a fulminant and life-threatening infection. The PWA with PCP may be mildly symptomatic or very symptomatic. Early in the course of PCP, respiratory rate is generally increased, but not dramatically so; paO2 is decreased (also not dramatically), and chest x-ray shows diffuse interstitial infiltrates (Kovacs & Masur, 1985). Although with respiratory symptoms there should be a high suspicion for PCP, definitive diagnosis requires seeing pneumocystis in bronchial secretions or lung tissue. This is obtained by bronchoscopy with lavage and/or biopsy, by induction of sputum, or in some cases by open lung biopsy (Armstrong et al., 1985; Kaplan et al., 1987; Kovacs & Masur, 1985; Volberding, 1985).

Toxoplasma gondii, another protozoan, causes a focal encephalitis in some PWAs, and occasionally disseminated infection. *Toxoplasma gondii* infection is probably the result of reactivation of a latent infection in the setting of an immunodeficiency (Kovacs & Masur, 1985). The patient presents with headache, seizures, lethargy, and focal neurologic signs. Many patients also experience a change in their personality and/or cognitive ability (Beckham & Rudy, 1986; Kovacs & Masur, 1985). Many of the symptoms in a PWA with *T. gondii* infection can be subtle and diffuse and require careful assessment and comparison with baseline data in order to detect them. On lumbar puncture, increased white blood cells (especially lymphocytes) and increased protein are usually found in the cerebrospinal fluid (CSF) (Beckham & Rudy, 1986; Durham & Cohen, 1987; Kovacs & Masur, 1985). On CT scan with contrast, a contrast-enhancing mass lesion or multiple lesions are usually demonstrated. Definitive diagnosis depends on brain biopsy and identification of the toxoplasma trophozoite in brain tissue (Lane & Fauci, 1987; Kovacs & Masur, 1985).

Cryptosporidiosis is an intestinal infection with the cryptosporidium, a protozoan. It is manifested by watery diarrhea, malaise, nausea, and abdominal cramps. In AIDS, the diarrhea can be voluminous, with some patients losing 10–15 liters of stool per day. The person with cryptosporidium gastroenteritis may go

Table 3–5. Opportunistic Infections and Diseases Commonly Associated with HIV Infection

A. *Infections*	*Body System Affected*
PATHOGENS	
1. Protozoal	
Pneumocystis carinii	respiratory
Toxoplasma gondii	neurologic and disseminated
Cryptosporidium	gastrointestinal
Isospora belli	gastrointestinal
2. Bacterial	
Mycobacterium avium intracellulare	disseminated
M. tuberculosis	respiratory, neurologic, or disseminated
3. Fungal	
Candida albicans	gastrointestinal (mouth and/or esophagus)
	disseminated
Cryptococcus neoformans	neurologic or disseminated
Histoplasma capsulatum	disseminated
4. Viral	
Herpes simplex	integumentary (mouth, genital, perianal)
Varicella-zoster	integumentary
Cytomegalovirus	neurologic (eyes) disseminated
Jakob-Creutzfeldt Papovavirus	neurologic
(causing progressive multifocal	
leukoencephalopathy)	

B. *Neoplastic Diseases Associated with HIV Infection*

1. Kaposi's sarcoma (epidemic form)
2. Burkitt's lymphoma
3. Non-Hodgkin's lymphomas
4. Hodgkin's disease
5. Chronic lymphocytic leukemia
6. Carcinoma of the oropharynx
7. Hepatocellular carcinoma
8. Adenosquamous carcinoma of the lung

C. *Autoimmune Disorders*

1. *Neurologic*
   Chronic demyelinating neuropathy
   Inflammatory myopathy
2. *Vascular*
   Vasculitis
3. *Hematologic*
   Immune thrombocytopenic purpura
   Leukopenia
   Coombs'-positive anemia
   Lupus-like anticoagulants
4. *Pulmonary*
   Lymphocytic interstitial pneumonitis
5. *Renal*
   Focal sclerosing glomerulonephritis

Developed by P. Ungvarski, 1988.
Adapted from: Masur et al., 1985; Safai & Koziner, 1985; Hollander, 1987.

**Table 3–6. Summary of Common Laboratory Abnormalities
Associated with HIV Infection and AIDS**

Anemia
Leukopenia
Lymphopenia (helper T cells: $400/mm^3$)
T4 helper/T8 suppressor ratio = 1.0
Thrombocytopenia
Anergy to skin tests
Mild elevation of liver enzymes
Elevated sedimentation rate

Developed by P. Ungvarski, 1988.

on to develop severe weight loss, fluid and electrolyte imbalance, malnutrition, and debility (Kaplan et al., 1987; Lane & Fauci, 1987). Cryptosporidiosis is diagnosed by demonstrating the organism in feces either via direct fecal wet mount or a sugar flotation method (Kovacs & Masur, 1985; Lane & Fauci, 1987).

Candida albicans (a fungus) infections of the mouth and esophagus are very common in PWAs (Armstrong et al., 1985; Durham & Cohen, 1987; Kovacs & Masur, 1985; Lane & Fauci, 1987). Oral candida may be present in an HIV-infected individual before the development of an opportunistic infection diagnostic of AIDS. Patients with oral candida usually complain of food tasting "funny" and sometimes pain in the mouth or difficulty swallowing. On examination, a white, thick cottage-cheesy exudate can be seen. The patient with candida esophagitis usually complains of difficulty swallowing as well as retrosternal burning and pain. Diagnosis of candida is done by microscopic examination of scrapings or swabs of infected lesions (Kovacs & Masur, 1985). For esophagitis, endoscopy with biopsy may be necessary.

Cryptococcus neoformans is a fungus that causes meningitis or disseminated disease in PWAs. Meningitis presents as an acute meningeal infection with fever, headache, nausea and vomiting, blurred vision, stiff neck, and confusion (Beckham & Rudy, 1986; Kovacs & Masur, 1985; Lane & Fauci, 1987). In AIDS, symptoms are often initially mild, so again careful assessment and comparison with baseline data is critical. Some patients with cryptococcal meningitis will present with focal neurologic signs, seizures, and obtundation. Cryptococcal meningitis is diagnosed by doing a lumbar puncture and looking for a pleocytosis (increased white blood cells), low glucose, high protein, positive India ink test, and a measurable cryptococcal antigen titer in CSF (Durham & Cohen, 1987; Kovacs & Masur, 1985). Even with treatment, cryptococcal disease often relapses in PWAs (Kaplan et al., 1987).

Cytomegalovirus (CMV), a member of the herpesvirus family, is a very common infection and cause of disease in PWAs. Although approximately one-half of persons in the general population have been infected with CMV and have antibody to it, the virus appears to remain in a latent, non-problematic form unless the person becomes immunocompromised. CMV is transmitted sexually and via blood and blood products. The incidence in healthy homosexual men (85%) is much greater than in the general population, and CMV is probably very common among drug users and blood recipients, although little data are available (Kovacs & Masur, 1985; Lane & Fauci, 1987). CMV can cause fever, malaise, weight loss, fatigue, and lymphadenopathy, but in AIDS it is probably just one of several infections that contributes to these symptoms. In AIDS, CMV causes major damage in multiple organ systems, especially in the retina, lung, and large intestine (Durham & Cohen, 1987; Kovacs & Masur, 1985; Lane & Fauci, 1987). Most commonly seen in AIDS is CMV retinochoroiditis. Patients initially complain of mildly impaired vision. On fundoscopic exam, areas of hemorrhage, exudate, and/or necrosis are seen. Lesions may be unilateral or bilateral, but can and do sometimes lead to total bilateral blindness. CMV in the gastrointestinal tract usually results in watery diarrhea and weight loss. CMV in the lungs presents as scattered pulmonary infiltrates on chest x-ray with symptoms of hypoxemia, dyspnea, tachypnea, and chest pain (Kovacs & Masur, 1985). CMV in the central nervous system may cause confusion, headaches, and dementia. Disseminated CMV can contribute to fever, general malaise, weight loss, and pancytopenia. The presence of CMV is determined by positive cultures from blood, urine, or throat washings. The diagnosis of CMV organ disease is made by biopsy and histopathologic evidence of intranuclear or intracytoplasmic inclusion bodies and an appropriate inflammatory response (Kovacs & Masur, 1985; Lane & Fauci, 1987). CMV seems to be one of the leading causes of death in AIDS; on autopsy, invasive CMV is a frequent finding.

Perirectal mucocutaneous disease caused by herpes simplex virus (HSV), usually HSV type II, is a fairly common occurrence in PWAs. Less commonly, genital or oral lesions are seen. Early lesions are vesicular, but with time the vesicles burst, collapse, and in the genital or perirectal area usually ulcerate (Kovacs & Masur, 1985). Lesions may range from minute, close to the anal sphincter, to lesions that are many centimeters in diameter. Patients with perirectal HSV ulcers usually complain of severe rectal pain, bleeding, tenesmus, hematochezia, or rectal discharge (Kovacs & Masur, 1985; Lane & Fauci, 1987). The pain associated with herpes lesions can be extraordinary, itself necessitating assessment and intervention. Presumptive diagnosis can often be made by clinical evaluation. Definitive diagnosis is established by culture of the lesions and/or biopsy (Kovacs & Masur, 1985).

Varicella-zoster virus (VZV) is also a herpesvirus. VZV is the cause of common childhood chickenpox. VZV also causes shingles, which occurs primarily in immunocompromised or older individuals. VZV occurs in AIDS, but not as commonly as other herpesvirus infections. VZV presents as vesicular eruptions that have a dermatomal distribution, characteristically unilateral (Kovacs & Masur, 1985; Lane & Fauci, 1987). The eruptions are usually accompanied by and sometimes preceded by itching or a tingling sensation and sometimes severe pain (Kovacs & Masur, 1985). The vesicles rupture and form a crust; this usually occurs within the first week and then the crusts persist for two to three weeks. Herpes zoster can also be a disseminated infection in patients with AIDS. VZV is diagnosed by clinical evaluation and culture of the vesicular lesions.

Epstein-Barr virus (EBV), another herpesvirus, is found frequently in AIDS patients. Almost all PWAs show serologic evidence of past infection with EBV. EBV causes a proliferation of atypical polyclonally activated B cells (Kovacs & Masur, 1985; Lane & Fauci, 1987). Normally T lymphocytes would destroy EBV infected B cells, and signs and symptoms of a mononucleosis-like syndrome including leukocytosis, lymphadenopathy, and splenomegaly occur. PWAs, probably because of defective T cell function, have high levels of circulating EBV infected B cells. EBV may also enhance the ability of HIV to infect lymphocytes (both T and B) (Margolick et al., 1987). Signs and symptoms caused by EBV include low-grade fever, malaise, pharyngitis, and lymphadenopathy (Kovacs & Masur, 1985). These symptoms in AIDS are attributed to several different organisms; to what extent EBV contributes to the clinical picture is unknown.

Mycobacterium avium intracellulare (MAI) is an environmental bacterium that only rarely caused significant infection in humans prior to the emergence of AIDS. Even in patients with severely compromised immunity, other forms of mycobacterial infection are more common than MAI (Kovacs & Masur, 1985). In AIDS, MAI is relatively common and occurs usually as a disseminated infection (Kaplan et al., 1987; Kovacs & Masur, 1985; Lane & Fauci, 1987). Patients have fever, weight loss, abnormal liver function tests, and progressive pancytopenia. MAI can be cultured from blood as well as from a number of body organs, including bone marrow, lymph nodes, liver, and spleen. MAI is also usually found in the sputum or bronchoscopic washings of patients with disseminated disease (Lane & Fauci, 1987). Whether or not MAI causes or contributes to specific organ disease is not known. The clinical contribution of MAI is also unclear, because persons infected with MAI are usually multiply infected.

Mycobacterium tuberculosis (MTB) is a more familiar disease that occurs as an opportunistic infection in PWAs. It is seen more frequently in PWAs in the developing world, but does occur in the United States. AIDS-associated tuberculosis is often extrapulmonary and can disseminate to virtually any organ system, particularly the lymph system, meninges, genitourinary system, pericardium, gastrointestinal tract, peritoneum, bones, joints, larynx, and pleura (Kaplan et al., 1987; Kovacs & Masur, 1985; Lane & Fauci, 1987). Symptoms vary with the organ affected, but fever is generally present. Diagnosis is made by detecting acid fast bacillus in specimens collected from the affected organs (Kovacs & Masur, 1985). A summary of the symptoms of AIDS-related diseases is contained in Table 3–7.

Malignant Neoplasms. Kaposi's sarcoma (KS), the most common neoplasm in AIDS, occurs in approximately 30% of PWAs (Safai et al., 1985). KS is a multifocal systemic neoplasm of the vascular endothelium. Classically, Kaposi's sarcoma is associated with immunodeficiency and may even contribute to progressive

Table 3–7. Signs and Symptoms of AIDS-Related Diseases

Symptoms	Possible Causes
fever, malaise, weight loss, myalgias, lymphadenopathy	HIV infection CMV infection disseminated MAI EBV lymphoma
shortness of breath, cough, fever, dyspnea, chest tightness, or discomfort	*Pneumocystis carinii* pneumonia CMV pneumonitis interstitial pneumonitis pulmonary Kaposi's sarcoma
mouth pain, difficulty swallowing, "funny" taste to food —without retrosternal burning —with retrosternal burning	oral candidiasis oral KS lesions oral HSV lesions esophageal candida
abdominal discomfort, diarrhea, weight loss	cryptosporidiosis isosporiasis CMV colitis Giardia, amoeba KS of GI tract HIV infection lymphoma
headache, disorientation, personality changes, apathy, confusion, seizures	toxoplasmosis cryptococcosis CMV encephalitis progressive multifocal leukoencephalopathy lymphoma HIV infection psychosis/depression
skin lesions	Kaposi's sarcoma herpes simplex varicella-zoster cryptococcal disease mycobacterial disease secondary syphilis

immunodeficiency. Even so, in general the immune profiles of PWAs with KS are better than those with AIDS-related opportunistic infections (Lane, 1987). The incidence of KS in homosexual men with AIDS is higher than in other AIDS-affected groups. Although KS has diverse clinical presentations, the most common presentation is a single or a few cutaneous lesions. These lesions are usually purplish-red in color, discrete, palpable, and not painful or pruritic. Lesions may appear on any part of the body, with the trunk, arms, head, and neck being frequent sites of lesions in AIDS (Durham & Cohen, 1987; Safai & Koziner, 1985). In certain places, KS lesions can be quite painful, for example on the foot, on or near the eyes, and on a beltline or collar edge. There is a higher incidence of extracutaneous KS in AIDS than in the classical form of KS (Kaplan et al., 1987; Lane, 1987; Safai et al., 1985). Common extracutaneous sites include the mucous membranes, lymph nodes, gastrointestinal tract, and lungs. Initially, the patient with KS presents with a suspicious lesion which was usually found by inspection. Some patients present with malaise, lymphadenopathy, fever, weight loss, and intermittent diarrhea, which may be due to KS. Others have no prodromal symptoms. AIDS-KS is a progressive disease; beginning with a few skin lesions, it often develops into a diffuse skin disease with gastrointestinal or lymph node involvement, and eventually pulmonary involvement (Fauci, 1987; Lane, 1987; Safai & Koziner, 1985). Kaposi's sarcoma is diagnosed by biopsy of suspicious cutaneous lesions or lymph nodes (Safai & Koziner, 1985).

Although less common than KS, there are other neoplasms that are seen with increased frequency in AIDS. Malignant lymphomas of the central nervous system, otherwise relatively rare, are seen in PWAs, as well as non-Hodgkin's lymphoma and Burkitt's-like lymphomas (Durham & Cohen, 1987; Volberding, 1985). In general these diseases in AIDS have an aggressive course, are not very responsive to therapy, and have a short survival time.

Summary

HIV is a retrovirus that selectively infects the T4 lymphocyte. The T4 lymphocyte is the central cell, the inducer cell in the immune response, sending induction signals to other cells of the immune system. HIV infection of T4 cells causes a progressive quantitative depletion of T4 cells and an abnormal function of T4 cells, both of which contribute to abnormalities in the function of the B cells, T8 cells, NK cells, and monocytes/macrophages. The PWA presents with an opportunistic infection or a malignancy that is indicative of a cell mediated immunodeficiency without any reason to be immunodeficient except for infection with HIV, and which therefore is diagnostic for AIDS. In dealing with AIDS, health care providers face a unique and variable disease. Patients may present with one or more of the aforementioned diseases and may have rapid progression of disease and a short survival. Alternatively, a patient may present with KS alone, or with one infection that is successfully treated, and then have one to two years or more of relative wellness with intermittent bouts of infection, symptoms, or new lesions.

References

Armstrong, D., Gold, J., Dryjanski, J., et al. (1985). Treatment of infections in patients with the acquired immunodeficiency syndrome. *Annals of Internal Medicine*, 103(5), 738–743.

Beckham, M., & Rudy, E. (1986). Acquired immunodeficiency syndrome: Impact and implication for the neurological system. *Journal of Neuroscience Nursing*, 18(1), 5–10.

Bellanti, J. (1985). *Immunology: basic processes*. Philadelphia: W.B. Saunders.

Bennett, J. (1986). AIDS: What we know. *American Journal of Nursing*, 86, 1016–1021.

Bowen, D., Lane, H., & Fauci, A. (1985). Immunopathogenesis of the acquired immunodeficiency syndrome. *Annals of Internal Medicine*, 5(103), 704–709.

Centers for Disease Control (1986). Classification system for human T-lymphotropic virus III/lymphadenopathy associated virus infections. *Mortality and Morbidity Weekly Report*, 35, 335.

Centers for Disease Control (1988). AIDS due to HIV-2 infection. *Mortality and Morbidity Weekly Report*, 37(3), 33–35.

Clavel, F., Mansinho, K., Chamaret, S., et al. (1987). Human immunodeficiency virus type 2 infections associated with AIDS in West Africa. *New England Journal of Medicine*, 316(19), 1180–1185.

Coffin, J., Haase, A., Levy, J., et al. (1986). What to call the AIDS virus? *Nature*, 321(6065), 10.

Durham, J., & Cohen, F. (1987). *The person with AIDS: Nursing perspectives*. New York: Springer Publishing Company.

Fauci, A. (1984). Immunologic abnormalities in the acquired immunodeficiency syndrome. Delivered at the American Federation for Clinical Research Meeting, Washington, D.C., May 1984.

Fauci, A.S. (1987). Personal Communication.

Gallo, R. (1987). The AIDS virus. *Scientific American*, 256(1), 46–56.

Halliburton, P. (1986). Impaired immunocompetence. In Carrieri, V.K., Lindsey, A.M., & West, C.M. (Eds.), *Pathophysiologic phenomena in nursing: Human responses to illness*. Philadelphia: W.B. Saunders.

Ho, D. (1985). Isolation of HTLV-III from cerebral spinal fluid and neural tissues of patients with neurological syndromes related to acquired immunodeficiency syndrome. *New England Journal of Medicine*, 313, 1493–1497.

Hollander, H. (1987). Human immunodeficiency virus infection: Diagnostic and treatment issues in an expanding spectrum. *Postgraduate Medicine*, 81, 79–84.

Impact of routine HTLV-III antibody testing on public health (1986, July). Report of the NIH Consensus Development Conference, Washington, D.C.

Kaplan, L., Wofsy, C., & Volberding, P. (1987). Treatment of patients with acquired immunodeficiency syndrome and associated manifestations. *Journal of American Medical Association*, 257(10), 1367–1374.

Kovacs, J., & Masur, H. (1985). Opportunistic infections. In J. Gallin, & A. Fauci (Eds.), *AIDS: advances in host defense mechanisms*, Chapter 5. New York: Raven Press.

Lane, H.C. (1987). Personal communication.

Lane, H.C., & Fauci, A.S. (1985). Immunologic abnormalities in the acquired immunodeficiency syndrome. *Annual Review of Immunology*, 3, 477–500.

Lane, H.C., & Fauci, A.S. (1987). Infectious complications of AIDS. In S. Border (Ed.), *AIDS*, Chapter 11. New York: Marcel Dekker Inc.

Laurence, J. (1985, December). The immune system in AIDS. *Scientific American*, 253(6), 84–93.

Margolick, J., & Fauci, A. (1987). Immunopathogenesis of the acquired immunodeficiency syndrome. *Progress in Immunology*, 6th edition.

Margolick, J., Lane, H., & Fauci, A. (1987). Immunopathogenesis of HTLV III/LAV infection. *Viruses and Human Cancer* (pp. 59–70). New York: Alan R. Liss.

Masur, H., Kovacs, J.A., Ognibene, F., et al. (1985). Infectious complications of AIDS. In V.T. Devita, S. Hellman, & S.A. Rosenberg (Eds.), *AIDS: Etiology, diagnosis, treatment and prevention* (pp. 161–184). Philadelphia: J.B. Lippincott.

McArthur, J., & McArthur, J. (1986). Neurologic manifestations of acquired immunodeficiency syndrome. *Journal of Neuroscience Nursing*, 18(5), 242–249.

Pedersen, C., Nielsen, C., Vestergaard, B., et al. (1987, June). HIV antigenemia precedes the development of AIDS or ARC in patients with HIV infection. Third International Conference on AIDS, Washington, D.C.

Phair, J., Chmiel, J., Wallenmark, C., et al. (1987, June). HIV Third International Conference on AIDS, Washington, D.C.

Roitt, I., Brostoff, J., & Male, D. (1985). Immunology. St. Louis: C.V. Mosby.

Safai, B., Johnson, K.G., Myskowski, P.L., et al. (1985). The natural history of Kaposi's sarcoma in AIDS. *Annals of Internal Medicine*, 103(5), 744–749.

Safai, B., & Koziner, B. (1985). Malignant neoplasms in AIDS. In V.T. De Vita, S. Hellman, & S.A. Rosenberg (Eds.), *AIDS: Etiology, diagnosis, treatment and prevention* (pp. 213–222). Philadelphia: J.B. Lippincott.

Stites, R., Stobo, J., Fudenberg, H., et al. (1984). *Basic Clinical Immunology* (5th Ed.). Los Altos: Lange Medical Publishers.

Urba, W., & Longo, D. (1985). Clinical spectrum of human retroviral induced diseases. *Cancer Research*, 45(suppl.), 4637–4643.

Volberding, P. (1985). The clinical spectrum of the acquired immunodeficiency syndrome. *Annals of Internal Medicine*, 103(5), 729–733.

Chapter 4

Clinical Manifestations and Treatment

Peter Wolfe

It is important for nurses to have a solid understanding of the often bewildering diversity of infections and neoplasms to which patients with AIDS are prone, so as to provide optimal nursing care. Indeed, probably no other illness makes such demands on nursing care. There are often occasions in treating persons with AIDS when medical/technological resources are exhausted owing to the inexorable course of the disease. At these times (and before), the human values of compassion and caring which are closely associated with nursing become of paramount importance to the person with AIDS.

Definition: Diagnosis

The definition of AIDS is simple. A person is diagnosed as having AIDS when two criteria are met. First, he or she must have an illness predictive of an underlying cellular immune deficiency. Second, he or she must not have any predisposition to such immune deficiency, such as immunosuppressive drug therapy with steroids or cancer chemotherapy. This definition was formulated before the etiologic agent of the disease was discovered, and it has been modified only slightly with the passage of time. The most recent case definition for AIDS can be found in Appendix B (CDC, 1987).

The natural history of AIDS is now fairly well understood. The disease is caused by a novel retrovirus called human immunodeficiency virus (HIV). The virus gains access to the bloodstream via a breaching of the mucosal membrane or skin barriers during sexual intercourse or intravenous drug use and attaches to a type of white blood cell called the T helper lymphocyte. The virus penetrates into the interior of the T helper lymphocyte and begins to replicate. Eventually, enough progeny virus particles are formed to cause the death of the host cell, and the new viruses are released to infect other T helper lymphocytes.

The T helper lymphocyte population is crucial to the normal functioning of the immune system. If these cells are depleted in number and/or abnormal in function, the host falls prey to a number of otherwise harmless microorganisms and eventually succumbs (Lang et al., 1987).

As can be inferred from the foregoing, the routes of transmission determine the epidemiology of the disease. AIDS is primarily a sexually transmitted disease. Sixty-five percent of the cases in the United States result from homosexual transmission. Another 17% result from direct inoculation via contaminated needles used by IV drug abusers; 8% of cases occur in the homosexual male/IV drug abuser transmission category (CDC, 1988). Currently, relatively few cases result from heterosexual activity, blood product contamination, and transplacental spread. No cases have been shown to result from casual social contact, or insect vectors. There is no medical ground for civil rights discrimination against the HIV-infected individual, which is due instead to fear and bigotry.

It is still unknown what proportion of individuals infected with HIV will ultimately come down with full-blown AIDS. Estimates run from 15 to 50 percent or more (Goedert et al., 1987). It is clear that AIDS represents the most severe infectious disease threat to public health since the polio epidemics of the first half of the century.

Opportunistic Infections

Opportunistic infections are caused by a diverse spectrum of infectious agents (Table 4–1). In general, all of these agents have in common an inability to cause significant disease in persons with normal immune systems. For the most part, these organisms are widely distributed in nature; there is no hiding from them. Persons with defective immune systems, such as those with the acquired immunodeficiency syndrome, are unable to resist infection with these organisms.

In the next section, clinical aspects and treatment of the most common opportunistic infections seen in AIDS are described. Some of the more common drugs used in treatment are listed in Table 4–2. An extensive table (Table 4–3) summarizes medications and their side effects; it is important for nurses who administer these drugs to know their effects and side effects.

Pneumocystis Carinii Pneumonia (PCP). *Pneumocystis carinii* is a one-celled protozoan parasite that is ubiquitous in temperate climates. Serologic studies have shown that the majority of the population is infected with the organism by adolescence. Like most opportunistic infections, *Pneumocystis carinii* infection occurs only in people with impaired immune systems. In the immunosuppressed, this organism causes pneumonia. In fact, *Pneumocystis carinii* pneumonia is the most frequent presenting diagnosis for AIDS, accounting for

Table 4–1. Common Opportunistic Infections Seen in AIDS

Agents	Target Organ(s)
Bacteria	
Mycobacterium avium	Blood, reticuloendothelial system
Mycobacterium tuberculosis	Lungs, bone marrow
Salmonella spp.	GI tract, gallbladder, blood
Viruses	
Herpes simplex	Mucosa, skin
Varicella-zoster virus	Peripheral nerves, skin
Cytomegalovirus (CMV)	Retina, lungs, GI tract, brain
Protozoa	
Toxoplasma gondii	Brain, lymph nodes, muscle
Pneumocystis carinii	Lungs
Cryptosporidium spp.	GI tract
Fungi	
Cryptococcus neoformans	Brain, lungs, bone marrow, skin
Candida albicans	GI tract, especially esophagus, oral mucosa
Histoplasma capsulatum	Reticuloendothelial system, bone marrow, skin, lungs

Table 4–2. Drugs Commonly Used in the Treatment of Opportunistic Infections

Drugs	Active Against	Toxicities
Anti-fungal Drugs		
Ketoconazole	Candida	Liver toxicity
Amphotericin	Diverse fungi	Chills, renal damage, fevers
Anti-viral Drugs		
Acyclovir	Herpes simplex Herpes zoster	Generally well tolerated
Ganciclovir (DHPG)	Cytomegalovirus	Bone marrow suppression
Anti-protozoal Drugs		
Cotrimoxazole (trimethoprim-sulfa, Bactrim Septra)	*Pneumocystis carinii*	Fever, rash, nausea, bone marrow suppression
Pyrimethamine (Daraprim)	*Toxoplasma gondii*	Rash, bone marrow suppression
Sulfadiazine	*Toxoplasma gondii*	Rash, bone marrow suppression
Anti-mycobacterial Drugs		
Isoniazid (INH)	Mycobacterial infections	Liver damage
Rifampin		Liver damage
Ethambutol		Optic neuritis
Ethionamide		Nausea, liver damage
Clofazamine		Liver damage, bone marrow suppression

Table 4–3. Medications Most Often Used to Treat HIV Infection and Secondary Diseases

Trade Name	Generic Name	Treatment For	Side Effects
Adriamycin	Doxorubicin (systemic)	Kaposi's sarcoma	Leukopenia or infection (fever, chills, sore throat); stomatitis, esophagitis, flank, stomach or joint pain; pain at injection site; peripheral edema; fast or irregular heartbeat; shortness of breath; gastrointestinal bleeding; thrombocytopenia (unusual bleeding or bruising); changes in skin color; diarrhea, nausea, vomiting; skin rash or itching; hair loss and reddish color to urine
Ancobon	Flucytosine (systemic)	Cryptococcosis	Skin rash, leukopenia, thrombocytopenia, anemia, confusion, hallucinations, diarrhea, nausea and vomiting, dizziness, drowsiness, headache
Bactrim Septra	Sulfamethoxazole and trimethoprim (systemic)	*Pneumocystis carinii* pneumonia	Skin rash or itching; Stevens-Johnson syndrome (myalgia, arthralgia, redness, blistering, peeling or loosening of the skin); extreme fatigue, dysphagia, fever, leukopenia (sore throat); thrombocytopenia (unusual bleeding or bruising); hepatitis (dark urine, pale stools, yellow skin and/or sclera); cystalluria, hematuria, diarrhea, dizziness, headache, anorexia, nausea, and vomiting
Blenoxane	Bleomycin (systemic)	Kaposi's sarcoma	Cough, shortness of breath, pneumonitis, fever, chills, stomatitis, confusion, syncope, diaphoresis, changes in skin color and texture, rashes, swelling of fingers, nausea, vomiting and anorexia, weight loss, and hair loss
Daraprim	Pyrimethamine (systemic)	Toxoplasmosis; used with sulfadiazine; (see also Microsulfon)	Folic acid deficiency, alteration of taste, soreness, redness, swelling, burning or stinging of tongue, diarrhea, dysphagia, leukopenia, thrombocytopenia, anemia, skin rash, ataxia, seizures, tremors, anorexia, vomiting
DHPG	9-(1,3-dihydroxy-2 propoxymethyl) quanine (systemic)	Cytomegalovirus (CMV) (CMV retinitis and CMV colitis)	Under investigation Leukopenia, bone marrow depression, elevation of serum liver enzymes
			Neutropenia, eosinophilia, elevated liver enzymes, decreased platelet count, edema, nausea, myalgias, headache, anorexia, disorientation, hallucinations, rash, phlebitis

Continued, p. 62

**Table 4-3. Medications Most Often Used to Treat HIV Infection
and Secondary Diseases** *Continued*

Trade Name	Generic Name	Treatment For	Side Effects
Fungizone	Amphotericin-B (systemic)	Cryptococcosis	Fever, chills, hypokalemia (irregular heartbeat, muscle cramps or pain, extreme fatigue), pain at site of infusion, anemia, blurred or double vision, renal failure (increased or decreased urination), paresthesias, impaired hearing, tinnitus, seizures, shortness of breath, skin rash or itching, agranulocytosis or leukopenia, thrombocytopenia
Microsulfon	Sulfadiazine (systemic)	Toxoplasmosis; used with pyrimethamine; (see also Daraprim)	Same as sulfanomides (see Bactrin/Septra)
Mycelex	Clotrimazole (oral-local)	Candidiasis (oropharyngeal)	Abdominal or stomach cramping or pain, diarrhea, nausea or vomiting
Mycostatin	Nystatin (oral-local)	Candidiasis (oropharyngeal)	Diarrhea, nausea and vomiting, stomach pain
Nizoral	Ketoconazole (systemic)	Candidiasis (cutaneous, disseminated)	Hepatitis, gynecomastia, nausea, vomiting, decreased libido, diarrhea, dizziness, drowsiness, photophobia, skin rash or itching, somnolence
Oncovin	Vincristine (systemic)	Kaposi's sarcoma	See Velban; also: agitation, hallucinations, confusion, anorexia, seizures, somnolence, loss of consciousness, bed wetting, orthostatic hypotension, lack of sweating, stomatitis, bloating, diarrhea, weight loss, skin rash
Pentam 300	Pentamidine isethionate (systemic)	*Pneumocystis carinii* pneumonia (PCP)	Hypotension, nausea, vomiting, syncope, pain at injection site, abscess and/or necrosis with I.M. injection, azotemia, leukopenia, abnormal liver function tests, hypoglycemia
Retrovir (formerly AZT)	Zidovudine (formerly azidothymidine) (systemic)	Human immunodeficiency virus (HIV) infection	Anemia, leukopenia, neutropenia, anorexia, asthenia, diarrhea, dizziness, fever, headache, insomnia, malaise, myalgia, nausea, pain in abdomen, rash, somnolence, taste alteration
Velban	Vinblastine (systemic)	Kaposi's sarcoma	Leukopenia, flank or stomach pain, peripheral edema, pain or redness at site of injection, stomatitis, thrombocytopenia, gastrointestinal bleeding, dizziness, ataxia, drooping eyelids, depression, headaches, paresthesias, myalgias, nausea, vomiting, muscle weakness, loss of hair

Continued, p. 63

Table 4–3. Medications Most Often Used to Treat HIV Infection
and Secondary Diseases *Continued*

Trade Name	Generic Name	Treatment For	Side Effects
Ve Pesid	Etoposide (systemic)	Kaposi's sarcoma	Leukopenia, thrombocytopenia, stomatitis, ataxia, paresthesias, tachycardia, shortness of breath or wheezing, pain at site of injection, nausea, vomiting and loss of appetite, diarrhea, fatigue, loss of hair
Zovirax	Acyclovir (systemic)	Herpes simplex Herpes zoster Varicella	*Oral:* changes in menstrual period, skin rash, diarrhea, dizziness, headache, joint pain, nausea and vomiting, acne, anorexia, and somnolence *Parenteral:* skin rashes or hives, hematuria, lightheadedness, headache, diaphoresis, confusion, tremors, abdominal pain, difficulty breathing, decreased frequency of urination, nausea and vomiting, unusual thirst or extreme fatigue

Developed by: P. Ungvarski, 1988.
Adapted from: Collaborative DHPG Treatment Study Groups, 1986; Drake et al., 1985; Kaplan et al., 1987; Masur et al., 1986; Richman et al., 1987; Sands et al., 1985; Tocci et al., 1984; USP DI, 1987.

about 60% of newly diagnosed cases. Typical symptoms include fever, non-productive cough, and shortness of breath. The illness is more often than not subtle in presentation; frequently patients will have insidious symptoms lasting several weeks before the infection becomes severe enough for the patient to seek a physician's care.

Pneumocystis carinii pneumonia is not transmissible from person to person, unlike tuberculosis, for example. Respiratory isolation is not appropriate for patients with PCP.

The diagnosis of PCP is most often made on the basis of bronchoscopic biopsies or direct staining of sputum specimens. Fortunately, PCP is one of the easiest of the opportunistic infections to treat (Wharton et al., 1986). The drugs of choice are cotrimoxazole (Bactrim, Septra), sulfatrimethoprim, and pentamidine (Pentam). Cotrimoxazole is usually administered intravenously every 6 or 8 hours for seven days and then orally for another one to two weeks, for a total of about three weeks of treatment. Adverse reactions are common; about half of the patients given cotrimoxazole will develop rashes, drug fevers, and/or severe nausea and vomiting, most often a week or so into therapy. It is important for nurses to monitor carefully the patient's skin for signs of cutaneous hypersensitivity.

Pentamidine is a drug which, before the advent of AIDS, had been used primarily in treating sleeping sickness in Africa. It is also effective in treating PCP. Like cotrimoxazole, it is associated with a high frequency of adverse drug effects. If administered intramuscularly, it can cause sterile abscesses; for that reason it is usually given intravenously. If administered too rapidly, hypotension can result. Acute hypoglycemia is sometimes observed, followed weeks to months later by hyperglycemia. Renal insufficiency and liver function abnormalities have been observed. Nurses must be alert to the signs and symptoms of disturbance of glucose homeostasis in patients receiving pentamidine: sweating, weakness, and confusion with low blood sugar and polyuria, polydipsia, and altered mental status in hyperglycemic states.

Recently, there has been some interest in the administration of the drug via the aerosol route; preliminary data suggests it is effective and less toxic than parenteral administration (Montgomery et al., 1987). Some patients have airway irritation when the drug is administered by this route, and if the nurse detects wheezing in the course of such treatment, a bronchodilator should be ordered.

Perhaps no other AIDS-associated illness requires more careful monitoring than does PCP. The most important parameter to follow is respiratory status. Some patients, despite appropriate therapy, rapidly develop respiratory insufficiency. The nurse should be vigilant in monitoring the respiratory status of the patient, and must sound the alarm should worsening dyspnea, tachypnea, or decreased mental status be observed.

Mycobacterial Infections. *Mycobacterium avium intracellulare* (MAI) and *Mycobacterium tuberculosis* (MTB) infections are seen with some frequency in persons with AIDS. MTB is the etiologic agent of human tuberculosis. MAI is one of a dozen or so species of nontuberculous mycobacteria called "atypical mycobacteria." The atypical mycobacteria have in common a wide distribution in nature, a lack of transmissibility from person-to-person, and in general, a relative resistance to drugs commonly used to treat tuberculosis.

MAI infection is relatively common in AIDS (Hawkins et al., 1986). There is some controversy as to how significant a pathogen it is, as it is often recovered from asymptomatic patients. It can be isolated from blood, lymph nodes, liver, spleen, and lung. In some patients, infection is overwhelming; the reticuloendothelial system is completely packed with MAI. In such patients, it is hard not to believe that the organisms are not pathogenic. Patients may have fevers, weakness, and cachexia; patients with AIDS may of course have concurrent infections producing the same symptoms, so it is hard to be sure these symptoms are attributable to MAI itself. Four, five, and even six drug combinations have been advocated in treating MAI; so far, however, no drug regimen seems effective in reducing the total body burden of MAI in infected individuals.

MTB has been seen with increasing frequency in patients infected with HIV, especially in minority groups and immigrant populations. The classic symptoms of pulmonary tuberculosis (fevers, productive cough, and systemic wasting) are usually present; less frequent presentations include tuberculous lymphadenitis (scrofula) and tuberculous enteritis. There is preliminary evidence that tuberculosis in the context of AIDS is more refractory to treatment than is tuberculosis in the immunocompetent person. The main significance of MTB in the context of

AIDS is that it represents virtually the only indication for respiratory isolation for AIDS patients, and even this is temporary: isolation can be discontinued after a few days of appropriate treatment.

Cryptococcosis. *Cryptococcus neoformans* is a common yeast, often found in nature in association with birds and their droppings. It has long been recognized as a cause of meningitis and pneumonia (Zuger et al., 1986). Infection with this organism is seen in both the immunocompetent and the immunosuppressed individual. In AIDS, it most frequently presents with high fevers, severe headache, and decreased mental status.

Diagnosis is made on the basis of demonstrating the yeast forms in India ink-stained cerebrospinal fluid. Like PCP, cryptococcosis is not transmitted from person to person, and no special nursing precautions are necessary.

The primary treatment for this infection is intravenous amphotericin B. This drug has a bad reputation among those inexperienced with its use because it is associated with some occasionally severe adverse side effects. The drug is usually given as a test dose of 1 mg diluted in 5% dextrose in water (D5W), to which is added a small amount of heparin. If the test dose is tolerated, then the dose of the drug will be increased by increments of 5 mg/day or more to a total daily dosage of around 0.9 mg/kg/day as tolerated. The drug is infused over 3 to 4 hours. Patients given this drug sometimes have acute fevers, urticarial rashes, hypotension, and uncontrollable rigors during the administration of the drug, and for this reason, many physicians premedicate patients one-half hour before the drug is given with acetaminophen, steroids, and diphenhydramine; 25 or 50 mg of meperidine is quite effective in abolishing rigors during the administration of the drug.

A more serious toxicity than the foregoing is azotemia, which is seen with some frequency in patients receiving amphotericin B. When the serum creatinine level rises to greater than 3.0 mg/dl,, many physicians hold further administration of the drug until the serum creatinine level falls to below 2.5 mg/dl. Hypokalemia and hypomagnesemia are also seen.

Cryptosporidiosis. Cryptosporidia are one-celled protozoan parasites that can cause diarrhea and dehydration in the immunosuppressed and, occasionally, in immunocompetent individuals (Soave et al., 1985). In nature, they are most commonly associated with diarrhea in dairy animals and sheep; cryptosporidiosis is therefore an occupational disease of farmers. The organisms presumably enter the body via the oropharyngeal route and colonize the brush border of the intestines, where they interfere with water absorption. Because cryptosporidia infection in the immunocompetent person is often self-limited, the organism has to be recovered in the stool of an .infected individual for more than a month for a diagnosis of AIDS to be made.

In patients infected with HIV, this organism can cause chronic, life-threatening diarrhea with resultant fluid imbalance and electrolyte disturbances. These patients are often a practical challenge for nurses as they sometimes put out gallons a day of watery stool; nurses must be vigilant for the signs of serious fluid volume depletion and hypokalemia and hyponatremia.

Unfortunately, there is no drug effective in eradicating the organism from the host. Spiramycin, a chemical relative of erythromycin, not available in the U.S. at the time of this writing, has had isolated success in reducing the frequency of diarrhea, but not in eliminating it completely. Most often, symptomatic control with opiate anti-peristaltic agents is the best that can be accomplished.

Toxoplasmosis. *Toxoplasma gondii* is a widely distributed protozoan parasite that can cause a serious central nervous system (CNS) infection in patients with defective immune systems (Luft et al., 1984). As with pneumocystis, many people have been infected with toxoplasma cysts, yet few ever have any symptoms from their infection. In persons with AIDS, however, it is another story.

The route of entrance of the toxoplasma organisms into the body is via the gastrointestinal (GI) tract. The cysts penetrate the wall of the GI tract, enter the bloodstream, and are carried to the brain, muscle, and heart, among other tissues. In the immunosuppressed person, the organisms can multiply in the brain, resulting in multiple brain abscesses, which can be clearly seen on computed tomography (CT) scans or magnetic resonance imaging (MRI) scans of the head. The symptoms of CNS toxoplasmosis, as would be expected, consist of focal neurologic deficits: weakness of one or more extremities, seizures, headaches, confusion, and fevers (Wong et al., 1984). Nurses should be alert for changes in the neurologic examinations of their patients.

The drugs for treatment for this infection include pyrimethamine and sulfadiazine, both of which are given orally. In persons with sulfa allergy, clindamycin or spiramycin is sometimes substituted for the sulfadiazine. Frequently, anticonvulsant drugs such as phenytoin (Dilantin) or phenobarbital are given as well. Treatment must often be continued indefinitely to avoid the danger of relapse.

Cytomegalovirus Infections

Cytomegalovirus (CMV) infection is extremely common among sexually active adults. For most people, the infection is asymptomatic. Occasionally, a mononucleosis-like illness is seen with fatigue and generalized lymphadenopathy, which may take months to resolve. In the immunosuppressed individual, however, the virus causes much more serious illness.

CMV involvement of the retina causes blindness; infection of the lungs can cause a virulent pneumonia; and infection of the colon can lead to perforation of the colon and peritonitis. Of these complications, CMV retinitis is by far the most common in patients with AIDS. This infection generally presents with progressive visual field deficits and can cause retinal detachment. The patient typically might notice he or she can see only one-half of a column of newsprint, for example.

Diagnosis can be made by an ophthalmologist from the characteristic appearance of the inflamed retina. Untreated CMV retinitis will progress to bilateral blindness.

Recently, an experimental drug called gancilovir (DHPG, a relative of acyclovir) has been shown to halt the progression of the retinitis. It is currently before the Federal Drug Administration (FDA) for final approval at the time of this writing. It is given once or twice a day via the intravenous route. Unfortunately, it is associated with bone marrow toxicity; leukopenia and neutropenia often prevent the chronic treatment necessary to prevent progressive blindness.

Malignancies

AIDS-related Kaposi's sarcoma. Kaposi's sarcoma (KS) is a skin cancer first described over 100 years ago by the Hungarian physician Moritz Kaposi. He documented the occurrence of an indolent, mild, multifocal skin cancer affecting primarily old men of Mediterranean descent. In most cases, this cancer did not have any effect on lifespan. In the 1960s, the same cancer was observed to occur in certain tribes in Africa, albeit in a much more aggressive form.

The American variety of KS associated with HIV infection resembles the aggressive African form. It accounts for about 20% of newly diagnosed cases of AIDS; interestingly, it almost never is seen in heterosexuals. It appears as raised, purplish spots, most often painless and nonpruritic, scattered over the limbs, trunk and face. The lesions are usually oval and are 1 cm or so in diameter; occasionally, they become confluent. KS lesions have a distressing predilection for acral parts of the body, such as the tips of the ears and nose. Usually, a previously well individual will inadvertently notice lesions while showering or sunbathing. For most people, KS lesions gradually become more numerous over months and even years; less often, some patients will have many lesions appear all over their body rapidly. Rarely, KS can involve internal viscera such as the GI tract (causing internal bleeding) or the lungs (causing respiratory distress).

A rare and very unfortunate complication of KS is involvement of the lymphatic system of the lower extremities. This causes painful lymphedema of the legs, which results in immobility; the pain can sometimes be controlled only by continuous morphine sulfate infusion. Radiation therapy to the inguinal nodes can sometimes reduce the lymphatic swelling.

Most oncologists do not recommend therapy for KS unless the lesions are on cosmetically unacceptable parts of the body (face and hands), or unless the lesions are appearing quite rapidly (Safai and Koziner, 1985). Simple excision is ineffective because the cancer is multifocal in origin. Radiation therapy has been used successfully to treat local lesions. In the past, multiple agent chemotherapy was attempted using four or more drugs, but these regimens were quickly found to be much too toxic. Currently, one- or two-agent therapy is most commonly given (Lewis et al., 1983). Vinca alkaloids such as vincristine, vinblastine, and VP-16, as well as doxorubicin (Adriamycin) and bleomycin, are useful. Alpha-interferon is sometimes used as well.

AIDS-related Lymphomas. An excess of lymphomas have been noted in patients infected with HIV (Ziegler et al., 1984). These have been represented by non-Hodgkin's lymphomas (NHLs) as well as primary lymphoma involving the brain.

NHLs are solid tumors that involve the lymphatic tissue; typically, the tumor may be found in peripheral (axillary, cervical, inguinal) node groups as well as in deeper (mediastinal, mesenteric, retroperitoneal) nodes as well. Bone marrow and the liver and spleen are usual sites of involvement. Diagnosis is made by biopsy of enlarged nodes, bone marrow, or liver.

Symptoms of NHL relate primarily to obstruction of vital structures by tumor masses; in addition, constitutional symptoms of fatigue, fever, night sweats, anorexia, and weight loss are frequent. Hemolytic anemias and lowered platelet counts are seen occasionally.

Primary lymphoma of the brain, as its name suggests, is a neoplasm which arises in the central nervous system. Quite rare before the AIDS epidemic, it is now seen with some degree of regularity at major referral centers. It presents very much like toxoplasmosis (see earlier discussion): focal neurologic deficits and/or seizures. This tumor resembles toxoplasmosis on CT scanning, and sometimes a brain biopsy is needed to establish a definitive diagnosis.

Neurologic Dysfunctions. It has been recently recognized that HIV can infect not only the helper T lymphocyte, but it also can infect cells of the central and peripheral nervous system, producing a variety of neurologic disorders. Most often, these neurologic disorders present late in the course of illness, but sometimes they are the first manifestation of HIV infection (Gabuzda & Hirsch, 1987).

Clinically the most important neurologic symptom of HIV infection is dementia. This is often subtle at first, with difficulties of memory, word-finding, and personality changes gradually progressing to a profound dementia. Early on, the symptoms can be confused with organic depression, and indeed it is often difficult to distinguish depression from AIDS dementia. Psychometric testing has shown that some degree of impaired mental functioning is demonstrable in many patients with ARC who are otherwise healthy and functional.

Another common neurologic syndrome is attributed to the direct effects of HIV on the peripheral nerves. Some patients develop a peripheral neuropathy which is indistinguishable from that seen in chronic alcoholism. They have pain, numbness, and tingling of their hands and feet; these symptoms can sometimes be relieved by Tegretol, Dilantin, or phenothiazines.

HIV Wasting Syndrome. The "wasting syndrome" is characterized by relentless weight loss, cachexia, fevers, and diarrhea. Findings of profound involuntary weight loss greater than 10% of baseline body weight, plus either chronic diarrhea (2 stools or more per day for 30 days or more), or chronic weakness and documented fever characterize this syndrome. Patients are often more ill than those with opportunistic infections or neoplasms and many die without ever developing a major opportunistic infection.

This syndrome is often accompanied by mucocutaneous fungal infections involving skin and the mucous linings of the mouth. Thrush is the most common manifestation: it is a whitish coating of the tongue caused by the yeast *Candida albicans*. It can easily be controlled by nystatin oral suspensions, clotrimazole troches, or systemic anti-fungal chemotherapy with ketoconazole.

Lymphadenopathy Syndrome (LAS) and ARC. As mentioned earlier, only a small minority of people infected by HIV meet the Centers for Disease Control's definition for the diagnosis of AIDS. The majority have no symptoms at all. Perhaps several hundred thousand people have signs and symptoms suggestive of minor immunodeficiency: for want of a better term, such people are often said to have AIDS-related complex or ARC (Abrams et al., 1983).

Clinically, the major syndrome that is often recognized is persistent generalized lymphadenopathy (PGL). PGL is characterized by diffuse adenopathy, involving at least two extra-inguinal node groups, which persists more than two to three months. Often these swollen nodes are completely asymptomatic and are noticed incidentally on physical examination. The nodes may wax and wane with the passage of time. PGL patients are at increased risk of developing AIDS (Kaplan et al., 1987a).

PGL is often accompanied by thrush and hairy leukoplakia. In contrast to thrush, hairy leukoplakia involves the lateral margins of the tongue (Greenspan et al., 1987). It appears to be caused by a virus and fortunately it does not seem to be associated with serious complications. The significance of thrush and of hairy leukoplakia are that both are predictors of future opportunistic infections: once either of these conditions is seen, there is about a 50% chance of AIDS developing within two years.

Another condition seen in HIV infection associated with an increased risk of developing AIDS is herpes zoster, or shingles. This is a painful skin inflammation usually involving one dermatome (although occasionally it is generalized). The rash is vesicular and is often secondarily infected with skin flora such as staphylococcus and streptococcus. It is caused by the same virus that causes chickenpox, and indeed, it represents a reactivation of the varicella-zoster virus in a person who had been infected with this virus in the past. Shingles is most commonly seen in the elderly and the immunosuppressed person, although apparently healthy young people can get it too. Nurses who have not had chickenpox, especially if they are pregnant, should avoid close contact with herpes zoster patients; if a nurse has already had chickenpox, however, there is no danger.

Therapy Directed Against HIV Infection

The recognition of the human immunodeficiency virus by Montagnier and Gallo in 1983 and 1984, together with the resultant understanding of the patho-

Table 4–4. Drugs Used in Treating HIV Infection

Drugs	Comments
Anti-viral agents (drugs that interfere with HIV replication)	
Zidovudine (AZT, Retrovir)	Only licensed drug to treat HIV infection
Ribavirin	Unknown efficacy, under investigation
Dideoxycytidine (DDC)	Analogue of ziodvudine, may be neurotoxic
Ampligen	Test-tube activity demonstrated
Suramin	Unacceptable toxicity
HPA-23	Efficacy studies unimpressive
Membrane-active agents (agents which interfere with HIV attachment to T cells)	
AL721	Unknown efficacy
Immune modulators (probably these drugs are not useful as single agents)	
Interleukin-2	Causes T cell growth in test tube
Immuthiol (DTC)	Unknown efficacy, under investigation
Isoprinosine	No benefits demonstrated
Interferons (alpha, gamma)	May be useful in treating Kaposi's sarcoma

physiology of HIV infection, provided the first rational basis for attempts at therapy for AIDS and ARC (Barre-Sinoussi et al., 1983; Gallo et al., 1984). Since AIDS is an infectious disease of the immune system, two obvious avenues of therapy suggested themselves: immune restoration and specific anti-viral chemotherapy (Gottlieb et al., 1985). Some of these drugs are listed in Table 4–4.

While only one drug, zidovudine, has been released by the FDA for treatment of AIDS and AIDS-related conditions, a large number of drugs are "in the pipeline" for future testing and evaluation. It is important to have an idea of the rationale for and the side effects of these drugs.

In general, immune-stimulating drugs have been disappointments. Although a large number of agents having test-tube effects on various cells of the immune system have been found, with one partial exception none so far have been found to have any beneficial effects in patients infected with HIV. The partial exception has been alpha-interferon, which seems to cause some slowing of disease progression of Kaposi's sarcoma. Interestingly, alpha-interferon possesses direct anti-retroviral activity in the laboratory.

Compounds such as isoprinosine, gamma-interferon, interleukin-2, and thymic extracts have shown no benefit despite extensive (noncontrolled, for the most part) study. A trip to any health food store will reveal extensive marketing campaigns directed toward HIV-infected individuals and those at risk promoting various expensive vitamins, plant extracts and the like to "boost" the immune system. There is not one scintilla of evidence that any of these preparations do anything more than enrich the manufacturers.

The reason immune-modulators as single agents have not proved efficacious may be that direct action must be taken against the causative virus for any positive results to be observed. For this reason, a number of anti-viral agents have been used in AIDS and ARC patients.

A number of possible ways of interfering with the virus's replicative cycle have been proposed: blocking viral attachment to the T cell, preventing penetration of genome into the cytoplasm and/or nucleus, and inhibiting the nucleic acid replication process itself. Zidovudine (AZT, azidothymidine, Retrovir, Compound S) has been found to block the replication of viral RNA and DNA in the test-tube. In a recently concluded placebo-controlled trial, the drug was shown to prolong life and reduce the frequency of opportunistic infections in selected patients with AIDS (Fischl et al., 1987). The data were convincing enough for the Federal Drug Administration to initially release the drug to patients meeting one of two criteria: history of PCP or having less than 200 T helper cells per cubic millimeter of blood. It seems certain that zidovudine does not cure the immunodeficiency, but it does have a beneficial effect on quality of life and length of life for some individuals.

It is very likely that many patients with AIDS whom nurses will care for in the future will be taking zidovudine or a similar drug. It is important for nurses therefore to be aware of the drug's adverse effects, so problems may be recognized early. Zidovudine is known to have short- and medium-term toxicities. The short-term toxicities (days to a few weeks) include headache, nausea and vomiting, and, rarely, fevers. Apart from the fevers, these toxicities are ephemeral and can be easily managed symptomatically. The medium-term toxicities are more serious and mainly target the blood-forming cells. Macrocytic anemia is very common in patients taking the drug longer than three or four months; usually, this can be managed by judicious transfusions and dosage modifications. The most serious problem appears to be leukopenia; rare patients develop aplastic anemia while on the drug, which is often fatal. It appears that hormones such as erythropoietin and granulocyte-monocyte colony stimulating factor (GM-CSF) potentially might be able to mitigate the hematologic toxicities of the nucleoside analogues.

Summary

AIDS, as unwelcome as it is, is immutably a part of the medical landscape, and will be so for the foreseeable future. While much research is going on in the area of treatment, it is clear that some medical means of prevention will be necessary as well to completely eradicate the disease. Work is progressing on the development of a vaccine to prevent AIDS in people not already infected with HIV, but it is likely such a vaccine will take years for development. A global vaccination campaign similar to the one mounted against smallpox will be needed.

Above and beyond the purely medical aspects of the disease, AIDS presents a challenge to all members of the health care team to re-examine attitudes toward death and dying, as well as homosexuality, drug abuse, and other forms of societally nonsanctioned behavior. Judgmental attitudes and avoidance behavior have no place in health care for any disease. While it is only human to shy away from the unknown, so much has been learned about AIDS that there is now no rational basis for fear. Nurses should look at AIDS as an opportunity to excel in their profession's traditional strengths: caring and compassion.

References

Abrams, D.I., Lewis, B.J., Beckstead, J.H., et al. (1983). Persistent diffuse lymphadenopathy syndrome in homosexual men: Endpoint or prodrome? *Annals of Internal Medicine*, 100, 801–808.

Barre-Sinoussi, F., Chermann, J., Rey, F., et al. (1983). Isolation of a T-lymphotropic retrovirus from a patient at risk for acquired immunodeficiency syndrome. *Science*, 220, 868–871.

Centers for Disease Control. (1987). Revision of the CDC Surveillance case definition of acquired immunodeficiency syndrome. *Morbidity and Mortality Weekly Report*, 36, 1–15.

Centers for Disease Control. (1988, February). *AIDS Weekly Surveillance Report*, United States AIDS Program, Atlanta, GA.

Collaborative DHPG Treatment Study Groups. (1986). Treatment for serious cytomegalovirus infections with 9-(1, 3-dihydroxy, 2-propoxymethyl) guanine in patients with AIDS and other immunodeficiencies. *New England Journal of Medicine*, 314, 801–805.

Drake, S., Lampasona, V., Nicks, H.L., et al. (1985). Pentamidine isethionate in the treatment of *Pneumocystis carinii* pneumonia. *Clinical Pharmacy*, 4, 507–516.

Fischl, M.A., Richman, D.D., Grieco, M.H., et al. (1987). The efficacy of azidothymidine (AZT) in the treatment of patients with AIDS and AIDS-related complex. A double-blind, placebo-controlled trial. *New England Journal of Medicine*, 317, 185–191.

Gabuzda, D.H., & Hirsch, M.S. (1987). Neurologic manifestations of infection with human immunodeficiency virus. Clinical features and pathogenesis. *Annals of Internal Medicine*, 107, 383–391.

Gallo, R.C., Salahuddin, S.Z., Popovic, M., et al. (1984). Frequent detection and isolation of cytopathic retroviruses (HTLV-III) from patients with AIDS and pre-AIDS. *Science*, 224, 500–503.

Goedert, J.J., Biggar, R.J., Melbye, M., et al. (1987). Effect of T4 count and cofactors on the incidence of AIDS in homosexual men infected with human immunodeficiency virus. *Journal of the American Medical Association*, 257, 326–330.

Gottlieb, M.S., Wolfe, P.R., Mitsuyasu, R. (1985). Immunotherapy of the acquired immune deficiency syndrome. *Advances in Host Defense Mechanisms*, 5, 149–170.

Greenspan, D., Greenspan, J.S., Hearst, N.G., et al. (1987). Relation of oral hairy leukoplakia to infection with the human immunodeficiency virus and the risk of developing AIDS. *Journal of Infectious Diseases*, 155, 475–481.

Hawkins, C.C., Gold, J.M.W., Whimbey, E., et al. (1986). *Mycobacterium avium* complex infections in patients with acquired immunodeficiency syndrome. *Annals of Internal Medicine*, 105, 184–188.

Kaplan, J.E., Spira, T.J., Fishbein, D.B., et al. (1987b). Lymphadenopathy syndrome in homosexual men: Evidence for continuing risk of developing the acquired immunodeficiency syndrome. *Journal of the American Medical Association*, 257(3), 335–337.

Kaplan, L.D., Wofsy, C.B., & Volberding, P.A. (1987). Treatment of patients with acquired immunodeficiency syndrome and associated manifestations. *Journal of the American Medical Association*, 257, 1367–1374.

Lang, W., Anderson, R.E., Perkins, H., et al. (1987). Clinical, immunologic, and serologic findings in men at risk for acquired immunodeficiency syndrome. *Journal of the American Medical Association*, 257, 326–330.

Lewis, B., Abrams, D.I., Ziegler, J., et al. (1983). Single agent or combination chemotherapy of Kaposi's sarcoma in acquired immune deficiency syndrome. Abstract C–232, in ASCD Abstracts Annual Meeting. San Diego, American Society of Clinical Oncology.

Luft, B.H., Brooks, R.G., Conley, F.K., et al. (1984). Toxoplasmic encephalitis in patients with the acquired immune deficiency syndrome. *Journal of the American Medical Association*, 252, 913–915.

Masur, H., Kovacs, J.A., Ognibene, F., et al. (1985). Infectious complication of AIDS. In V.T. Devita, S. Hellman, & S.A. Rosenberg (Eds.), *AIDS: Etiology, diagnosis, treatment and prevention* (pp. 161–184). Philadelphia: J.B. Lippincott.

Montgomery, A.B., Debs, R.J., Luce, J.M., et al. (1987). Aerosolized pentamidine as sole therapy for *Pneumocystis carinii* pneumonia in patients with the acquired immunodeficiency syndrome. *Lancet, 2,* 480.

Richman, D.D., Fischl, M.A., Grieco, M.H., et al. (1987). The toxicity of azidothymidine (AZT) in the treatment of patients with AIDS and AIDS-related complex. *The New England Journal of Medicine, 317,* 192–197.

Sands, M., Kron, M.A., Brown, R.B. (1985). Pentamidine: a review. *Review of Infectious Diseases, 7,* 625–633.

Safai, B., Koziner, B. (1985). Malignant neoplasms in AIDS. In V.T. DeVita, S. Hellman, S.A. Rosenberg (Eds.), *AIDS: Etiology, diagnosis, treatment and prevention* (pp. 213–222). Philadelphia, PA: J.B. Lippincott.

Soave, R., Danner, R.L., Honig, C.L., et al. (1985). Cryptosporidiosis in homosexual men. *Annals of Internal Medicine, 102,* 593.

Tocci, M.J., Livelli, T.J., Perry, H.C., et al. (1984). The effects of the nucleoside analog 2'—nor—2'deoxy-guanosine on human cytomegalovirus replication. *Antimicrobial Agents and Chemotherapy, 25,* 247–252.

USP Dispensing Information (USP DI) drug information for the health care provider (1987). Easton, PA: Mack Printing.

Wharton, M., Coleman, D.L., Fitz, G., et al. (1986). Trimethoprim-sulfamethoxazole or pentamidine for *Pneumocystis carinii* pneumonia in the acquired immunodeficiency syndrome. *Annals of Internal Medicine, 105,* 37–44.

Wong, B., Gold, J.W.M., Brown, A.E., et al. (1984). Central nervous system toxoplasmosis in homosexual men and parenteral drug abusers. *Annals of Internal Medicine, 100,* 36–42.

Ziegler, J.L., Beckstead, J.A., Volberding, et al. (1984). Non-Hodgkin's lymphoma in 90 homosexual men: Relation to generalized lymphadenopathy and the acquired immunodeficiency syndrome. *New England Journal of Medicine, 331,* 565.

Zuger, A., Louie, E., Holzman, R.S., et al. (1986). Cryptococcal disease in patients with the acquired immunodeficiency syndrome. *Annals of Internal Medicine, 104*(2), 234–240.

Chapter 5

Nursing Management of the Adult Client

Peter J. Ungvarski

The major responsibility of the professional nurse with regard to human immunodeficiency virus (HIV) infection is health maintenance. This can be best described as nursing activities directed toward: (1) concerns of individuals and groups about potential health problems and (2) reactions of individuals and groups to actual health problems (ANA, 1980).

When considering the planning of nursing care for the person with, or at risk for, HIV infection, it is important to consider the entire spectrum of this illness and not to simply just focus on acquired immunodeficiency syndrome (AIDS), which represents only "the tip of the iceberg" (Fauci, 1986). In order to clarify and facilitate communication about the responses of individuals with, or at risk for, HIV infection, and to identify the appropriate nursing activities, a three-tiered model can be utilized (Table 5–1).

Primary Health Maintenance

This category of nursing care focuses on an organized, systematic approach to health appraisal in order to (1) identify individuals with risk behaviors associated with HIV transmission; (2) detect signs and symptoms that may indicate the presence of HIV infection or an opportunistic disease that is indicative of AIDS; (3) determine the need for health teaching to reduce the risk of acquiring HIV infection; and (4) determine the need for secondary and/or tertiary levels of health maintenance and nursing care (Pender, 1987).

Because the majority of persons with HIV infection will be members of already stigmatized groups within our society, that is, homosexual/bisexual men and/or intravenous drug users, it is imperative that when taking a health history

**Table 5–1. Levels of Health Maintenance
Related to HIV Infection**

Primary Level:	Nursing activities directed toward the health appraisal of persons concerned about or with HIV infection.
Secondary Level:	Nursing activities directed toward health protection for persons with HIV infection.
Tertiary Level:	Nursing activities directed toward minimizing the residual disabilities related to advancing HIV infection or AIDS, and maximizing the quality of life for persons with these illnesses.

Adapted from Pender, 1987.

the nurse be aware of his or her own feelings regarding these life styles. History taking should be performed, as much as possible, in a truly nonjudgmental manner (Ungvarski, 1984).

The Health History

The health history should include a social history beginning with exploration of the person's sexual activities. The major pitfall to be avoided when taking a sexual history is to jump to conclusions based upon a single answer to the simple question of sexual preference. If the client is homosexual and has been in a monogamous relationship with another man for the past 25 years, and neither has participated in sexual activities with other persons, they are no more at risk for HIV infection than a monogamous married heterosexual couple about to celebrate their silver wedding anniversary! Sexual preference and sexual behavior are two different things. Sexual behaviors can be classified as risk-free, low-risk, and high-risk with regard to the potential for HIV transmission (Bjorklund, 1987; Carr & Gee, 1986; Ungvarski, 1983). It is the specific sexual behaviors that increase the risk of HIV transmission between two individuals (Barnes, 1986; Darrow et al., 1987; Guinan & Hardy, 1987; Leads from *MMWR*, 1985; Marmor et al, 1986; Winkelstein et al., 1987).

The question of condom use should be raised with both male and female clients. Questioning should also address the brand or type of condom since research has demonstrated that only latex condoms should be used (Van de Perre, et al., 1987). The nurse should ascertain from the discussion whether or not the client has knowledge of the proper use of condoms (Hatcher, 1987).

When asking about the use of drugs, the nurse should explore their relationship to sexual activities since drugs such as alcohol or marijuana will tend to reduce inhibitions and increase high-risk activities during sex (Carr & Gee, 1986; Ungvarski, 1983). When inquiring about the use of drugs the nurse should avoid the question "Do you ever use drugs?" Instead, the question should correctly be phrased "Have you ever used drugs?" since the client may through previous IV drug use or drug/sex behaviors been at risk for infection with HIV.

Questions of drug use will lead to questions about needle exposure. Although the obvious exposure, as seen with the IV heroin addict, is clear, nurses should be aware of other types of needle exposure, such as tattoos that are done on the street or in neighborhood shops, sharing of estrogens that are self-administered intramuscularly by individuals who would like to eventually have transsexual surgery, and self administration of steroids and body builders. In the early days of AIDS, epidemiologic studies in Haiti revealed dirty needle exposure related to untrained persons giving intramuscular injections (Pape et al., 1985).

When reviewing the past medical history, the nurse should include a review of past illnesses that are likely to recur in the person with HIV infection, as the immune system's ability to fight disease decreases. Most noteworthy are past infections due to the herpes simplex virus (HSV) and the varicella-zoster virus (VZV), both of which remain dormant in the body after the initial infection. Recurrent chronic HSV infection and/or the secondary appearance of VZV, commonly referred to as shingles, should be appropriately monitored. Both HSV and VZV are members of the herpesvirus family, which are frequent causes of chronic, often severe diseases in persons with AIDS (Masur, et al., 1985; Quinnan et al., 1984).

The last part of the health history, the review of systems, is a detailed look for signs and symptoms of HIV infection and possibly of an associated opportunistic infection or disease. After completion, careful review of the history with the client will provide the opportunity to discuss what the client and nurse would like to change. This will provide the basis for nursing care planning and health teaching. Table 5–2 provides a detailed outline for taking a health history.

The Physical Examination

The physical examination findings are as diversified as is the spectrum of HIV infection. Findings range from a normal exam in an asymptomatic HIV-infected person, to evidence of the presence of an opportunistic disease or infection that is associated with a diagnosis of AIDS (Masur et al., 1985; Kaplan & Volberding, 1986). Autopsy findings have demonstrated that the manifestations of HIV infection are even more protean than clinically suspected (Cammarosano & Lewis, 1985; Welch et al., 1984). Organ system involvement has been found to include: (1) the central nervous system; (2) lungs; (3) gastrointestinal tract; (4) liver; (5) lymphoid system including the spleen, thymus and lymph nodes; (6) endocrine system, including the adrenals, thyroid, and parathyroid; (7) genitourinary

Table 5–2. Primary Health Maintenance:

Table 5–2. Primary Health Maintenance:
Health Appraisal Specific for HIV Infection and Related Illnesses

Health History

A. Social History
  1. Sexual Activities
     a. Absolutely safe: abstinence, mutually monogamous with non-infected partner.
     b. Very safe: body massage; hugging; body to body rubbing without penetration (frottage); mutual masturbation; use of sex toys that are *not* shared; social (dry) kissing.
     c. Possibly safe: French (wet) kissing; anal or vaginal intercourse with a condom; fellatio with a condom (condoms can tear); cunnilingus; use of shared sex toys when washed and covered with a condom.
     d. Risky behaviors: anal or vaginal intercourse without a condom, fellatio without a condom and exposure or ingestion of semen or seminal fluid; cunnilingus at the time of menses; sharing unclean, unprotected sex toys; anilingus; sexual activities that involve mucocutaneous contact with other body fluids, secretions or excretions such as blood, urine, or feces.
     e. Use of condoms including application/removal and use of lubricants.
     f. Engaging in sex with multiple partners.
     g. Use of mood-affecting drugs prior to sexual activities.
     h. Has any person with whom the client has had sexual contact developed AIDS?
  2. Use of Mood-Affecting Drugs
     a. Drugs such as alcohol, marijuana, cocaine, crack, LSD, Quaaludes, amphetamines, barbiturates, tranquilizers, amyl or butyl nitrate (called poppers), and/or heroin.
     b. The route of administration should be questioned also; oral, inhalation (including sniffing, snorting, and/or smoking), and/or intravenous.
     c. Any current or previous treatment for substance abuse.
  3. Needle Exposure
     a. Use of drugs via intravenous route, sharing of needles, syringes, and other drug paraphernalia.
     b. Other needle-exposure activities such as tattoos, acupuncture, treatment by unlicensed individuals or "folk doctors," or sharing prescribed drugs between friends.
     c. Has any person with whom the client has shared needles developed AIDS?
  4. Travel
     a. Within the past ten years.
     b. Sexual activities when traveling in areas where the number of AIDS cases is high, such as New York, California, New Jersey, Texas, Florida, or countries such as Haiti or Zaire.
B. Medication History
  1. Current or previous use of medication that suppresses the immune system, such as steroids and/or antibiotics. Current treatment for drug addiction if applicable.
C. Medical History
  1. Major diseases including (but not limited to) tuberculosis; hepatitis A or B or non A/B; mononucleosis; hemophilia and receiving treatment with clotting replacements, such as factor VIII.
  2. Treatment for psychiatric/emotional disorders.
  3. Transfusion donor or recipient.
D. Surgical History
E. Childhood Diseases
  1. Including but not limited to varicella.
F. Sexually Transmitted Diseases (STDs)
  1. Including (but not limited to) syphilis; gonorrhea; amebiasis; herpes simplex (oralis or genitalis); *Giardia lamblia* enteritis and/or lymphogranuloma venereum.

Continued, p. 78

Table 5–2. Primary Health Maintenance:
Health Appraisal Specific for HIV Infection and Related Illnesses *Continued*

G. Review of Systems
1. General: A comment from the client concerning a self-appraisal of his or her current state of health should be elicited.
2. Skin: eruptions, lesions, itching, dryness, redness, rashes, lumps, color changes, changes in hair and/or nails.
3. Head: headaches, lightheadedness, or other sensations.
4. Eyes: blurred vision or diplopia.
5. Ears: impaired hearing or tinnitus.
6. Nose and Sinuses: obstruction, pain, discharges, or nose bleed.
7. Mouth and Throat: creamy white patches, lesions, bleeding gums, dysphagia, odynophagia, changes in taste, or sore throat.
8. Respiratory: dyspnea with or without certain activities, coughing, wheezing, chest pain, cold or "flu-like" symptoms, as well as the date of last chest x-ray and tuberculin test and results.
9. Cardiovascular: chest pain, palpitations, edema, or known hyper/hypotension.
10. Gastrointestinal: changes in appetite, involuntary weight loss, abdominal pain or cramping, changes in bowel habits, diarrhea, blood in stool, rectal or perianal pain or itching.
11. Genitourinary: dysuria, nocturia, pain, itching, discharges or lesions.
12. Gynecologic: changes in menstruation, dyspareunia, vaginal discharge, breast problems, obstetric history and contraception.
13. Musculoskeletal: arthralgia or myalgia.
14. Neurologic and Emotional: problems with memory, nervousness, personality changes, confusional states, stiff neck, photophobia, tremors, paresthesias, seizures, or syncope.
15. Endocrine: polyuria, polyphagia, polydipsia, fevers, or night sweats.
16. Hematopoietic: lymphadenopathy, bruising or bleeding, history of anemia.

system; (8) cardiovascular system; and (9) integumentary system (Cammarosano & Lewis, 1985; Welch et al, 1984). Therefore a complete exam should be performed and any deviations from normal findings should be considered significant in relation to HIV infection.

Table 5–3 provides guidelines for conducting the physical exam. Tables 5–2 and 5–3 reveal the more common significant findings when performing a health appraisal specific for HIV infection. They are not intended as a complete review and do not preclude the need for a more detailed history and physical examination based on the individual needs of each client.

Secondary Health Maintenance

The secondary level of health maintenance should be implemented as soon as an individual is diagnosed as having HIV infection. This category of nursing care focuses on activities directed toward health protection for persons with HIV infection. Basic to planning is an awareness by the professional nurse that the leading cause of morbidity in the immunodeficient person is infection (Schimpff, 1980). The depressed activity of the T4 lymphocytes in the person with HIV infection leaves them vulnerable to a variety of infections (Gurevich & Tafaro, 1985; Jacobs & Piano, 1987; Nelson, 1987; Schimpff, 1980; Ungvarski, 1984, 1987). Therefore, infection prevention should be considered a pragmatic necessity

Table 5–3. Primary Health Maintenance:
Appraisal Specific for HIV Infection and Related Illnesses

Physical Examination

A. Neurologic Examination
  1. Cerebral Functions: impaired cognitive functions, decreased level of consciousness, anger, inattentiveness, depression and/or denial.
  2. Cranial Nerve Examination
      a. C-II (optic nerve): papilledema, cotton-wool patches (exudate); visual field deficiencies and/or blurred vision.
      b. C-III, C-IV, C-VI (oculomotor, trochlear, abducens nerves): impaired extraocular movements, unequal pupils, diplopia, ptosis and/or nystagmus.
      c. C-V (trigeminal nerve): photophobia.
      d. C-VII (facial nerve): hemiparesis.
      e. C-VIII (acoustic nerve): tinnitus, vertigo and/or impaired hearing.
      f. C-IX, C-X (glossopharyngeal and vagus nerves): dysphagia and/or dysarthria.
  3. Motor Examination: hemiparesis.
  4. Sensory examination: dysesthesia, and/or areas of anesthesia.
  5. Cerebellar Examination: ataxia, dysmetria and/or intention tremors.
  6. Reflexes: abnormal reflexes and/or a positive Babinski sign.
  7. Meningeal Signs: nuchal rigidity, Brudzinski's sign and/or Kernig's sign.
B. Mouth and Throat Examination
  1. Lesions, discoloration, or exudates.
C. Cardiovascular Examination
  1. Heart: disturbances in cardiac rate, rhythm and the presence of a pericardial friction rub.
  2. Peripheral Vascular: edema, decrease in peripheral pulse(s).
D. Respiratory Examination
  1. Tachypnea: on palpation note lag on excursion, dullness to percussion and the presence of rales (crackles) and/or rhonchi (wheezes).
E. Lymphatic Examination
  1. Lymphadenopathy
F. Abdominal Examination
  1. Masses or tenderness, hepatomegaly, or splenomegaly or hyperactive bowel sounds.
G. Examination of genitalia and perianal region
  1. Lesion or discharges.
H. Musculoskeletal Examination
  1. Pain on range of motion.

rather than just an abstract concept (Ungvarski, 1985). The tendency to acquire opportunistic infections by the person with HIV infection is further increased when they are treated with antimicrobial or antineoplastic agents, many of which induce leukopenia and cause some degree of cellular or mucosal damage. Critical to infection development in the person with HIV is an interaction of multiple predisposing factors, such as (1) local colonization of potentially pathogenic organisms from normal flora or the environment; (2) local damage to the integument or mucosa that allows entry of these organisms; and (3) a decrease in the number of T helper cells, which results in rapid progression of the infectious process (Schimpff, 1980; Ungvarski, 1984). Thus the focus of health protection on a secondary level is the maintenance or improvement of the individual's level of wellness through health teaching as well as instruction on limiting the spread of HIV from the client to others. Table 5–4 illustrates the key elements to be covered with the HIV positive individual.

Table 5–4. Secondary Health Maintenance:
Health Protection for the Person with HIV Infection

Current Health Activities	Encourage	Discourage	Individual is at Risk for:
1. Skin Care	-showering daily -use mild soap -damp drying -using emollient cream such as petroleum jelly	-tub baths -drying, perfumed soap -creams, lotions that have alcohol content and are drying	secondary skin infections or transfer of infections from one part of the body to another
2. Hair Care	-washing hair infrequently -using mild shampoo -using conditioner -covering head while in bed -combing hair	-washing hair daily -drying, perfumed shampoo -brushing hair	excessive hair loss related to chronic infection (HIV) and/or decreased nutritional intake
3. Mouth Care	-using soft toothbrush -non-abrasive toothpaste (or baking soda) -using Toothettes for mucosal surface cleaning -performing mouth care t.i.d.	-using firm or hard toothbrush -using abrasive toothpaste -brushing mucosal surfaces -performing only q.d or b.i.d	secondary oral infections, especially thrush
4. Handwashing	-frequent washing after activities of daily living -using soap in a pump dispenser -rinsing well -applying emollient cream to protect the skin -wearing rubber/latex gloves when cleaning -demonstration of handwashing	-using hot water -using bar soap -teaching handwashing without demonstrating correct method	secondary infections related to poor handwashing practices
5. Nutrition	-high-protein, high-calorie diet -balanced diet -small frequent feedings -low microbial diet (washing/peeling fruits and vegetables; cooking meats well-done)	-skipping meals -attempting to eat three large meals per day -eating unpasteurized dairy products -eating unwashed/ unpeeled or organic fruits and vegetables	secondary infections related to inadequate protein and calorie intake or contaminated foods

Continued, p. 81

Current Health Activities	Encourage	Discourage	Individual is at Risk for:
5. Nutrition (Continued)	-demonstration of ability to select/ plan 24 hour diet	-eating raw fish or meats cooked rare -using standard dietary instruction sheets that may be irrelevant to client's dietary preferences	
6. Environmental Cleaning	-using household bleach (5.25% sodium hypochlorite) diluted 1:10 with water for cleaning -discarding solution daily and remixing when necessary -cleaning up blood or body fluids with this solution -using household bleach for laundry soiled with blood or body fluids -using double plastic bags to discard disposable items contaminated with blood or body fluids -changing filters on air conditioners frequently	-using expensive ineffective (for disinfection) household detergents -using cleaning solutions beyond 24 hours after mixing -discarding soiled disposable items without using double plastic bags	secondary infections related to unclean environment; contamination of environment with HIV
7. Pet Care	-at best should not be performed by person with HIV infection -when necessary wear gloves and wash hands when finished	-handling pet excreta or cleaning litter boxes, bird cages, or aquariums	secondary infections related to microbes in pet excreta
8. Health Care Follow-up	-establishing a pattern for health care follow-up (physician, visiting nurse, clinic, etc.) -establishing a relationship with health care	-changing patterns of health care follow-up -seeking health care from health care professionals with knowledge deficits of HIV infection	delayed health care intervention when secondary complications develop

Continued, p. 82

Current Health Activities	Encourage	Discourage	Individual is at Risk for:

8. Health Care Follow-up (Continued)	professional knowledgeable about HIV infection
	-watching for signs and symptoms indicating secondary complications of HIV infection including but not limited to:
	  1. skin lesions, rashes, lumps or bruising
	  2. swollen lymph nodes
	  3. lesions or exudate in mouth
	  4. persistent fever
	  5. extreme fatigue even when getting plenty of rest
	  6. weight loss
	  7. changes in digestion and/or diarrhea
	  8. shortness of breath, persistent coughing
	  9. headaches, photophobia, forgetfulness, dizziness
	  10. unusual bleeding e.g., bleeding gums
		-ignoring warning signs	

9. Sexual Practices	-risk-free sexual practice (see Table 5-2)	-low- or high-risk sexual practice	sexually transmitted diseases and transfer of HIV to a non-infected person
10. Procreation	-contraception	-conception	perinatal transmission of HIV
11. Intravenous Drug Use	-cessation of drug use -not sharing drug paraphernalia with others -disinfecting drug paraphernalia before sharing equipment (if client persists in sharing)	-continued use of recreational drugs -sharing of contaminated drug paraphernalia	secondary infections related to contaminated "works" and transmission of HIV to others

Continued, p. 83

Table 5–4. Secondary Health Maintenance:
Health Protection for the Person with HIV Infection *Continued*

Current Health Activities	Encourage	Discourage	Individual is at Risk for:
12. Stress Management Coping	-joining support groups from community-based AIDS organizations or professional guidance -meditation -using visualization, relaxation techniques -use of therapeutic touch	-continued stress -relying on friends, gossip, or the media for the "latest" information about AIDS	stress and continued use of recreational drugs such as alcohol and tobacco further diminish the immune system and increase the potential for secondary infections/ diseases
	-getting factual answers to health care concerns related to HIV infection from reliable sources, such as health care professionals knowledgeable about HIV infection		-undue stress related to hysterical media reports
	-review of financial status and health insurance as well as Medicaid eligibility	-delays in accessing required health care due to lack of financial planning	delays in obtaining health care related to inability to pay
13. Additional Considerations	-using own personal care items (e.g., razors, toothbrushes, make-up, etc.) -refraining from donating blood or organs -informing health care professionals that one is HIV positive	-sharing of personal care items -donating blood or making plans to donate body organs -not telling health care professionals that one is HIV positive	transmitting HIV to others

Health teaching by the nurse should include the client's lover, spouse, friends, or family (whomever the client designates as significant others), and should include the sharing of printed materials that they can use as a reference source. This is especially true of the initial diagnosis of HIV infection. Weisman (1979) best describes this period as a period of existential plight. It is a period of acute psychological turmoil that is precipitated by the overwhelming impact of the initial diagnosis, and it can last for several weeks. Personal experience has demonstrated that minimal, if any, retention of information takes place at this time; however, this may be the only contact the nurse will have with the client. Providing printed material and sharing information with the client and significant others will ensure, to some degree, that the information has been provided and made available. It is also important, at this time, that the nurse provide printed information for health care follow-up as well as community-based organizations for professional and peer support.

Tertiary Health Maintenance

The tertiary level of nursing activity is concerned with minimizing the residual disabilities that are the consequences of advancing HIV infection or AIDS-diagnosed opportunistic diseases, infections, and neoplasms. It is also concerned with maintaining and improving the quality of life for individuals in the later stages of illness.

Since an entire chapter covering the psychosocial and neuropsychiatric manifestations of HIV infection and AIDS is included in this text, only the most commonly encountered psychological responses will be presented (see Chapter 8). The focus here is on nursing management, exclusive of medical orders. The material contained within this chapter is not intended to be representative of an exhaustive list of responses to illness and potential treatments.

Nursing Care Planning

Planning and implementing the client's nursing care involves assessment, diagnosis, goals, interventions and health teaching, referrals, and evaluation (Carpenito, 1983; McDonnell & Sevedge, 1986). It is organized around the symptoms of weight loss, dry skin/skin lesions, fatigue, diarrhea, shortness of breath, cough, impaired vision, dry/painful mouth, bleeding/bruising, fever, and pain.

Symptom: WEIGHT LOSS
  Etiology:
      A. Inadequate intake of nutrients to meet caloric demands of chronic HIV infection
      B. Stomatitis due to:
          1. *Candida albicans*
          2. Herpes simplex
      C. Candida esophagitis
      D. Secondary opportunistic infection of the gastrointestinal tract causing diarrhea (see etiology for Diarrhea)

    E. Buccal cavity or esophageal invasion by Kaposi's sarcoma

    F. Inability to pay for, obtain, or prepare food

    G. Knowledge deficit regarding proper nutrition and/or caloric needs with a chronic infection

    H. Anemia

    I. Fatigue

    J. Nausea and vomiting

Nursing Assessment:

    A. Subjective Data

        1. History of problem

        2. Amount of weight loss

        3. Present dietary patterns

        4. Ability to pay for and obtain food

        5. Living arrangement and ability and interest in preparing food

        6. Response to stress as related to eating (increase or decrease)

        7. Basic knowledge of nutrition

        8. Medical/surgical history

        9. Current drug therapy

    B. Objective Data

        1. Height and weight

        2. Anthropometric measurements

        3. Examination of skin, nails and oral cavity

        4. Examination of cranial nerves: C-I, olfactory; C-V, trigeminal; C-IX, glossopharyngeal; C-X, vagus

        5. Evaluation of the ability to feed self

Nursing Diagnosis:

    Alterations in nutrition: less than body requirements related to anorexia, difficulty in chewing or swallowing, and/or inability to obtain food.

Goals:

    After discussing and validating the findings of assessment and the nursing diagnosis, the client and nurse will select interventions to:

    A. Identify contributing factors associated with weight loss

    B. Increase nutritional intake and reduce weight loss

Interventions and Health Teaching:

    A. Minimize factors contributing to anorexia

        1. For alteration in the sense of smell

            a. hyperosmia (increased sense of smell)—avoid cooking odors by keeping windows open and the home well aerated; encourage meals that include cold foods

            b. hyposmia (decreased sense of smell)—use spices to enhance smell such as basil, oregano, rosemary, thyme,

cloves, mint, cinnamon, or lemon juice
2. For alterations in sense of taste (especially related to distaste for red meat)
   a. marinate red meat before cooking in commercial marinade, wine, or vinegar
   b. substitute red meat with other protein sources, such as eggs, peanut butter, cheeses, poultry or fish
3. For person living alone or experiencing fatigue
   a. explore the use of complete frozen dinners that can be prepared in oven or microwave
   b. use of easily prepared foods such as canned creamed soups, and liquid nutritional supplements
   c. explore the availability of community resources that provide meals and social gatherings for persons with AIDS
   d. explore the availability of community volunteers to assist with meal preparation at home, e.g., "Meals on Wheels"
   e. plan for rest periods before meals
4. For nausea and/or vomiting
   a. avoid odors, keep home well aerated
   b. if possible have someone else prepare food
   c. restrict liquids before, during, and immediately after meals
   d. avoid lying down after meals if immobilized and in bed, keep head of bed elevated
   f. encourage taking antiemetic on a scheduled basis rather than p.r.n.
B. Minimize factors related to difficulty chewing, dysphagia (difficulty swallowing), or odynophagia (painful swallowing)
   1. Avoid:
      a. rough foods such as raw fruits and vegetables
      b. spicy, acid or salty foods
      c. alcohol and tobacco
      d. excessively hot or cold foods
   2. Eat foods at room temperature
   3. Eat dry grain foods such as bread and crackers after adding to soups or broths
   4. Eat Jello, puddings, and applesauce
C. Minimize factors related to inability to obtain food
   1. Evaluate financial resources and the need for referral for Medicaid, food stamps, etc.
   2. Evaluate the environmental ability to prepare/obtain food,

looking for such factors as:

    a. absence of cooking facilities, e.g., living in a shelter or hotel for the homeless

    b. needs for alternate housing arrangements

  3. Explore community resources that provide free meals

D. Discuss nutritional requirements for persons with HIV infection, including the following (Ungvarski, 1987):

  1. High-protein sources and ways to increase protein intake by:

    a. adding skim milk powder to regular whole milk

    b. preparing canned creamed soups with heavy cream instead of water or milk

    c. increasing intake of peanut butter and eating whole wheat bread

    d. adding pasteurized processed cheeses to soups and vegetables

    e. eating hard boiled eggs for snacks

  2. Increasing caloric intake by:

    a. using extra peanut butter, cream cheese, sugar, honey, sour cream, and mayonnaise

    b. substituting heavy cream for milk in coffee, tea, soups, etc.

    c. eating sweets for snacks

    d. drinking liquid dietary supplements

    e. drinking Borden's Frosted Shakes or adding Carnation Instant Breakfast to milk

    f. eating small frequent meals instead of a few large meals

  3. Eating a low microbial diet:

    a. using canned or bottled commercial products (canned fruits and vegetables are cheaper than fresh and do not have to be prepared or washed)

    b. using only pasteurized dairy products

    c. washing and peeling fresh fruits and vegetables

    d. avoiding the use of organically grown fruits and vegetables

    e. broiling or baking meats until well done

  4. Reviewing a balanced diet selection for a 24 hour menu plan

Referrals:

A. Dietitian

B. Social Worker

C. Clinical Nurse Specialist in HIV Infection

D. Visiting Nurse

E. Community-based AIDS program that provides meals

Evaluation:

The client will:

A. Demonstrate weight maintenance or gain
B. Identify factors related to anorexia, difficulty chewing, dysphagia, or odynophagia
C. Identify sufficient resources to obtain and prepare food or social service intervention has been established
D. Identify means of increasing protein and calorie intake
E. Identify key concepts in planning a low microbial diet
F. Select a balanced 24 hour menu

Symptom: DRY SKIN/SKIN LESIONS

Etiology:

A. Infection of the skin due to: .
   1. Herpes simplex
   2. Varicella-zoster
   3. *Candida albicans*
   4. *Mycobacterium avium intracellulare*
B. Dry skin secondary to diaphoresis and febrile states associated with HIV infection
C. Anemia
D. Cutaneous invasion by Kaposi's sarcoma
E. Immobility
F. Malnutrition
G. Cutaneous reactions to drug therapy

Nursing Assessment:

A. Subjective Data
   1. History of symptoms
   2. Usual patterns of bathing and skin care
   3. Bathing facilities in home
   4. Current nutritional history
   5. Past medical/surgical history
   6. Exercise/rest patterns
   7. Current drug therapy
B. Objective Data
   1. Examination of skin, paying particular attention to:
      a. areas under skin folds
      b. pressure points
      c. sites of invasive procedures (i.e. incisions, biopsy sites, venipuncture sites, etc)
      d. genital, perineal, and perianal regions
   2. Palpate skin for temperature, texture, pain, turgor, moisture, circulation, and/or edema

Nursing Diagnosis:

Impairment of skin integrity related to dryness, pruritus, immobility, malnutrition, or skin lesions.

Goals:

After discussing and validating the findings of assessment and the nursing diagnosis, the client and nurses will select interventions to:

A. Maintain the integrity of healthy skin

B. Reduce the potential for secondary infections of the skin

C. Reduce or relieve symptoms of inflammatory process

Interventions and Health Teaching:

A. Keep skin clean and well moisturized:
   1. Shower or bed bath daily
   2. Use mild soap in pump dispenser
   3. Damp dry
   4. Apply emollient cream

B. Prevent dissemination of infection and/or secondary infection:
   1. Avoid tub baths or sitz baths
   2. Avoid bar soap
   3. Use separate wash cloth to bathe areas with infectious lesions

C. Maintain skin integrity for immobile persons:
   1. Turn and reposition frequently
   2. Massage bony prominences frequently
   3. Institute a schedule of both active and passive range of motion exercises
   4. Use pressure-relieving devices such as egg crates, sheep skin, foam protectors and alternating pressure devices
   5. Use a "pull-sheet" for turning and positioning
   6. Apply skin barriers such as Skin-prep to bony prominences and before applying tape to skin
   7. Use a foot board to prevent sliding
   8. When out of bed, use a reclining chair that supports legs and alternate the chair positions frequently
   9. For comatose persons, use pillows and/or blanket in a normal or neutral position

D. Provide adequate nutrition and hydration:
   1. Hydrate with 2.5 to 3 liters of fluid per day
   2. Provide high-calorie, high-protein diet; see also "Weight Loss"

E. Provide incontinent care:
   1. For confused clients
      a. observe incontinent periods to determine a pattern of occurrence

      b. establish a schedule of toileting to prevent incontinence

      c. use an external catheter and/or adult diaper for ambulatory female

   2. When incontinent, wash with soap and water, rinse well, and apply protective cream

   3. Consider the use of external catheter and fecal incontinence collecting bags when situation cannot be controlled

  F. Implement specific skin care regimens in collaboration with physician's orders

NOTE WELL:

Occlusive dressings such as Stomahesive, Op-site, and Duo Derm are contraindicated for immunocompromised patients. These dressings require the presence of WBCs to collect under the dressing and clean out the wound (McDonnell & Sevedge, 1986, p. 572).

Referrals:

  A. Physical Therapist

  B. Clinical Nurse Specialist in HIV Infection

  C. Visiting Nurse

Evaluation:

The client will:

  A. Describe factors that contribute to dry skin and secondary skin infections

  B. Demonstrate the ability to provide special skin care

  C. Change position frequently when immobilized

  D. Plan a diet high in protein and calories for a 24 hour period

  E. Retain intact mucocutaneous surfaces without evidence of redness, dryness, or secondary infection

Symptom: FATIGUE

Etiology:

  A. Chronic HIV infection

  B. Secondary opportunistic infections(s) and/or malignancies

  C. Anemia

  D. Malnutrition

  E. Diarrhea

  F. Prolonged immobility

Nursing Assessment:

  A. Subjective Data

    1. History of symptom

    2. Associated symptoms

    3. Current ability to perform activities of daily living

    4. Medical/surgical history

    5. Current drug therapy

6. Nutrition history

B. Objective Data

1. Assess activity tolerance by taking vital signs before and immediately after the performance of an activity such as bathing, dressing, ambulating, etc.

2. Assess for associated symptoms such as pallor, diaphoresis, or complaints of dyspnea or dizziness

Nursing Diagnosis:

Activity intolerance related to insufficient oxygen transport, nutritional deficiencies, diarrhea and fluid loss, prolonged immobility, and/or knowledge deficit regarding need for rest and pacing activities of daily living.

Goals:

After discussing and validating the findings of assessment and nursing diagnosis, the client and nurse will select interventions to:

A. Identify contributing factors associated with fatigue

B. Identify methods that will increase activity tolerance and promote independence in activities of daily living

Interventions and Health Teaching:

A. Minimize factors contributing to fatigue

1. See "Shortness of Breath"

2. See "Weight Loss"

3. See "Diarrhea"

4. For prolonged immobility or the potential for prolonged immobility:

a. plan a schedule of turning, positioning, and active and passive range of motion exercises

b. plan a schedule of getting out of bed daily in a recliner if possible and/or as necessary (even if intubated while in hospital)

c. increase activities gradually when recovering from an acute episodic period of immobilization

5. Encourage the use of assist devices when necessary to mobilize and promote independence and teach safe use of:

a. trapeze bar while in bed

b. wheelchair

c. walker or crutches

d. cane

e. bath/shower chair, tub bars, hand held shower, etc.

B. Assist by planning to pace activities of daily living:

1. Plan a 24 hour schedule for activities of daily living that incorporates short activities with rest periods

2. Evaluate individual needs and point out ways to conserve

energy
- a. sitting down while dressing, shaving, or preparing food
- b. sitting in shower chair while bathing
- c. using disposable items for eating so there is no clean up

Referrals:

A. Physical Therapist
B. Occupational Therapist
C. Clinical Nurse Specialist (CNS) in HIV Infection or CNS in Rehabilitation
D. Visiting Nurse
E. Community-based AIDS Program that provides visitors or "buddies"

Evaluation:

The client will:

A. Identify causative factors that increase fatigue
B. Demonstrate the ability to plan a schedule of paced activity for a 24 hour period
C. Demonstrate the ability to safely use assist devices
D. Verbalize a decrease in the amount of fatigue experienced over a 24 hour period

Symptom: DIARRHEA

Etiology:

A. Gastrointestinal infection due to:
    1. HIV
    2. *Giardia lamblia*
    3. *Entamoeba histolytica*
    4. Salmonella
    5. Shigella
    6. Campylobacter
    7. *Isospora belli*
    8. Cryptosporidium
    9. *Mycobacterium avium intracellulare*
    10. Cytomegalovirus
B. Kaposi's sarcoma in the gastrointestinal tract
C. Gastrointestinal reaction to medications
D. Lactose intolerance
E. Inappropriate dietary intake
F. Intolerance to dietary supplements with a high osmolarity

Nursing Assessment:

A. Subjective Data:
    1. Usual pattern of elimination
    2. Usual pattern of nutrition

3. Food intolerance
4. History of diarrhea
5. Associated symptoms
6. Current drug therapy
7. Sexual activities involving anal intercourse or oral-anal contact
8. Current past medical/surgical history
   B. Objective Data:
1. Observation of fecal material
2. Assessment of mucocutaneous surfaces (hydration status)
3. Assess blood pressure for orthostatic hypotension
4. Auscultation/palpation of abdomen
5. Examination of perianal region

Nursing Diagnosis:
   A. Alteration in bowel elimination: diarrhea related to untoward side effects
   B. Fluid volume deficit related to abnormal fluid loss

Goals:
   After discussing and validating the findings of assessment and the nursing diagnosis, the client and the nurse will select interventions to:
   A. Reduce symptoms and facilitate the restoration of usual bowel patterns
   B. Prevent associated potential complications, such as dehydration and/or skin breakdown

Interventions and Health Teaching:
   A. Low-residue, high protein, high calorie diet (Culhane, 1984).
1. Including:
   a. cottage cheese, cream cheese, and mild processed cheeses
   b. cooked eggs
   c. low-fat milk, yogurt, and buttermilk
   d. clear broth and bouillon
   e. baked, broiled, or roasted fish, poultry or lean ground beef
   f. gelatin, pudding, custard
   g. cooked cream of wheat or rice cereal
   h. bananas, applesauce, peeled apples, apple juice, grape juice, or avocados
   i. white bread, toast or crackers made from refined flour
   j. noodles, pasta, or white rice, cooked vegetables such as baked potatoes, carrots, squash, peas, green or wax beans
   k. cream soups
2. Excluding:

       a. whole grain bread, cereals, or rice
       b. nuts, seeds, popcorn, pretzels, potato chips, and similar snacks
       c. fried foods
       d. fresh fruits (except those listed above), dried fruits
       e. raw vegetables and fresh salads
       f. rich pastries
       g. strong spices such as chili powder or curry
       h. foods that increase flatus such as cabbage, broccoli, onions, etc.
       i. coffee, tea, colas, chocolate
       j. carbonated beverages
       k. alcoholic beverages
       l. tobacco

B. Hydrate with at least 2.5 to 3 liters of fluid per day including:
   1. Water
   2. Gatorade
   3. Non-carbonated drinks or sodas that have been opened and are relatively "flat" (with minimum carbonation left)
   4. caffeine-free drinks

C. Provide small frequent meals and dietary supplements

D. Avoid foods that are very hot, very cold, or spicy

E. In the presence of lactose intolerance use lactose free dairy products

F. Provide skin care by washing perianal region with soap and water, damp drying, and applying creams or ointments

G. For ambulatory persons:
   1. use plastic squeeze bottle filled with warm water and use soap to wash perianal area, while sitting on toilet, after each bowel movement
   2. carry Tucks to clean perianal area when not at home
   3. wear "panty liners" (sanitary napkins) to protect clothing and prevent embarrassment from accidental incontinence or staining of fecal liquid, or from creams applied to perianal region; if severe, adult diaper may be used
   4. assess for orthostatic hypotension and teach gradual assumption of upright position

H. Avoid anal intercourse or oral-anal sexual activities

I. Encourage the use of antidiarrheal agents on a scheduled basis, not p.r.n.

Referrals:
A. Dietitian
B. Clinical Nurse Specialist (CNS) in HIV Infection or CNS in

Ostomy Care
  C. Visiting Nurse
Evaluation:
  The client will
    A. Identify factors that contribute to diarrhea
    B. Plan a 24 hour menu of foods that are low residue, high protein and high in calories
    C. Demonstrate the ability to provide proper skin care after each bowel movement
    D. Verbalize the need to avoid anal sexual practices
    E. Verbalize a decrease in the number of bowel movements over a 24 hour period

Symptom: SHORTNESS OF BREATH/BREATHLESSNESS/DYSPNEA
  Etiology:
    A. Infections of the respiratory system due to:
      1. *Pneumocystis carinii*
      2. Cytomegalovirus
      3. *Cryptococcus neoformans*
      4. *Mycobacterium avium intracellulare*
      5. *Mycobacterium tuberculosis*
      6. *Histoplasma capsulatum*
      7. *Candida albicans*
      8. Cryptosporidium (Ma et al., 1984).
    B. Respiratory tract invasions by:
      1. Kaposi's sarcoma
      2. Lymphomas
    C. Autoimmune manifestation of HIV infection:
      1. Lymphocytic interstitial pneumocystosis
    D. Anemia
    E. Exercise intolerance
  Nursing Assessment:
    A. Subjective Data:
      1. History of problem
      2. Associated symptoms
      3. Presence of associated contributing factors such as smoking, drug use, pain, etc.
      4. Medical/surgical history
      5. Current drug therapy
    B. Objective Data:
      1. Detailed respiratory assessment including observation, palpation, and auscultation
      2. Cardiovascular assessment including blood pressure, pulse,

and skin color
3. Evaluation of cardiovascular and respiratory system in relation to client's response to simple activities of daily living

Nursing Diagnosis:
Impaired gas exchange related to acute and/or chronic tissue
hypoxia.

Goals:
After discussing and validating the findings of assessment, the
client and the nurse will select interventions to:
A. Identify causative factors related to the perception of breathlessness
B. Develop and implement a plan of care that will allow maximum independence through pacing activities of daily living to
conserve energy

Interventions and Health Teaching:
A. Minimize factors contributing to the client's perception of
shortness of breath
1. For smoking:
a. if client has need to continue, discourage smoking
before eating and before, during, and immediately after
performing activities of daily living
b. discuss a daily reduction schedule in cigarettes smoked
c. consider use of commercial filters to reduce the amount
of tar, nicotine, and carbon monoxide inhaled (especially
if the client uses marijuana)
2. For inadequate pulmonary hygiene and/or immobility:
a. change position frequently
b. for immobilized clients, develop a regimen of frequent
coughing and deep breathing exercises
c. if necessary and not contraindicated, consider the use of
incentive spirometer and chest physical therapy
d. provide adequate hydrating; 2.5 to 3 liters of fluid per
day
e. in the presence of productive cough and/or copious
secretions, see "Cough"
B. Develop a plan of care that will minimize the client's perception of breathlessness
1. See "Fatigue"

Referrals:
A. Physical Therapist
B. Occupational Therapist
C. Clinical Nurse Specialist (CNS) in HIV Infection or CNS in
Respiratory Disorders

D. Visiting Nurse

Evaluation:

The client will

A. Identify the contributing factors related to breathlessness

B. Develop a plan of self care by pacing activities of daily living

C. Verbalize a decrease in the number of times per day breathlessness is experienced

Symptom: COUGH

Etiology:

A. See "Shortness of Breath"

B. Post bronchoscopic procedures

Nursing Assessment:

A. See "Shortness of Breath"

B. Observation of client with chronic coughing

Nursing Diagnosis:

Ineffective airway clearance related to chronic, nonrelieved cough,
pain or fear of pain, and/or viscous secretions.

Goals:

After discussing and validating the findings of assessment and the
nursing diagnosis, the client and nurse will select interventions to:

A. Promote optimum respiratory function

B. Minimize the discomfort associated with chronic cough

Interventions and Health Teaching:

A. Minimize discomfort associated with chronic nonrelieved
cough:

1. Encourage client to take cough medications on a scheduled
basis rather than p.r.n. and to schedule appropriately between, and not with, meal times

2. Encourage use of cough drops and tea with lemon and
honey

3. Consider warm, saline gargle frequently to soothe sore
throat

B. Minimize factors that contribute to cough suppression:

1. If chest pain is present from chronic, nonrelieved cough,
medicate on a scheduled basis and not p.r.n.

2. Demonstrate splinting techniques to minimize pain associated with coughing

C. Minimize cough related to viscous secretions:

1. Hydrate with 2.5 to 3 liters of fluid per day

2. Assist client in controlled coughing exercise schedule

Referrals:

A. Clinical Nurse Specialist (CNS) in HIV Infection and CNS in

Respiratory Disorders
B. Visiting Nurse
Evaluation:
A. Identify effective cough remedies
B. Demonstrate the ability to cough effectively
C. Verbalize a decrease in the amount of cough experienced daily

Symptom: EDEMA
Etiology:
A. Lymphatic occlusion due to:
1. HIV
2. Kaposi's sarcoma
3. *Mycobacterium avium intracellulare*
4. Cryptococcus
5. *Histoplasma capsulatum*
6. Epstein-Barr virus
7. Cytomegalovirus
8. *Toxoplasma gondii*
B. Vascular invasion by Kaposi's sarcoma
Nursing Assessment:
A. Subjective Data:
1. History of edema
2. Contributing or causative factors
3. Current drug therapy
4. Dietary intake
5. Limitations of activities of daily living related to immobility
B. Objective Data:
1. Observation of edematous areas
2. Palpation of:
a. lymph nodes
b. skin for edema
c. arterial pulses
3. Assess condition of skin over edematous areas
4. Weigh patient routinely
Nursing Diagnosis:
Alteration in tissue perfusion related to anemia, decreased O_2 exchange, Kaposi's sarcoma lesions, third space syndrome, and decreased cardiac output.
Goals:
After discussing and validating the findings of assessment and the nursing diagnosis, the client and the nurse will select interventions to:
A. Identify causative factors and methods of reducing the edema

B. Develop a plan of care to protect the skin over the edematous areas

Interventions and Health Teaching:

    A. Avoid excessive sodium intake:
        1. Read labels; look for low-sodium canned products
        2. Avoid convenience snack foods and frozen foods
        3. Substitute salt by using other spices
    B. Avoid dependent venous pooling:
        1. Keep edematous areas above level of heart
            a. extremities should be extended, not flexed
            b. affected arm(s) should be in abduction
            c. affected leg(s) should be completely supported avoiding pillow placement at pressure points especially behind knees
            d. if face is edematous, keep head elevated while in bed
        2. Reduce potential impediments to venous return:
            a. discourage leg or ankle crossing
            b. avoid constrictive garments such as girdles, garters, knee-length socks, or stockings
        3. Consider the use of elastic bandages, support hose applied in the morning before getting out of bed
    C. Protect the affected area from injury:
        1. Examine skin over edema regularly for circulation and skin discolorations or breakdown
        2. See "Dry Skin"

Referrals:

    A. Physical Therapist
    B. Clinical Nurse Specialist (CNS) in HIV Infection or CNS in Cardiovascular Disorders
    C. Visiting Nurse

Evaluation:

The client will:

    A. Identify factors that increase edema
    B. Plan a low-sodium menu for a 24 hour period
    C. Demonstrate the ability to provide special skin care to edematous areas
    D. Exhibit decrease in edema

Symptom: IMPAIRED VISION
Etiology:

    A. Chorionretinitis due to:
        1. Cytomegalovirus
        2. *Toxoplasma gondii*

   B. Central nervous system malignancy such as:
      1. Kaposi's sarcoma
      2. Lymphoma

Nursing Assessment:
   A. Subjective Data:
      1. Previous health history related to vision
      2. History of visual impairment
      3. Description of visual impairment limitations on activities of daily living especially noting:
         a. housing
         b. egress to home
         c. assistance needed
         d. ability to summon assistance
         e. ability to feed, bathe, dress, toilet, and medicate self
      4. Current drug therapy
   B. Objective Data:
      1. Examination of cranial nerves: C-II, optic, C- III, C-IV, and C-VI, oculomotor, trochlear and abducens, C-V, trigeminal
      2. Evaluation of ability to
         a. negotiate immediate surroundings
         b. feed self
         c. bathe self
         d. dress self
         e. toilet self
         f. medicate self

Nursing Diagnosis:
   A. Potential for injury, related to sensory (visual) deficit
   B. Self-care deficit related to inability to feed, bathe, dress, toilet, and medicate self

Goals:
   After discussing and validating the findings of assessment and the nursing diagnosis, the client and the nurse will select interventions to:
   A. Identify potential hazards in the environment and methods to avoid injury
   B. Maintain maximum independence in activities of daily living

Interventions and Health Teaching:
   A. Provide for safety
      1. Orient to unfamiliar surroundings:
         a. explain call system and assess the client's ability to use it
         b. keep bed in lowest position
         c. assess frequently at night and keep a night light on at all times

      d. encourage client to ask for assistance at night especially when first adjusting to impaired vision

  2. Discuss general safety measures for the home:

      a. avoid changing furniture arrangements

      b. remove hazards such as small, unsecured area rugs, exposed sharp objects, etc.

      c. smoking when alone or unsupervised

B. Accommodate clients with unilateral visual loss by:

  1. assigning to a bed in which the intact visual field is toward the approach entry of staff (door)

  2. place overbed table, telephone, call light, etc. on the appropriate side of person's bed

C. Minimize sensitivity to light by:

  1. encouraging the use of sunglasses

  2. keeping environment dimly lit

  3. wearing brimmed hats when out of doors

  4. keeping television at low level of brightness

D. Promote independence and assist in relearning activities of daily living:

  1. feeding self

      a. describe location of utensils when serving food

      b. describe location on a plate referring to clock (e.g., the potatoes are at 12 o'clock, meat at 6 o'clock, etc.)

      c. use "finger foods" for snacks

      d. use cups or mugs for liquids such as soups

  2. Bathing and grooming self

      a. arrange equipment in preference of client and replace in same location when finished with toileting

      b. consider use of assist devices such as bath bar, shower chair, etc.

      c. provide supervision until client is comfortable performing alone

      d. encourage short hair styles that require a minimum of care and grooming

      e. encourage the use of electric shavers

  3. Dressing self

      a. assist in planning location of clothing with client

      b. place matching clothing on same hanger

  4. Toileting self

      a. if bedpan or urinal is necessary, keep accessible at all times

      b. if diarrhea is present, evaluate usefulness of bedside commode

  c. if confusion is present, consider use of external catheter with drainage bag or leg or the use of adult diapers

 5. Medicating self

  a. develop a plan for medication

  b. frequently review side effects of drugs that may further increase the potential for injury such as narcotic analgesics and the need to restrict activities

Referrals:

 A. Occupational Therapist

 B. Clinical Nurse Specialist (CNS) in HIV Infection or CNS in Neurologic Disorders

 C. Visiting Nurse

Evaluation:

 The client will:

  A. Identify potential hazards in the environment

  B. Demonstrate the ability to safely move about the environment

  C. Demonstrate the ability to feed, bathe, dress, and toilet self

  D. Describe a plan for assistance with medication administration and other activities of daily living

Symptom: DRY/PAINFUL MOUTH

 Etiology:

  A. Secondary infections due to:

   1. *Candida albicans*

   2. Herpes simplex

  B. Malnutrition

  C. Dehydration

  D. Reaction to drug therapy or local radiation therapy

  E. Poor-fitting dentures due to weight loss

  F. Mouth breathing

  G. Inadequate oral hygiene

  H. Continued alcohol and/or tobacco use

Nursing Assessment:

  A. Subjective Data:

   1. History of symptoms

   2. Associated symptoms

   3. History of recent nutritional intake

   4. History of oral hygiene

   5. Use of alcohol and/or tobacco

   6. Medical/surgical history

   7. Current drug therapy

  B. Objective Data:

   1. Assessment of lips, tongue, buccal mucosa, teeth and dental

appliances.

Nursing Diagnosis:

Alteration in oral mucous membrane related to Kaposi's sarcoma lesions, infectious lesions, treatment-induced stomatitis, or malnutrition.

Goals:

After discussing the findings and the nursing diagnosis, the client and the nurse will select interventions to:

    A. Establish a routine oral hygiene regimen

    B. Minimize the potential for or severity of stomatitis

Interventions and Health Teaching:

    A. Implement an oral hygiene regimen:

        1. Perform oral hygiene with a mirror over sink or with an emesis basin if in bed

        2. Remove dental appliances

        3. Examine oral cavity with adequate lighting

        4. Brush teeth using soft toothbrush, avoid brushing mucosal surfaces

        5. Use sodium bicarbonate made into paste with water in place of toothpaste

        6. Use a sponge on a stick (Toothette) dipped in hydrogen peroxide diluted with water to cleanse mucosal surfaces

        7. Rinse thoroughly with cool water

        8. Floss between teeth

        9. Establish this routine after meals and before sleep at night

        10. Consider the use of denture adhesive for poorly fitting dentures

    B. Provide adequate nutrition and hydration

        1. See "Weight Loss"

Referrals:

    A. Clinical Nurse Specialist in HIV Infection

    B. Visiting Nurse

Evaluation:

The client will:

    A. Demonstrate the ability to assess oral cavity before and after hygiene

    B. Demonstrate the ability to perform an oral hygiene routine

    C. Demonstrate moist pink mucosal surfaces

    D. Verbalize a decrease in perceived symptoms

Symptom: BLEEDING/BRUISING

    Etiology:

        A. Autoimmune responses to HIV infection:

            1. Immune thrombocytopenic purpura

        2. Lupus-like anticoagulants
     B. Vascular invasion by Kaposi's sarcoma
     B. Bone marrow suppression due to drug therapy

Nursing Assessment:
     A. Subjective Data:
         1. History of symptoms
         2. Associated symptoms
         3. History of skin care and oral hygiene
         4. Medical/surgical history
         5. Current drug therapy
     B. Objective Data:
         1. Examination of mucocutaneous surfaces for bleeding, bruises and/or petechiae

Nursing Diagnosis:
Potential for injury related to a lack of measures to minimize bleeding.

Goals:
After discussing the findings of the physical assessment and the nursing diagnosis, the client and the nurse will select interventions to:
     A. Minimize the potential for injury that may result in bleeding
     B. Prevent environmental contamination of HIV related to bleeding

Interventions and Health Teaching:
     A. Maintain skin integrity; see "Dry Skin/Skin Lesions"
         1. Wear loose clothing
         2. Avoid heavy objects especially those that may rest and bump against the body (e.g., over the shoulder bags)
     B. Maintain good oral hygiene
         1. Clients with bleeding gums should not use a toothbrush; use non-waxed dental floss and Toothettes only
         2. See "Dry/Painful Mouth"
     C. Maintain nutrition and hydration; see "Weight Loss"
     D. Avoid medications that increase the potential for bleeding, such as aspirin products, anticoagulants, phenothiazines, indomethacin, and alcohol (Gannon, 1984).

NOTE:
Clients with Hickman/Broviac catheters, who require low-dose anticoagulant therapy, need additional observation and teaching for bleeding.
     E. Prevent environmental contamination with HIV
         1. For clients with continuously bleeding gums:
            a. an oxygen face tent, lined with several layers of gauze,

        can be used to prevent blood splash when ambulating
and when talking
2. Clean up splash/spills with 1:10 dilution of household
bleach (5.25% sodium hypochlorite)

Referrals:

A. Clinical Nurse Specialist in HIV Infection

B. Visiting Nurse

Evaluation:

The client will:

A. Identify factors that increase the potential for bleeding

B. Identify appropriate interventions to decrease bleeding potential

C. Identify the methods for minimizing environmental contamination and the correct method for cleaning up splash/spills

Symptom: FEVER

Etiology:

A. Chronic HIV infection

B. Secondary opportunistic infection(s)

C. Diarrhea

D. Dehydration

Nursing Assessment:

A. Subjective Data:

1. History of symptoms

2. Associated symptoms

3. Medical/surgical history

4. Current drug therapy

B. Objective Data:

1. Elevated temperature

2. Assess for dehydration

a. vital signs

b. mucocutaneous surfaces

Nursing Diagnosis:

Fluid volume deficit related to abnormal fluid loss.

Goals:

After discussing the findings of assessment and the nursing
diagnosis, the client and the nurse will select interventions to:

A. Control fever

B. Replace fluid loss and maintain electrolyte balance

Interventions and Health Teaching:

A. Maintain near normal body temperature

1. Predetermine with physician the antipyretic of choice
(acetaminophen is contraindicated in client taking Retrovir

and aspirin is contraindicated in clients with severe thrombocytopenia)
2. Tepid water sponge bath
3. Eliminate excessive clothing and bed covers
4. Keep on bed rest when fever occurs
5. Keep room well aerated and cool
6. Provide plenty of cool liquids to drink: 2.5 to 3 liters per
day
7. Provide dry clothes and bed linens and prevent chills and
shaking
8. Assess client's ability to take and record temperature
Referrals:
A. Clinical Nurse Specialist in HIV Infection
B. Visiting Nurse
Evaluation:
The client will:
A. Identify appropriate measures to be taken in the presence of
fever
B. Demonstrate the ability to initiate and maintain adequate hydration
C. Demonstrate the ability to accurately take and record the tem-
perature

Symptom: PAIN
Etiology:
A. Localized pain in bone, nerve, viscera due to:
1. Tumor invasion
2. Opportunistic infection(s)
B. Generalized arthralgia and myalgia associated with chronic
HIV infection
C. Autoimmune response to HIV infection resulting in:
1. Vasculitis
2. Chronic demyelinating neuropathy
3. Inflammatory myopathy
Nursing Assessment:
A. Subjective Data:
1. History of symptom
2. Associated symptoms
3. Non-drug remedies
4. Limitations of activities
5. Medical/surgical history
6. Current drug therapy
B. Objective Data:

    1. Assess vital signs
    2. Assess affect
    3. Observe the ability and/or willingness to participate in activities of daily living

Nursing Diagnosis:

    Alteration of comfort: pain related to knowledge deficit of pain control measures.

Goals:

    After discussing the findings of assessment and the nursing diagnosis, the client and the nurse will select interventions to:
    A. Identify factors that increase the perception of pain
    B. Reduce the pain experience and improve mobility

Interventions and Health Teaching:

    A. Identify aggravating factors
        1. Ask client to identify activities of daily living that appear to increase the type and amount of pain perceived
        2. Use a visual analog scale to rate and record the perception of pain (on a scale of 0 to 10) relating to activities identified in #1
    B. Maximize comfort and pain control by:
        1. Explaining the need for controlling the pain versus the pain controlling the client and medicate on a scheduled basis rather than p.r.n.
        2. Explore the use of non-medicinal techniques such as relaxation, visualization, and/or distraction
        3. Encourage client to plan activities of daily living in relation to therapeutic schedule; e.g., bathing after taking analgesic or performing relaxation techniques
        4. Institute comfort measures such as
            a. using egg crates, air mattresses, etc.
            b. frequent massage and back rubs
            c. warm soaks to painful muscles/joints
            d. ice bag or cold wash for headaches
            e. positioning when in bed or up in a chair
            f. use "pull-sheet" to move patient and change position
        5. Encourage the family or significant other to bring in familiar objects such as:
            a. pillows, blankets
            b. pictures
            c. religious articles
            d. clothing
            e. colognes, make-up, powders, etc.

Referrals:

    A. Occupational Therapist

Table 5–5. Reducing the Risk of Infection for the Immunocompromised Client

A. Reduce the frequency of invasive and/or traumatic procedures.
  1. Restrict the use of urinary catheters to clinical situations that require these devices, such as renal impairment or shock.
  2. Intravenous lines should be left in place only during treatment and changed according to CDC guidelines.
  3. All dressings, wounds, and IV insertion sites should be changed according to CDC guidelines.
B. Reduce the risk of acquisition of new potential pathogens.
  1. Compromised hosts should not be placed in rooms with clients who have dissimilar infections.
  2. Routine care of ventilatory equipment should be established:
      a. oxygen masks, nasal cannulae, etc., as well as tubing, should be dated and changed according to CDC guidelines;
      b. nebulizer solutions should be changed using sterile water;
      c. measures should be taken to limit condensation accumulation in oxygen tubing.
  3. Suctioning should be performed aseptically using sterile catheters, gloves and techniques.
  4. Education of all personnel regarding the importance and technique of handwashing should be repeated on a routine basis.
  5. Isolation precautions should be reviewed with the concept of client protection as well as health worker protection. Most notably is staff's lack of knowledge regarding changing gloves, (e.g., the need to change after emptying excreta and proceeding with personal care such as bathing or mouth care).

    B. Physical Therapist

    C. Clinical Nurse Specialist (CNS) in HIV Infection and/or CNS in Mental Health

    D. Visiting Nurse

Evaluation:

    The client will:

    A. Identify aggravating or precipitating factors related to the pain experienced

    B. Identify measures to control pain

    C. Verbalize a decrease in the amount and type of pain experienced over a 24 hour period

For the hospitalized client, nursing goals directed toward infection control can be based upon the recognition of factors that predispose the immunosuppressed individual to infection in this setting (Table 5–5) (Schimpff, 1980; Ungvarski, 1984).

Summary

According to Dr. Anthony S. Fauci, Director of the National Institute of Allergy and Infectious Diseases: "There has been no disease in the recent memory that has occupied the attention and stimulated the concern of the biomedical community and lay public as has the acquired immunodeficiency syndrome"

(Fauci et al., 1985). Professional nurses can meet this challenge by: (1) obtaining the requisite knowledge and education regarding the etiology and epidemiology of HIV infection and the plethora of opportunistic diseases that occur with AIDS; (2) practicing infection control techniques that are based on scientific evidence and available to all health care workers; (3) providing the necessary care for persons with HIV infection and AIDS in a competent, dignified, and nonjudgmental manner; (4) providing health teaching regarding behaviors that increase the potential for development of the disease not only to the predominant groups at risk, but also to the population at large; and (5) keeping themselves up to date on changes and developments in knowledge, teaching, and care of persons with HIV infection.

References

American Nurses Association. (1980). *Nursing—A social policy statement* (Report No. NP–63 22M 11/84R). Kansas City, MO: American Nurses' Association.

Barnes, D.M. (1986). Grim projections for AIDS epidemic. *Science, 232*, 1589–1590.

Bjorklund, E. (1987). Prevention: reducing the risk of AIDS. In J.D. Durham & F. Cohen (Eds.), *The person with AIDS: Nursing perspectives* (pp. 178–191). New York: Springer.

Callen, M. (Ed.) (1987) *Surviving and thriving with AIDS: Hints for the newly diagnosed.* New York: People with AIDS coalition.

Cammarosano, C., Lewis, W. (1985). Cardiac lesions in acquired immune deficiency syndrome (AIDS). *Journal of American College of Cardiology, 5*, 703–706.

Carpenito, L.J. (1983). *Nursing diagnosis: application to clinical practice.* Philadelphia: J.B. Lippincott.

Carr, G.S., Gee, G. (1986). AIDS and AIDS-related conditions: Screening for populations at risk. *Nurse Practitioner, 11*, 25–26, 29, 32–34, 36, 41–47.

Culhane, B. (1984). Diarrhea. In J.M. Yasko (Ed.), *Nursing management of symptoms associated with chemotherapy* (pp. 41–47). Reston, VA: Reston Publishing.

Darrow, W.W., Echenberg, D.F., Jaffe, H.W., et al. (1987). Risk factors for human immunodeficiency virus (HIV) infections in homosexual men. *American Journal of Public Health, 77*, 479–483.

Fauci, A.S. (1986). Current issues in developing a strategy for dealing with the acquired immunodeficiency syndrome. *Proceedings of the National Academy of Science, 83*, 9278–9283.

Fauci, A.S., Masur, H., Gelmann, E.P., et al. (1985). The acquired immunodeficiency syndrome: An update. *Annals of Internal Medicine, 102*, 800–813.

Gannon, C.T. (1984). Bleeding due to thrombocytopenia. In J.M. Yasko (Ed.), *Nursing management of symptoms associated with chemotherapy* (pp. 77–83). Reston, VA: Reston Publishing.

Guinan, M.E., Hardy, A. (1987). Epidemiology of AIDS in Women in the United States. *Journal of the American Medical Association, 257*, 2039–2042.

Gurevich, I., Tafaro, P. (1985). Nursing measures for the prevention of infection in the compromised host. *Nursing Clinics of North America, 20*, 257–260.

Hatcher, R. (1987). Some advice on using condoms against STD's: what every man (and woman) should know. *Journal of the American Medical Association, 257*, 2266.

Jacobs, K.S., Piano, M.R. (1987). The clinical picture of AIDS: underlying pathological processes. In J.D. Durham & F. Lashley Cohen (Eds.). *The person with AIDS: Nursing perspectives* (pp 52–80). New York: Springer.

Kaplan, L.D., Wofsy, C.B., Volberding, P.A. (1987). Treatment of patients with acquired immunodeficiency syndrome and associated manifestations. *Journal of the American Medical Association, 257*, 1367–1374.

Leads from *MMWR* (1985). Heterosexual transmission of human T-lymphytropic type III/lymphadenopathy associated virus. *Journal of the American Medical Association, 254*, 2051–2054.

McDonnell, M., Sevedge, K. (1986). Acquired immune deficiency syndrome. *Journal of the American Medical Association, 252*, 1298–1301.

Ma, P., Villaneuva, T.G., Kaufman, D., et al. (1984). Respiratory cryptosporidiosis in acquired immune deficiency syndrome. *Journal of the American Medical Association, 252*, 1298–1301.

Marmor, M., Weiss, L.R., Lyden, M., et al. (1986). Possible female to female transmission of human immunodeficiency virus. *Annals of Internal Medicine, 105*, 969.

Masur, H., Kovacs, J.A., Ognibene, F., et al. (1985). Infectious complications of AIDS. In V.T. DeVita, S. Hellman & S.A. Rosenberg (Eds.). *AIDS: Etiology, diagnosis, treatment and prevention* (pp. 161–184). Philadelphia: J.B. Lippincott.

Masur, H., Lane, H.C., Palestine, A., et al. (1986). Effect of 9-(1,3 dihydroxy-2-propoxymethyl) guanine on serious cytomegalovirus disease in eight immunosuppressed homosexual men. *Annals of Internal Medicine, 104*, 41–44.

Nelson, W.J. (1987). Nursing care of the acutely ill person with AIDS. In J.D. Durham & F. Lashley Cohen (Eds.). *The person with AIDS: Nursing perspectives* (pp. 95–109). New York: Springer.

Pape, J.W., Liautraud, B. Thomas, F. et al. (1985). The acquired immunodeficiency syndrome in Haiti. *Annals of Internal Medicine, 103*, 674–678.

Pender, N.J. (1987). Part I. The quest for health: Health-protecting (preventive) behavior. In *Health promotion in nursing practice* (pp. 37–56). Norwalk, CT: Appleton & Lange.

Quinnan, G.V., Masur, H., Rook, A.H., et al. (1984). Herpesvirus infections in the acquired immune deficiency syndrome. *Journal of the American Medical Association, 252*, 72–77.

Schimpff, S.C. (1980). Infection prevention with cancer and granulocytopenia. In M.H. Grieco (Ed.): *Infections in the abnormal host* (pp. 926–950). New York: Yourke Medical Books.

Ungvarski, P.J. (1983). Acquired immune deficiency syndrome. *Nursing Mirror, 157*, 17–20.

Ungvarski, P.J. (1984). Infection control in the patient with AIDS. *The Journal of Hospital Infection, 5* (A), 111–113.

Ungvarski, P.J. (1985). Learning to live with AIDS. *Nursing Mirror, 160*, 20–22.

Ungvarski, P.J. (1987). *Living with AIDS: A Care Givers Guide*. New York: National Center for Homecare Education and Research.

Van de Perre, P., Jacobs, D., Sprecher-Goldberger, S. (1987). The latex condom, an efficient barrier against sexual transmission of AIDS-related viruses. *AIDS, 1*, 49–52.

Weisman, A.D. (1979). A model for psychological phasing in cancer. *General Hospital Psychiatry, 1*, 187–195.

Welch, K. Finkbeiner, W., Alpers, C.E., et al. (1984). Autopsy findings in the acquired immune deficiency syndrome. *Journal of the American Medical Association, 252*, 1152–1159.

Winkelstein, W., Samuel, M., Padian, N.S., et al. (1987). The San Francisco men's health study: III. Reduction in human immunodeficiency virus transmission among homosexual/bisexual men, 1982–1986.*American Journal of Public Health, 76*, 685–689.

Chapter 6

Infants, Children & Adolescents

Keeta DeStefano Lewis
Helen Bosson Thomson

As of February 1988, 789 cases of AIDS in children under 13 years of age were reported to the Centers for Disease Control (CDC). This figure represented only those children who met the AIDS case definition for national reporting. The number of children who were HIV antibody positive is not known. Of those reported, 86% were under the age of 5 years and 77% were due to perinatal transmission. The majority of the children were Black and Hispanic and the greatest percentages of reported cases were from New York, Florida, New Jersey, and California. At the same time CDC reported 203 cases of AIDS in adolescents. Adolescence covers the age span from 13–19 years. AIDS in this population is defined under the same criteria as in adults.

The primary mode of HIV transmission to children is perinatal and parenteral (transfusion of blood or blood products). In 1985 American blood banks initiated a system for screening donated blood for HIV and this has virtually eliminated the potential for infection through transfusion. In the adolescent the primary source of infection is sexual activity (homosexual and bisexual) and intravenous drug use. A source of infection for both children and adolescents is sexual abuse.

Case Definitions

In August 1987, CDC issued a revised case definition for surveillance of AIDS (CDC, 1987b). The revised definition included both adults and children, whereas previously each had had its own definition. The criteria required for an illness to be diagnosed as AIDS were greatly broadened, making the revision more effective than the original definition in tracking the morbidity associated with HIV infection. (See Appendix B for revised CDC Surveillance case definition for AIDS.)

Application of the revised CDC case definition for children differs from that of adults in two ways. First, multiple or recurrent serious bacterial infections and lymphoid interstitial pneumonia/pulmonary lymphoid hyperplasia are accepted as indicative of AIDS among children but not among adults. Second, for children less than 15 months of age whose mothers are thought to have had HIV infection during the child's perinatal period, the laboratory criteria for HIV infection are more stringent, since the presence of HIV antibody in the child is, by itself, insufficient evidence for HIV infection because of the persistence of passively acquired maternal antibodies less than 15 months after birth (CDC, 1987b).

A classification system has been developed by CDC for HIV infection in children under 13 years of age. The system is designed primarily for public health purposes, including epidemiologic studies, disease surveillance, prevention programs, and health care planning and policy. Two definitions for infection in children are necessary, one for infants and children under 15 months with perinatal infection and another for older children with perinatal infection and those infants and children under age 13 years acquiring the virus by other means (Table 6–1). Those 13 years and above are classified under the adult classification system. This classification system is not to be used for reporting purposes. Children must meet the criteria of the CDC case definition to be reported as having AIDS.

Children fulfilling the definition of HIV infection may be classified according to the presence or absence of clinical signs and symptoms. Further subcategorization is based on the presence or absence of immunologic abnormalities

---

Table 6–1. Summary of the Definition of HIV Infection in Children

Infants and children under 15 months of age with perinatal infection:
  1. Virus in blood or tissues
     or
  2. HIV antibody
     and
     evidence of both cellular and humoral immune dysfunction
     and
     one or more categories in Class P-2 (symptomatic infection)
     or
  3. Symptoms meeting CDC case definition for AIDS

Older children with perinatal infection and children with HIV infection acquired through other modes of transmission:
  1. Virus in blood or tissues
     or
  2. HIV antibody
     or
  3. Symptoms meeting CDC case definition for AIDS

Source: *Morbidity and Mortality Weekly Report*, 1987a.

**Table 6–2. Summary of the Classification of
HIV Infection in Children under 13 Years of Age**

Class P-0. Indeterminate infection.

Class P-1. Asymptomatic infection.

    Subclass A. Normal immune function.
    Subclass B. Abnormal immune function.
    Subclass C. Immune function not tested.

Class P-2. Symptomatic infection.

    Subclass A. Nonspecific findings.
    Subclass B. Progressive neurologic disease.
    Subclass C. Lymphoid interstitial pneumonitis.
    Subclass D. Secondary infectious diseases.

        Category D-1. Specific secondary infectious diseases listed in the CDC surveillance definition for AIDS.
        Category D-2. Recurrent serious bacterial infections.
        Category D-3. Other specified secondary infectious diseases.

    Subclass E. Secondary cancers.

        Category E-1. Specified secondary cancers listed in the CDC surveillance definition for AIDS.
        Category E-2. Other cancers possibly secondary to HIV infection.

    Subclass F. Other diseases possibly due to HIV infection.

Source: *Morbidity and Mortality Weekly Report*, 1987a.

and specific disease patterns. Indeterminate infection refers to those cases in children who have been exposed perinatally, are age 15 months and younger, and cannot be classified as definitely infected according to definition but have antibodies to HIV (Table 6–2).

Pregnancy and AIDS

The major source of HIV infection in children occurs as vertical transmission from the infected mother to the fetus or to the newborn. HIV infection can be transmitted from an infected woman to her infant in utero, during parturition, or during post-partum breast feeding. The efficiency of perinatal transmission seems to be high; however, this varies among women (Jovaisae et al., 1985; Scott et al., 1985; Surgeon General, 1986; Ziegler et al., 1985).

As a large percentage of HIV-infected women do transmit HIV to their newborns, it is important to identify and counsel those women who are infected or who are at high risk for infection. Women considered to be at risk for infection are prostitutes, IV drug abusers, those with multiple, previous sexually transmitted diseases, Haitians and Central Africans, and women who have had sexual contact with IV drug abusers, hemophiliacs, bisexuals, Haitians and Central Africans, and those persons who are seropositive and asymptomatic (Guinan & Hardy, 1987). Those within these groups should be tested for the presence of HIV antibodies and, if positive, advised to avoid pregnancy until further information is available regarding transmission to the infant and how the pregnancy may affect the progression of the mother's infection (CDC, 1985b; Rogers, 1987; Rutherford et al., 1987). Seropositive women who become pregnant are more likely to have an acceleration of the disease and develop AIDS-related complex (ARC) or AIDS (Wofsy, 1987; Loveman et al., 1986).

Though not identified in the categories noted, another group of women is at some risk of transmitting HIV infection to infants: women who have had artificial insemination. In Australia four of eight women developed HIV infection following insemination from an infected donor (Stewart et al., 1985). Case studies involving transmission by artificial insemination also point to the reality that, in some situations, a single encounter with HIV is sufficient to infect.

The psychosocial impact of AIDS on the child-bearing woman cannot be separated from the disease itself. Many women who are HIV antibody positive face the dilemma of whether to heed advice not to have children or gamble that their child will be one of the fortunate and escape infection with HIV. Their own well-being also is in conflict with their desire to bear a child. The infected pregnant woman or the one who seroconverts during the pregnancy must face a mixture of feelings about delivering a child who will be affected by a debilitating and fatal disease. In addition, she must face her own mortality. Spouse and children will be affected by the emotional turmoil and, in some instances, they, too, may be infected.

In caring for and counseling these women and families, the nurse will be called upon to meet many needs and, at times, the nurses' emotional resources will be drained. Compassion and non-judgmental attitudes are certainly essential ingredients in dealing with the problems related to pregnancy and the HIV-infected woman. Above all, the nurse must keep informed regarding the syndrome if comprehensive and quality nursing care and counseling are to be provided.

Pediatric AIDS

HIV has invaded the child and adolescent population in ever-increasing numbers. Two different sources pose a risk for HIV infection in children: (1) during the perinatal period, the infected mother can transmit the virus to the fetus or newborn; and (2) blood transfusions or blood products received through 1985 are possible sources of infection for the pre-school and school-aged child (for example, children with hemophilia and leukemia).

Over 70% of children with AIDS have mothers who are either at high risk for HIV infection or have AIDS. These mothers may be unaware of their antibody status and exhibit no symptoms of the disease. Studies suggest that between 65% and 91% of infants born to infected mothers eventually seroconvert to HIV positive status (Scott et al., 1985; Surgeon General, 1986). Maternal antibodies cross the placenta and newborns are not fully immunocompetent, therefore, serologic methods for rapidly detecting HIV in newborns are not efficient (Harnish et al., 1987). More sophisticated studies may need to be done; however, current tests for detecting the virus or its antigens are expensive, not standardized, and are not readily available (CDC, 1987a). Some believe that all children born to HIV-positive mothers should be considered infected until proved otherwise. Benefits of early confirmation of HIV infection are close medical supervision, early family education, and prompt response to signs of infection and of growth and development delays. Questions still remain unanswered regarding the rate of perinatal transmission and the health status of children who escape perinatal HIV infection and are still living with an infected and ill mother, as well as those children born to high-risk mothers who are unaware of their HIV status (Thomas et al., 1987).

Clinical Signs. Infants and children diagnosed as having HIV infection demonstrate a full range of responses from asymptomatic to overt clinical AIDS (McCance-Katz et al., 1987; Marion et al., 1986; 1987). It is not clear what proportion of infected children will develop clinical disease, nor what the long-term natural history of childhood HIV infection will be. Infants who are born to high-risk mothers and are small for gestational age, premature, or later fail to thrive can alert the nurse to possible HIV infection. Common symptoms of HIV infection include hepatosplenomegaly, lymphadenopathy, recurrent bacterial infections, persistent oral candidiasis, chronic diarrhea, recurrent fevers, eczema-like rash, parotitis, interstitial pneumonitis, and encephalopathy. Rarely seen in children are Kaposi's sarcoma and B cell lymphoma. Additionally, a loss or plateau of developmental milestones may occur due to the encephalopathy (Church et al., 1986; Klug, 1986).

Infections are a prominent feature of HIV-infected children. Bacterial infections seen in the HIV-infected child are otitis media, sinusitis, septicemia, recurrent pneumonia, and enterocolitis. Viral infections also occur, such as those caused by cytomegalovirus, hepatitis B, and Epstein-Barr viruses (Church et al., 1986).

An increased risk of infection with unusual opportunistic microorganisms is characteristic of AIDS. These organisms represent most major microbial groups, including bacteria, mycobacteria, fungi, viruses, and parasites. As with adults, children with HIV infection eventually develop opportunistic infections. The most serious of these is *Pneumocystis carinii* pneumonia (PCP), which requires an open lung biopsy for definitive diagnosis.

Serologic and culture abnormalities of the T cells associated with HIV infection are found in both pediatric, and adult, AIDS cases. In maternally transmitted and transfusion-associated AIDS this occurs later in the clinical course. Abnormal B lymphocyte activity seems to occur early in pediatric AIDS. B cell numbers are generally increased and immunoglobulin levels, particularly IgG and IgA, are drastically increased. Circulating immune complexes are also elevated (Church et al., 1986).

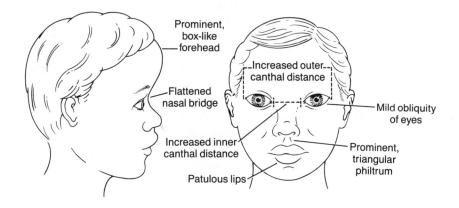

Figure 6–1. Fetal Acquired Immunodeficiency Syndrome. These dysmorphic features have been observed in children infected in utero with HIV. The features differ from fetal alcohol syndrome and may be the first indication of fetal AIDS. (Marion, et al., 1986)

Infants and children with positive serologic tests for HIV infection at birth are noted to have similar features. This similarity of features has been termed fetal AIDS syndrome (Marion et al., 1986; 1987). As yet it is undetermined whether the features are a consequence of direct infection of the craniofacial primordia with HIV or whether the features are a secondary effect of intrauterine HIV infection. Features include growth failure, microcephaly, and craniofacial abnormalities consisting of ocular hypertelorism, prominent box-like appearance of the forehead, flat nasal bridge, mild upward or downward obliquity of the eyes, long palpebral fissures with blue sclerae, short nose with flattened columella, well-formed triangular philtrum, and patulous lips (Figure 6–1). These dysmorphic features have been observed in children infected during utero with HIV. The features differ from fetal alcohol syndrome and may be the first indication of fetal AIDS (Marion et al., 1986; 1987).

Immunization. The CDC has made recommendations to help health care providers develop policies for the immunization of children infected with HIV (Table 6–3). Each policy may vary according to the prevalence of HIV infection, incidence of vaccine-preventable diseases in the community, individual assessment of a child's health status, and benefits and risks of immunization in a particular situation. The current CDC recommendations are reasonable within the limits of present knowledge and will change as more information becomes available regarding the risks and benefits associated with immunization of HIV-infected and high-risk children (CDC, 1986).

There is concern regarding the immunization of symptomatic HIV-infected children due to immunologic abnormalities associated with the infection. Serious

Table 6–3. CDC Recommendations for Immunization
of Children with HIV Infection and Household Members

Vaccine	Symptomatic HIV Infection	Diagnosed Asymptomatic HIV Infection	Not Known to be Infected with HIV Infection	Residence in Household of Patient with AIDS
Measles, Mumps, Rubella* (MMR)	No	Yes†	Yes†	Yes
Oral Polio Vaccine* (OPV)	No	Questionable due to the fact that other family members may have HIV/AIDS	Yes	No
Bacille Calmette-Guérin (BCG)	No			
Inactivated Polio Vaccine (IPV)	Yes†	Yes		Yes
Haemophilus Influenzae Type B (HIB)	Yes†	Yes†	Yes†	
Diphtheria, Tetanus, Pertussis (DTP)	Yes†	Yes†	Yes†	
Pneumococcal Vaccine (PV)	Yes Over 2 Years		Yes†	
Inactivated Influenza Vaccine	Yes Over 6 months		Yes	

*Live vaccines and live bacterial vaccines.
†Immunization is recommended in accordance with U.S. Public Health Advisory Committee on Immunization Practice (ACIP) recommendations.
Note: Children born to women who are at risk for HIV infection, or known to be infected, should be evaluated for HIV infection with the virus.
Adapted from *Morbidity and Mortality Weekly Report*, 1986.

adverse events may follow immunization of immunodeficient persons with live attenuated vaccine viruses. Close contact with household members and others who have received oral polio vaccine (OPV) poses a threat to an immunosuppressed person. OPV is excreted by those who have received the vaccine, and the immunodeficient person has a higher risk of developing vaccine-associated poliomyelitis than the normal individual. Siblings and household contacts should receive inactivated polio vaccine (IPV) for routine immunization. Extensive studies show that live attenuated measles, mumps, and rubella (MMR) vaccine viruses are not transmitted from vaccinated individuals to others. Therefore, MMR may be given to a child and others residing in the household of the individual with AIDS (CDC, 1986).

Medical Management. Antimicrobial therapy, antitumor therapy, and nutritional support have prolonged the lives of some pediatric and adult AIDS patients. Interferon, interleukin-2, thymic factors, and bone marrow transplants have been tried with little success. The onset of opportunistic infections generally indicates extreme irreversible immunologic compromise, and intravenous immunoglobulin therapy has been used for these bacterial infections. High-dose biweekly immunoglobulin treatments may not only prevent bacterial infection, but prohibit or reverse immunologic deterioration in certain pediatric patients. Viral infections, such as PCP, are treated with sulfamethoxazole/trimethoprim or pentamidine, and possibly both, although not always successfully, and corticosteroid therapy has been helpful in treating lymphoid interstitial pneumonitis in children with AIDS. Long-term prognosis for these children remains unknown (Church et al., 1986).

Other than avoidance of pregnancy, there is no known way to prevent pediatric AIDS (PAIDS) in the child of an infected mother. PAIDS acquired through blood transfusion and by blood products can be eliminated by screening out HIV positive donors. However, a small number of infected donors may be seronegative at the time of donation. It should be stressed that the likelihood of this occurring is not common and the benefits of transfusion would outweigh the possible risks.

Nursing Care. Hospitalized children with AIDS warrant the use of precautions, and infection control techniques should be followed as stipulated by individual hospital policy and CDC guidelines. Nursing care needs to be supportive and non-judgmental. Major concerns are nutritional, hematologic, respiratory, and psychosocial.

When a child identified as having PAIDS is discharged from the hospital, successful transition occurs when clear communication exists between the hospital, home health agency, social agencies, and the family or other caregiver. Statistics indicate that many infants with AIDS are from lower income families, and single parent homes, and they often have mothers who are prostitutes and/or IV drug users (CDC, 1985b). When parents are unable to care adequately for the child, the child may be placed in a foster home situation. These foster caregivers need to be included in the transition and education process.

During the initial home visit, the nurse will assess the environment, as well as the physical, psychological, and social needs of the family (Boland & Klug, 1986; CDC, 1985c). Assessment of the child should include physical growth, level of development, and cognitive ability. The initial home visit also includes identification of others who may be at risk for developing AIDS, as well as how informed the parent(s)/caregivers are regarding the diagnosis, treatment, and prognosis of the disease. A nursing care plan should be developed from this interview. Education of the natural parents or caregivers is of primary importance and must include specific information for meeting the physical needs of the child, infection control techniques to prevent the spread of HIV infection to others living in the home, signs and symptoms of opportunistic infections, and measures for controlling these infections. The parent(s) or caregivers also need to be told of the danger to the immunosuppressed child if exposed to common childhood infectious diseases such as chickenpox, measles, respiratory infections, and other viral infections. They must be made aware of recommendations regarding immunizations and discuss these with their physician.

Family members are to routinely follow prevention recommendations regarding blood and secretions as detailed in Chapter 7, particularly handwashing. If environmental barriers exist that prevent the family from following preventive measures, such as no running water, the nurse needs to make sure that the family understands the hygienic dilemma and the need to engage social agencies for assistance.

Parents are going to experience a number of conditions associated with PAIDS and will need guidance in managing these problems in the home setting. Children with AIDS will have chronic problems with anorexia, diarrhea, malabsorption, oral lesions, and recurrent infections. Secondary encephalopathy can cause hypertonia or hypotonia, and physical therapy may be indicated. Neurologic involvement can also cause speech difficulties and feeding problems. Pain may be a major problem and result from a variety of sources. Parent(s) and caregivers must pay attention to non-verbal indicators of pain, as small children cannot always express their needs. Behavioral clues such as crying, restlessness, posturing, or acting out become important signs. Older children may display behaviors inappropriate to age and situation in response to pain.

Adolescents

AIDS/HIV infection is one of the most serious health problems of modern times and a major threat to the adolescent population. Young people 13 to 19 years of age are considered adolescents. The primary sources of HIV infection among adolescents are sexual activity and sharing of needles during drug use. Statistics regarding sexually transmitted disease and teenage pregnancy clearly show that a large percentage of adolescents are sexually active. Also, many are experimenting with drugs, a number of which can be used intravenously. Adolescents are at risk for HIV infection also because of ignorance and risk taking. Accurate information and informed counseling needs to reach these young people before risky health habits are adopted or firmly established.

The number of adolescent AIDS cases reported to CDC is small compared to the numbers reported for children and adults. These numbers do not mean that AIDS is any less of a threat to this group than it is to adults and children. HIV infection can be contracted during the adolescent years, but, due to the possible long incubation period of 5 to 7 years, clinical signs may not develop until the adult years (Quackenbush & Sargent, 1986).

Nurses working with adolescents face a challenge. They must be knowledgeable about AIDS in order to: (1) teach which behaviors put adolescents at risk and the means of prevention; (2) provide support for those with the infection, their family, and friends; (3) develop a health program for those who are HIV-infected, both asymptomatic and symptomatic; (4) participate in AIDS/HIV infection curriculum planning and policy development; and (5) protect the rights and privacy of the infected person.

Guidelines for Schools, Child Care Facilities, and Foster Care Settings

Placement in the School and Child Care Setting. As the number of pediatric AIDS cases has steadily increased, so have the legal issues surrounding educational and child care settings (Black, 1986; Price, 1986; Schuster et al., 1986). The rights of the child who is HIV-infected to an education, privacy, and quality of life must be protected while simultaneously protecting the rights and health of others. The CDC has responded to this dilemma by issuing guidelines for use by state and local health and education departments in developing policies relating to the education and day care,* and foster care of the HIV-infected child. It should be noted that no identified cases of HIV infection in the United States have been transmitted in school, day care, or foster care settings (CDC, 1985a).

CDC has recommended that most school-aged infected children be allowed to attend school (1985a). AIDS is not known to be transmitted by casual contact, and evidence indicates the type of contact that ordinarily would occur among school children does not transmit HIV. Also, immunologically normal classmates are not susceptible to the opportunistic infections that affect the immunodeficient child with AIDS.

A more restricted environment is advised by CDC for infected preschool-age children, children who have uncoverable, oozing lesions, and for those neurologically handicapped who have behaviors such as mouthing objects, biting, and lack of control over body secretions. Restrictive environment refers to one that will, "minimize exposure of other children to blood and body fluids" (CDC, 1985a).

Every school district should establish guidelines for dealing with children and employees who are HIV-infected (City of S.F., 1987; Committee on School Health, 1986; Rubenstein, 1986; S.F. Epidemiologic Bulletin, 1987). These guidelines need to be reviewed periodically and revised as necessary. CDC has recommended that decisions regarding school, day care, and foster care be made on a case-by-case basis. Each case will be reviewed by a team composed of the student's parent(s) or guardian, the student's physician, public health representatives, and appropriate school personnel. The team will consider the child's behavior, physical condition, and neurologic development; the child's expected type of interaction with others in the school and care setting; and the effect attendance will have on other children, as well as the infected child. When a decision is made by the team not to allow a child to attend classes or participate in school activities,

---

*Day care includes nursery schools, day care centers, Head Start programs, and after-school programs.

efforts must be made to provide the infected child with an adequate alternative education (CDC, 1985a; NEA, 1986).

School nurses need to be involved in the development of AIDS guidelines for the school setting and members of the case review teams. School nurses' professional preparation, skills, and knowledge of the school environment make their input invaluable to these processes.

Whether or not a foster home should accept a child who is infected with HIV will depend on a number of factors, such as the number of other children in the home, the ability of the foster parents to handle ongoing medical problems, the possible social and psychological effects on the family of the foster parents, the foster parents' level of education in transmission and prevention of the disease, the willingness to follow prevention techniques, the expected type of interaction with others in the home, and the behavior and level of function of the child.

Any person involved in the education and care of the AIDS or HIV-infected child shall respect the individual's privacy. The number of persons aware of the infected individual's condition should be kept to a minimum and records kept confidential. Certain states have mandates to protect HIV-infected individuals' privacy and penalties for non-compliance are severe. The American Academy of Pediatrics has also issued guidelines for attendance in school, day care, and foster care settings, and these statements are similar to those of CDC.

Special precautions. When an HIV-infected child is part of a school program, day care facility, or multiple-client foster home, certain precautions must be taken to ensure the child's welfare. The child with AIDS is generally immunodeficient and is, therefore, at greater risk of developing severe complications if exposed to certain infections, such as those caused by varicella-zoster virus, cytomegalovirus, measles virus, and herpes simplex virus. Precautions must be followed, and exclusion of the AIDS child may be necessary if there is an outbreak of any of these conditions. The physician should be notified if exposure does occur and specific immune globulin given. School and day care entrance procedures require positive proof of certain vaccinations. However, live virus vaccines, such as polio, measles, mumps, and rubella, can be dangerous for some infected with HIV, and a medical exemption needs to be obtained (Committee on Infectious Diseases, 1987).

Precautions in handling blood and body fluids need to be practiced in school, day care programs, and foster care settings (CDC, 1983). Since a child may be HIV-infected yet asymptomatic, infection control techniques should be practiced routinely (Table 6–4).

Education. All teaching staff, day care personnel, and foster care providers would benefit greatly from periodic in-service programs covering transmission and prevention of HIV infection. Janitors, transportation providers, substitutes, and babysitters need to be included when in-service programs are held. The time spent in education will go far in alleviating fears, providing the best care and protection for the infected child, and minimizing the risk of transmission to others.

Table 6–4. Infection Control in Child Care Settings

1. Wash hands before and after working with each child.

2. Wear disposable gloves when handling blood and body excretions or secretions and for diapering and toileting. Gloves should also be worn for oral care or assessment and whenever the care provider has open cuts, eczema, or weeping lesions.

3. Double-bag or use bags with melt away linings for soiled diapers, sanitary napkins, Band-Aids, and other disposable articles soiled with body excretions and secretions.

4. Wash toys, furniture, and any other articles soiled with blood and body excretions with a cleaning agent, then wipe again using a solution of 1:10 household bleach and water or 70% alcohol. Prepare the bleach solution daily as bleach dissipates quickly once diluted.

5. Wear smocks if there is a possibility that clothing of staff members will be contaminated with blood or secretions/excretions.

6. Double bag or use bags with melt away linings for contaminated linen until laundered. Rinse in cold water with bleach added and then wash in hot water. Bleach loses its effectiveness when added to hot water.

7. Store toothbrushes separately and do not allow children to share eating utensils, plates, glasses, or cups.

From Lewis, K. and Thomson, H., 1986.

Effect of AIDS

Family. Most forms of chronic illness do not produce the level of response in the family and community that is generated by the label of AIDS (Hanson, 1986). Aside from the physical care and daily precautions, families are faced with numerous other problems, such as social isolation, inordinate medical bills, lack of confidence in parenting ability, and a sense of loss of control. Because of the complexity of the disease, the family must work with numerous agencies and health professionals, and some of these individuals may lack sensitivity due to fear and ignorance. In the midst of all the sorrow and pain, families will often turn to the nurse for support and guidance. The stability of the entire family is at risk as the disease progresses and as the physical and emotional needs of the child increase.

Parents and siblings experience a range of emotions. Parental guilt can be overwhelming when there has been perinatal transmission. Anger and frustration are inevitable when the parents of a hemophiliac learn that their child has been infected by transfused blood or blood components. Words cannot describe the grief all parents experience as they watch their child suffer and wither away with no hope of a cure. Dreams for their child are shattered. Some parents may even fear that they themselves will become infected. Brothers and sisters of the child with AIDS can develop psychological problems because the parents have less time and energy available for them. They, too, may fear they will become infected. Ambivalence toward the ill sibling often develops which can, in turn, produce feelings of guilt. Everyone in the family experiences loneliness and rejection as friends, relatives, playmates, and neighbors no longer visit or obviously avoid any physical contact. Marital conflicts can easily develop from the stress and emotional consequences of AIDS.

Families often face financial concerns when a parent must stay at home to care for the ill child. Even when the child is physically well, day care centers and sitters are not always an option, financially, for children diagnosed as having PAIDS and HIV infection.

Child and Adolescent. How the child will cope with illness will depend on age, cognitive development, social support network, reactions of others, and quality of care. At a time when the child and adolescent are trying to achieve developmental tasks, this illness leaves them weak and helpless. Feelings of isolation and rejection increase if they are not allowed to attend school. Numerous hospital admissions, gowned and gloved personnel, and a general dependency on others can be very disconcerting. In the older child and adolescent, feelings of guilt develop with the realization of the stress and costs the illness is inflicting upon the family.

Consideration should be given to providing counseling for the child and adolescent with HIV infection. The diagnosis of a fatal illness can lead to despair, personality changes, anger, insomnia, or even suicide. Family members would also benefit from professional help.

Many children with AIDS or HIV infection are living in foster homes. There are a number of reasons why a child would be placed outside of his or her own home: (1) the natural mother is taking drugs; (2) the mother and/or father are too ill from the disease to adequately care for the child; (3) parenting skills are poor or the parent(s) are unable to adequately follow through on the many medical appointments and concerns.

If placement in a foster home occurs prior to diagnosis, the family will have bonded with the child and, in most cases, will choose to continue to care for the child. The nurse will find little difference in the feelings and problems faced by these caregivers as compared to those of natural parents. However, when diagnosis is made prior to a placement, then finding a home willing to take the child may be difficult.

AIDS Education in the School

At the present time there is no cure or vaccine for AIDS and it appears that both are distant on the horizon. Awareness and avoidance of behavior that results in infection is the primary means of prevention at this time. This objective can be achieved only through education. AIDS affects all age groups; therefore, it is vital that AIDS education reach every segment of the community (Francis & Chin, 1987). The information must be clear, medically correct, and not based on prejudice and/or hysteria. The CDC and the Surgeon General have recommended AIDS prevention be taught in the schools, and some states have mandated this specific instruction.

Any student who is sexually active, using drugs, or sexually abused is at risk for contracting AIDS; however, the adolescent is generally considered most vulnerable. Adolescence is defined as a period between puberty and maturity. During this transition the young person is seeking a personal identity, establishing independence, developing morals and values, and adjusting to feelings associated with sexuality. Many teenagers are experimenting with sex and drugs and accurate information about AIDS must reach these young people before risky health habits are adopted or firmly established.

The most efficient means of disseminating information to young people is through the schools, beginning no later than the seventh grade (Fulton et al., 1987; USDHHS, 1987; Yarber, 1987). AIDS/HIV infection prevention curricula should include discussion of the causative virus, methods of transmission, precautions and techniques for prevention, need for abstinence, conditions and infections seen in the disease, a comparison of AIDS to other sexually transmitted diseases, and necessary changes in behavior, such as use of condoms and reducing the number of sexual partners. Information on the risks of IV drug use should include resources and counseling services. If the school provides a family life or sex education program, the AIDS material can be incorporated into this curriculum.

Though highly controversial, many believe AIDS education should begin at the early elementary level (Sex and schools, *Time*, 1986). The Surgeon General has recommended education about AIDS begin at the third grade. A number of communities throughout the nation presently offer outstanding programs that run from grades K through 12. Curricula at the younger levels include such basics as anatomy and physiology, recognition of the difference between wellness and illness, general health habits and the role of children in preventing illness and disease, types of infectious agents, and the concepts of communicable and noncommunicable diseases. In addition, the young students develop a sense of responsibility for their own health and how they can affect the health of others. Fifth and sixth graders are taught the basics of AIDS virus action, infection, and prevention. Various forms of lifestyles are presented at this level, and respect for the values and beliefs of others is encouraged.

The public frequently seeks out the nurse professional for information and guidance in health matters. Nurses must be knowledgeable regarding AIDS and willing to keep continually updated on new information. Changes are probable in the areas of epidemiology, transmission, antibody testing, vaccine, and treatment. Nurses need to be a part of AIDS curriculum planning and, whenever possible, should teach the prevention class. School health nurses are responsible for the educational needs of six groups: school board members; school administrators; parents; teachers and other school-related persons, including instructional assistants, psychologists, and speech therapists; transportation and janitorial staff; and students. Each of these groups has unique needs. The nurse must also be prepared to utilize counseling skills when a recommendation for HIV antibody testing is necessary and when called upon to help those with positive results cope with the disease and its prognosis.

Teaching about HIV infection requires discussion of sexuality, and some nurses may find it difficult to talk frankly about this subject. It is helpful to both teacher and students when "rules of behavior" are agreed upon during the first class. The following are suggestions: (1) it is not necessary to disclose personal opinions about sexuality or reveal experiences; (2) individual values are to be respected; (3) sharing in class of a personal nature is not to be discussed with others outside the class; (4) during discussion, participants are to clarify whether a statement is fact or personal opinion; and (5) any question is acceptable and embarrassment is understandable.

Periodic evaluation of content and effectiveness of class presentation is essential. One of the greatest signs of trouble is lack of class participation. Students will be unresponsive if the material is too technical and difficult to understand, there is anxiety regarding the sexual aspects of the material and discussion, the teacher is poorly prepared or uncomfortable, or there is guilt and hesitation because of parental disapproval. Teachers should select material geared to the capabilities of the class and be well prepared for each session. Speaking directly or in a matter-of-fact manner on sexual topics will lessen the student's anxiety and encourage the same type of response. Parental disapproval will be greatly reduced when anticipated and addressed prior to the first day of class.

Most parents are interested in what their children are being taught in school and become concerned if there is a chance the information will conflict with their personal beliefs and values. Before implementation of an AIDS curriculum, parents can be given the opportunity to review the material and express an opinion. Meetings can be scheduled at a time most parents are able to attend, with at least a two-week notice. If large numbers are expected, more than one meeting may be necessary to keep groups small enough for effective discussion and response to questions. Prior to presenting the proposed curriculum, the parents can be provided with information and handouts on AIDS.

There are parents who believe that any sex-related information, including AIDS prevention, should be taught in the home. These opinions should be respected and an AIDS program provided for this group of parents. It is hoped that the benefits of offering these educational programs to parents will be twofold: the parents will be well informed, and the information they give to their children will be current and medically correct.

Summary

AIDS is a major public health problem of near epidemic proportions. Statistics involving infants, children, and adolescents are rising steadily at an alarming rate. Education is the only hope at present for prevention of this physically, socially, and emotionally devastating disease. Nurses must keep themselves well informed and be willing to take a leadership role in providing this education to children, adolescents, and their parents.

References

Black, J. L. (1986, March). AIDS: Preschool and school issues. *Journal of School Health*, 56(3), 93–95.

Boland, M., Klug, R. (1986). AIDS: The implication for home care. *Maternal Child Nursing*, 11(6), 404–411.

Centers for Disease Control (1983, September). Acquired immunodeficiency syndrome (AIDS): Precautions for health-care workers and allied professionals. *Morbidity and Mortality Weekly Report*, 32, 450–451.

Centers for Disease Control (1985a, August). Education and foster care of children infected with human T-lymphotrophic virus type/III lymphadenopathy associated virus. *Morbidity and Mortality Weekly Report*, 34(34), 517–521.

Centers for Disease Control (1985b). Recommendations for assisting in the prevention of perinatal transmission of human T-lymphotrophic virus type III/lymphadenopathy-associated virus and acquired immunodeficiency syndrome. *Morbidity and Mortality Weekly Report*, 34, 721–732.

Centers for Disease Control (1985c, November). Recommendations for preventing transmission of infection with human T-lymphotropic virus type III/lymphadenopathy-associated virus. *Morbidity and Mortality Weekly Report*, 34, 681–686, 691–695.

Centers for Disease Control (1986). Immunization of children infected with human T-lymphotrophic virus type III/lymphadenopathy-associated virus. *Morbidity and Mortality Weekly Report*, 35, 595–598, 603–606.

Centers for Disease Control (1987a, April). Classification system for human immunodeficiency virus (HIV) infection in children under 13 years of age. *Morbidity and Mortality Weekly Report*, 36(15), 225–230.

Centers for Disease Control (1987b). Revision of the CDC surveillance case definition for acquired immunodeficiency syndrome. *Morbidity and Mortality Weekly Report*, 36(15), 3–15.

Church, J., Allen, J., Stiehm, E. (1986). New scarlet letter(s), pediatric AIDS. *Pediatrics*, 77(3), 423–427.

City and County of San Francisco, Department of Public Health, Perinatal and Pediatric AIDS Advisory Committee (1987, March). Education of children infected with human immunodeficiency virus. *San Francisco Epidemiologic Bulletin*, 3(1), 25–65.

Committee on Infectious Diseases (1987, March). Health guidelines for the attendance in day-care and foster-care settings of children infected with human immunodeficiency virus. *Pediatrics*, 79(3), 466–469.

Committee on School Health and Committee on Infectious Diseases (1986, March). School attendance of children and adolescents with human T-lymphotropic virus III/lymphadenopathy-associated virus infection. *Pediatrics*, 77(3), 430–432.

Francis, D. P., Chin, J. (1987, March). The prevention of acquired immunodeficiency syndrome in the United States; An objective strategy for medicine, public health, business and the community. *Journal of the American Medical Association*, 257(10), 1357–1365.

Fulton, G. B., Metress, E., Price, J. H. (1987, January). AIDS: Resource materials for school personnel. *Journal of School Health*, 57(1), 14–18.

Guinan, M. E., Hardy, A. (1987). Epidemiology of AIDS in women in the United States, 1981 through 1986. *Journal of the American Medical Association*, 257, 2039–2042.

Hanson, G. (1986, April). Social, psychological, and ethical aspects of AIDS in children. *Focus*, 1(5), 1.

Harnish, D., Hammerberg, O., Walker, I. R., et al. (1987). Early detection of HIV Infection in a newborn. *New England Journal of Medicine*, 316(5), 272–273.

Jovaisas, E., Kock, M. A., Schafer, A., et al. (1985). LAV/HTLV-III in 20-week fetus. Lancet, 2, 1129.

Klug, R. (1986, October). Children with AIDS. *American Journal of* Nursing, 86, 1126–1132.

Lewis, K., Thomson, H. (1986). *Manual of school health*. Menlo Park, CA: Addison-Wesley Publishing Company.

Loveman, A., Colburn, V., Dobin, A. (1986). AIDS in pregnancy. *Journal of Gynecological and Neonatal Nursing*, 15(2), 91–93.

Marion, R. W., Wiznia, A. A., Hutcheon, R. G., et al. (1987). Fetal AIDS syndrome score, correlation between severity of dysmorphism and age at diagnosis of immunodeficiency. *American Journal of Disease Control*, 141(4), 429–431.

Marion, R. W., Wiznia, A. A., Hutcheon, G., et al. (1986). Human T-cell lymphotropic virus type III (HTLV-III) embryopathy. *American Journal of Disease Control*, 140(7), 638–640.

McCance-Katz, E., Hoecker, J., Vitale, N. (1987). Severe neutropenia associated with antineutrophil antibody in a patient with acquired immunodeficiency syndrome related complex. *Pediatric Infectious Disease Journal*, 6(4), 417–418.

National Education Association (1986). Recommended guidelines for dealing with AIDS in the schools from the National Education Association. *Journal of School Health*, 56(4), 129–130.

Price, J. H. (1986, April). AIDS, the schools, and policy issues. *Journal of School Health*, 56(4), 137–139.

Quackenbush, M., Sargent, P. (1986). *Teaching AIDS, a resource guide on acquired immune deficiency syndrome*. Santa Cruz, CA: Network Publications.

Rogers, M. (1987). Controlling perinatally acquired HIV infection. *Western Journal of Medicine*, 147(1), 109–110.

Rubenstein, A. (1986). Schooling for children with acquired immunedeficiency syndrome. *Journal of Pediatrics*, 109(2), 242–244.

Rutherford, G., Oliva, G., Grossman, M., et al. (1987). Guidelines for the control of perinatally transmitted human immunodeficiency virus infection and care of infected mothers, infants, and children. *Western Journal of Medicine*, 147(1), 104–108.

San Francisco Epidemiologic Bulletin, City and County of San Francisco, Department of Public Health, Bureau of Communicable Disease Control (1987, March). *Education of Children Infected with Human Immunodeficiency Virus*, 3(1).

Schuster, C., Will, S., Luehr, R. E., et al. (1986, November/December). AIDS in children and adolescents—learning to cope with a harsh reality. *School Nurse*, 14–15, 18, 20, 22, 24–25.

Scott, G. B., Fischl, M. A., Klimas, N., et al. (1985). Mothers of infants with the acquired immunodeficiency syndrome: Evidence for both symptomatic and asymptomatic carriers. *Journal of the American Medical Association*, 253(3), 363–366.

Sex and schools. (1986, November). *Time*, 54–60, 63.

Stewart, G. J., Tyler, J. P. P., Cunningham, A. L., et al. (1985). Transmission of human T-cell lymphotrophic virus type III (HYTLV-III) by artificial insemination by donor. *Lancet*, 2(8455), 581–584.

Surgeon General. (1986, November). From the Surgeon General, U.S. Public Health Service. *Journal of the American Medical Association*, 256(20), 2783–2789.

Thomas, P., Lubin, K., Milberg, J., et al. (1987). Cohort comparison study of children whose mothers have acquired immunodeficiency syndrome and children of well inner-city mothers. *Pediatric Infectious Disease Journal*, 6(3), 247–251.

U.S. Department of Health and Human Services, Public Health Service (1987, March). *AIDS Information/Education Plan to Prevent and Control AIDS in the United States*. Washington, D.C.: U.S. Government Printing Office.

Wofsy, C. (1987). Human immunodeficiency virus in women. *Journal of the American Medical Association*, 257, 2074–2076.

Yarber, W. L. (1987). *AIDS, What Young Adults Should Know, Instructor's* Guide. Reston, VA: American Alliance for Health, Physical Education, Recreation, and Dance.

Ziegler, J. B., Cooper, D.A., Johnson, R. O., Gold, J. (1985). Postnatal transmission of AIDS-associated retrovirus from mother to infant. *Lancet*, 1(8434), 896–898.

Chapter 7

Infection Control

Nancy B. Parris

HIV infection is transmitted through sexual contact and exposure to blood and other body fluids from infected persons. It can also be transmitted perinatally from mother to neonate. It should be emphasized that HIV is not casually or easily spread. Although only blood, semen, vaginal secretions, and, possibly, breast milk have been implicated in the transmission of HIV by epidemiologic evidence, the virus has been isolated from many other body fluids such as saliva, tears, and urine. Therefore, all body fluids are presumed to be potentially infective when discussing precautions which should be taken when caring for persons who are HIV-infected. In order to discuss precautions taken in the workplace, blood and body fluid contact will be referred to since sexual contact is not relevant in this setting.

It is important for all nurses and other health care workers to consider the potential of any patient to be infected with HIV or other blood-borne pathogens when providing patient care. Therefore, appropriate and sensible infection control precautions should be taken at all times. This chapter will review those precautions which should be followed with all patients infected with HIV, regardless of whether they have clinical AIDS or not. However, the same precautions should be taken when in contact with any body fluids from all patients, so as to avoid percutaneous and mucous membrane exposure. Donning appropriate garb is not enough. Too often a needlestick injury has occurred when the nurse was in full isolation garb, feeling protected and comfortable, but became careless when handling the syringe and needle. Health care workers should use common sense in following the recommended guidelines but should never become lackadaisical in their approach to infection control, which can occur when they perform procedures by rote.

When caring for any person requiring isolation precautions or when taking precautions with any patient's body fluids, it is always important to consider the individual patient. Observing good infection control practices and thereby minimizing the risk of exposure to infectious diseases is completely consistent with the objective of providing high quality patient care.

Precautions for Nurses

Precautions have been established which protect nurses and other health care workers from potential exposure to blood and other body fluids from patients with AIDS and with HIV infection, thereby preventing the opportunity for transmission of HIV. Exposure refers specifically to percutaneous or mucous membrane contact with infected blood or other body fluids. It is important to distinguish exposure from casual contact since there is no risk of transmission of HIV from contact without exposure. Blood and body fluid precautions should be followed for all patients with diagnosed disease as well as those suspected of having AIDS, ARC (AIDS-related complex), and HIV infection (CDC, 1987b). The Centers for Disease Control (CDC) has suggested further that these precautions should be used consistently for all patients; the CDC has referred to these precautions as "Universal Blood and Body Fluid Precautions," "Universal Precautions," or "Body Substance Isolation." Use of these precautions is especially important in situations where the infection status of a patient is unknown.

The guidelines which follow in this chapter are similar to the CDC's Disease-Specific Isolation Precautions for patients with AIDS and outline the measures to be followed. The suggested precautions are aimed at preventing the transmission of HIV (Besner et al., 1986; CDC, 1985, 1987a,b; Eickhoff et al., 1984; Garner & Simmons, 1983; Gerberding et al., 1986; Harris, 1986; Jackson et al., 1986; Martin et al., 1985; Spire et al., 1984).

Since patients with AIDS are often infected with other organisms, appropriate precautions must also be taken for these other infections. For many of the other infections, no additional precautions are required because they are transmitted in the same way as HIV (e.g., hepatitis B), or because they are not transmitted person-to-person (e.g., toxoplasmosis). If the patient is infected with pulmonary tuberculosis and has not yet received appropriate treatment, additional precautions will be needed. However, precautions to be taken with other infections will not be discussed here; appropriate precautions should be followed as recommended by the CDC for other infections.

Guidelines for Precautions

Gloves. Appropriate barrier precautions (e.g., gloves, cover gown, mask, and protective eyewear) should be used routinely when contact with a patient's body fluids is anticipated to prevent percutaneous and mucous membrane exposure

Table 7–1. Barrier Precautions

Gloves prevent contact with and/or exposure to:
  body fluids
  items contaminated with body fluids
  mucous membranes
  non-intact skin

Gowns or aprons protect:
  clothes from soiling with body fluids

Masks and protective eyewear protect:
  mucous membranes
  non-intact skin from splashing or spraying body fluids

Handwashing prevents and/or reduces:
  transient colonization with non-resident microbial flora
  resident flora

(Table 7–1). Disposable examination gloves should be worn when handling any blood or other body fluids; however, they are not necessary for direct care of patients when there is no contact with body fluids. They are also needed when touching mucous membranes or non-intact skin and for handling items or surfaces contaminated with body fluids. For example, examination gloves should be worn when handling feces of an incontinent patient and when cleaning the patient following use of the toilet, but they would not be necessary when taking vital signs on that patient or any other patient. Gloves should be worn when starting an IV due to potential contact with blood, but not when changing the bottle, tubing or adding fluid to a buritrol. They are not needed when transporting a patient, as any drainage or secretions should be adequately contained prior to transport. When ambulating a patient, gloves will not be necessary, nor are they needed to bathe a patient. Gloves should be changed after each contact with each patient. Thorough handwashing following removal and disposal of the gloves is essential.

Disposable examination gloves are adequate in protecting the health care worker's skin from exposure to body substances and any microorganisms present so long as the gloves are not torn. It is not necessary to purchase special gloves exclusively for use with patients with HIV infection as they provide no additional protection and serve no practical purpose. The gloves should be properly fitted; rings which might tear through the glove should not be worn and nails should not be so long as to poke through the gloves. Some nurses find that a latex glove provides a better fit than vinyl gloves, and thereby allows them greater dexterity. This becomes an individual choice but has no bearing on the overall protection to the health care worker.

Handwashing. Intact skin is an effective barrier against infection for health care workers. Hands should be washed immediately after being soiled with any body fluids, as handwashing is the single most important means of infection prevention. This applies to all occasions when caring for patients with AIDS as well as patients with any other problem or illness. Good handwashing, including cleaning beneath fingernails, between fingers and beneath any allowable rings, is essential between any patient contact and immediately following removal of any type of gloves. Special antimicrobial soaps are not necessary; most important is having a soap that is acceptable to staff and that will be used.

Gowns. Protective gowns or aprons are recommended to be worn only for contact that would cause the health care worker's clothing to become soiled with body fluids. Since AIDS is not transmitted by fomites and therefore not transmitted via contaminated clothing, this is actually more of an issue of esthetics than of protection from infection. As with the examples given above in the section on gloves, a cover gown would not be needed routinely when taking vital signs, or when feeding or ambulating a patient. On the other hand, use of a gown or apron might be desirable when emptying a bedpan and cleaning a patient who is incontinent of urine and feces, when changing a dressing that involves a great deal of drainage, and when performing any procedures that may generate splashes of body fluids. Cover gowns are not necessary when a patient is transported because any drainage or secretions should be adequately contained prior to transporting the patient. Some institutions now require their health care workers to wear a protective water-resistant apron for protection of clothing, rather than the traditional cloth or disposable paper long-sleeved cover gown. Either is adequate so long as it protects clothes from contamination. Once worn a gown should be discarded into the proper receptacle and not re-used.

Masks and Protective Eyewear. Since AIDS is not transmitted by the airborne route, masks are not necessary as a routine precaution. There is, however, presently one documented case of HIV infection in a health care worker from an exposure involving blood from a patient with AIDS splashing into the health care worker's mouth. To prevent this type of exposure, a mask may be worn in certain instances as a barrier to cover the mouth and nose from any splashing body fluids. At the same time, protective eyewear or face shields should be worn, as a barrier to protect the eyes. Both should be worn to protect the eyes, mouth and nose during procedures which may generate droplets of body fluids. Such procedures would include suctioning a patient, assisting with bronchoscopy, and assisting with surgery that involves high-powered drills which may generate spraying particles. Except in the last example, where masks are not removed during surgery and removing eyewear becomes impractical, the masks and eyewear should be worn only while performing the procedure for which they are indicated. Protective eyewear not only should be such that it provides a shield in front of the eyes and is large enough to be worn over prescription eyeglasses, but should have protective sides and a top shield and be configured so that the bottom of the lenses angle toward the face for maximum protection. Goggles may be preferred by some, and should be vented, although an eyeglass which satisfies the foregoing criteria is often more acceptable and less offensive to both patients and staff. Masks are worn once and discarded; protective eyewear must be cleaned and dis-

Table 7–2. Procedure Precautions

Needles and Sharps:
> Do not re-cap, bend, or break
> Avoid accidental puncture injuries

Cardiopulmonary Resuscitation:
> Use resuscitator bag or
> Mask with one-way valve

Transport:
> Standard procedures are adequate

Dishes:
> Standard procedures are adequate

Laboratory Specimens:
> Standard procedures for all infective and potentially
> infective materials are adequate

infected following each use if disposable glasses or goggles are not used. This protects subsequent users of the eyewear not only from any organisms which may splash onto the front of the lenses, but also from any infection the previous wearer may have had.

Needles and Sharps Disposal. Nurses are involved on a frequent basis in several procedures and routines with patients in the hospital. Some of these situations require that special precautions be taken and others cause concern to nurses (Table 7–2). To date, of the few cases of HIV infection in health care workers, most have occurred as a result of improper handling of needles and sharps. Extreme caution should be taken to avoid any accidental injuries caused by needles, scalpels, or other sharp instruments or divides. Needles should never be re-capped, bent, or broken and should not be handled in such a manner as to cause a potential puncture injury. Once used, needles and sharps should be discarded immediately into a rigid puncture-proof container; they should never be left unattended on counter-tops or other surfaces. Containers should be placed at convenient and accessible sites to encourage their immediate use by nurses. Once filled, the sharps containers should be closed securely and discarded with no further handling of the contents.

Any accidental needlestick or puncture injury from articles contaminated with blood or other fluids from any patient should be immediately attended. The site should be bled initially, then washed well with an antimicrobial soap. The incident should be reported to the facility's Occupational Health Department with follow-up according to CDC's recommended protocol.

Cardiopulmonary Resuscitation (CPR). It is recommended that alternatives to mouth-to-mouth resuscitation be available for hospital staff for use not only with patients with HIV infection but for all patients. The available alternatives are a hand-held resuscitator bag or a protective mask with a one-way valve. This equipment must be readily and consistently available on every unit or in every patient room to be effective. The equipment is for protection against possible exposure to any communicable disease, not only HIV infection, since saliva has not been implicated in HIV transmission.

Transporting the Patient. Nothing special is required to transport the patient. Any open draining wounds should be adequately covered. If secretions and drainage are contained prior to transport, this will alleviate the need for a gown or gloves to be worn by transport personnel. It is not necessary for transport personnel to wear a mask or protective eyewear, nor does the patient with HIV infection need to wear a mask.

Dishes. It is not necessary to provide patients with HIV infection with any special dishes, glasses, or flatware for meals. Dishes, glasses and utensils can be washed following the routine procedures used with all other dishes.

Laboratory Specimens. Laboratory specimens from patients with AIDS/HIV infection do not need special handling beyond procedures followed for handling all infective and potentially infective specimens. In many hospitals all specimens are treated as such, as is the recommendation here. Some facilities may prefer that specimens from patients with AIDS be labeled as containing infective material; however, they should not be identified as "AIDS" specimens. Specimen containers should always be sealed securely to prevent leakage and placed in a plastic bag. The laboratory requisition should remain outside of the bag and not be contaminated by the specimen. Once the specimen is bagged, it is not necessary for the person transporting the specimen to wear gloves since there should be no contact with the contents by transport personnel.

Precautions for Other Infections. Since AIDS involves a deficiency in the immune system, many patients will present for treatment with other infections. These are often opportunistic infections in which event no additional precautions will be required. However, certain infections will require further precautions. It is essential that any additional isolation precautions required for the additional infections be observed. For example, if the patient has pulmonary tuberculosis, tuberculosis, or acid-fast bacilli (AFB), isolation procedures as recommended by the CDC are indicated. The patient with diarrhea will require enteric precautions in addition to precautions previously mentioned.

Pregnant Women. Many female nurses and health care workers have questioned whether it is appropriate for pregnant women to provide direct care for patients with AIDS. The pregnant health care worker is at no greater risk of contracting HIV infection than the non-pregnant health care worker. However, if a pregnant woman is infected with HIV, the infant is at risk of infection due to perinatal transmission. Meticulous adherence to the recommended precautionary techniques should be observed to prevent inadvertent exposure during routine patient care and subsequent risk of HIV infection.

Table 7–3. Environmental Precautions

Cleaning the Room:
   Standard cleaning procedures are adequate

Trash and Linen:
   Standard procedures for infective trash and linen are adequate

Sterilization and Disinfection:
   Standard procedures are adequate

Environmental Considerations

Procedures for cleaning and disinfecting the patient's environment are generally those in standard use for infective materials (Table 7–3).

Cleaning the Room. Standard cleaning procedures are recommended both while the room is occupied with a patient with HIV infection and when the patient leaves the room upon discharge, transfer, or death. Neither HIV nor other infections are transmitted as a result of soiled walls, ceilings, floors, counters, and other environmental surfaces, therefore terminal or other extraordinary cleaning is not necessary. Any articles or surfaces visibly soiled with body fluids should be cleaned as soon as possible after exposure with a germicide solution. Disinfectant fogging is neither necessary nor recommended.

Trash and Linen. Trash and linen contaminated with blood and body fluids from patients with HIV infection should be handled in accordance with the policy of the facility for all infective trash and linen. Infective trash and linen may be handled in the same manner as all soiled trash and linen. Handling may require the use of a specially marked bag. It is not necessary to use a double-bag procedure (i.e., two nurses removing the bag from the patient's room, one wearing protective garb and the other holding a cuffed outer bag into which the linen or trash bag is placed). Special handling of trash once it leaves the facility may be required by the applicable county or state regulations. This generally involves decontamination prior to final disposal in a landfill or incineration. It is important to emphasize that disposal of trash from a patient with AIDS/HIV infection is no different from routine handling of trash containing any infective material.

Soiled linen should be handled as little as possible. It should be placed directly into the linen hamper and not placed on the floor or on furniture in the patient's room. It should not be sorted or rinsed in the patient care areas. Any linen soiled with blood or other body fluids should be placed in a leak-proof bag.

All soiled linen should be handled in the laundry facility in such a manner as to protect the laundry room staff from any inadvertent exposure to any organisms contained in the soiled linen, although actual risk of disease transmission is negligible. This will require that all laundry personnel handling soiled linen wear protective garb, including gloves and water-resistant aprons. Linen washed in hot water with detergent or in cool water with germicide will be decontaminated during the laundering; therefore, once laundered, the linen can be used for any patient. There is no reason to dispose of or incinerate linen soiled with blood from a patient with AIDS/HIV infection.

Sterilization and Disinfection. Standard procedures for disinfection and sterilization of equipment, instruments and, other articles are recommended. No additional steps need be taken since, when properly followed, disinfection or sterilization procedures will destroy HIV. Studies have demonstrated that commonly used germicides will rapidly inactivate HIV with routine use (Eickhoff et al., 1984; Garner & Simmons, 1983; Gerberding & UCSF, 1986; Martin et al., 1985). It is neither necessary nor recommended that separate equipment or instruments be used exclusively for patients with AIDS/HIV infection.

Special Areas in the Hospital

Patient care may vary significantly in different areas of the hospital depending on the specific patient population (e.g., surgical units vs. pediatric, in-patient vs. out-patient) or procedure or purpose (e.g., operating room vs. delivery room vs. dialysis unit). Non-hospital settings can also be the sites of health care delivery. Precautions may differ depending on the area under consideration (Table 7–4).

In-patient Areas. All of the precautions described previously apply. As in-patients, persons with AIDS, ARC, or HIV infection do not routinely require a private room to prevent the spread of their disease to other patients. They may, however, because of their immunocompromised status, need to be protected from other patients who have infections. If their condition is such that they cannot contain bodily fluids, persons with AIDS may desire or prefer an individual room. For example, the need for a private room may be due to a fulminating diarrhea which

**Table 7–4. Precautions for
Special Areas in the Hospital**

Special Areas
    Inpatient units
    Outpatient clinics
    Emergency rooms
    Operating rooms
    Labor and delivery rooms
    Dialysis units

Precautions
    Universal blood and body fluid precautions
    Standard infection control procedures
    Availability of manual resuscitation equipment
    Special caution in handling sharps
    Routine cleaning procedures
    Plastic sleeve for dialysis

causes the patient to be incontinent of stool, or it may be due to central nervous system involvement which interferes with the patient's ability to handle personal secretions and excretions properly and hygienically. There are no special requirements for positive or negative air balance for the room because HIV is not airborne. Furthermore, there is no reason to restrict the patient to the room, unless the patient has pulmonary tuberculosis or some other infection requiring such restriction or cannot contain or control his or her excretions and secretions. The patient may ambulate in the halls, use common lounges, treatment rooms, cafeteria, and lobby area.

Separate toilet facilities are not required routinely for patients with AIDS, although they may be needed in certain instances, such as when the patient has diarrhea. No special procedure is needed for cleaning the toilet seat following its use by a patient with AIDS. Any toilet soiled with feces or urine should be cleaned using routine cleaning procedures before being used by another person, whether or not the person has AIDS.

Out-patient Departments. Essentially the same precautions apply in hospital out-patient departments as in in-patient units. Patients with AIDS/HIV infection may share a waiting area with other patients and may share bathroom facilities. No additional precautions need to be taken.

Operating Rooms. There are no additional precautions necessary for patients with AIDS when in the operating room. The patient can be safely admitted to a multi-patient pre-operative room without risk of infection to other patients. No special room is needed, nor is special equipment.

During surgery, no additional garb is required (e.g., double gloves or gowns). Precautions stated previously would apply. For example, a circulating nurse who is counting and handling bloody sponges should wear non-sterile gloves; protective eyewear should be worn by all persons scrubbed in on the case who are at risk of having blood or body fluids splash into their eyes. A glove which is torn should be removed and replaced as soon as possible.

Post-operatively, the patient may be admitted to the post-anesthesia room for recovery. Surgical instruments are washed and disinfected according to hospital policy for a "contaminated" or infected case; trash and linen are handled according to routine policy for infective trash and linen. Routine cleaning procedures are followed for cleaning the room before the next patient.

It is most important to be extremely cautious with all sharp instruments so as to avoid an accidental puncture injury resulting in potential exposure to the virus. In some hospitals, surgeons pick up their own instruments, rather than having them passed, in order to prevent accidental puncture injuries. This is an acceptable alternative to current practice. It should be noted that double-gloving is not a useful alternative since a needle will go through two gloves as easily as one, and this only provides a false sense of security.

Labor and Delivery Rooms. Recommendations similar to those for operating room nurses should be followed. In addition, a patient with AIDS may share a labor room with another patient if appropriate for that facility. During and following delivery, gloves and a gown should be worn when handling the placenta and the infant until the blood and amniotic fluid have been removed from the newborn infant's skin. These should be worn also for post-delivery care of the umbilical cord.

Emergency Rooms/Emergency Transport. Standard emergency room procedures and routines should be carried out with adequate and appropriate precautions taken for patients with infections of any kind, including HIV infection (Holloway, 1986). A patient with AIDS/HIV infection in an emergency room or in an emergent situation is treated no differently than one in an in-patient setting. The same precautions are indicated in the same instances. As mentioned previously, manual resuscitation equipment (masks, bags) should be available to staff at all times so that mouth-to-mouth resuscitation need not be performed in the event of a respiratory arrest.

Dialysis Units. When dialyzing all patients, universal blood and body fluid precautions should be followed routinely. The patient with HIV infection need not be isolated from other patients. Since there is a great deal more exposure to blood and it is not uncommon for accidents to occur which cause a great deal of blood splashing when a patient is placed on and taken off dialysis, additional measures should be taken. A clear plastic bag with a hole at both ends could be used to cover the arm and dialysis site (Corea, 1987). Then, if blood splashes, it is contained and should not contaminate anyone else, thus minimizing contact with blood and the potential for exposure. The dialyzer should be similarly covered with a plastic bag in the event that it ruptures and blood splashes. Routine care and cleaning of the dialysis equipment should be followed.

Non-Hospital (Acute Care) Settings

Psychiatric Facilities. Many patients with HIV infection may be treated in psychiatric facilities for either psychiatric disorders or problems resulting from central nervous system involvement with HIV. In this setting, no special restrictions need be placed on a patient with HIV infection (Table 7–5). They may share common rooms and dining facilities with other patients and staff. If the facility involves patients in their own food preparation, patients with HIV infection may participate and share responsibilities and duties with other patients. Laundry can be washed in machines provided for all patients. Patients with HIV infection should not be restricted from group events and activities or from using the facility's swimming pool. As in other health care settings, the patient may need to be evaluated for the presence of unacceptable behaviors or any changes which cause inappropriate actions, such as biting or lack of control of secretions and/or excretions. Psychiatric patients demonstrating these behaviors may need to be isolated or segregated from other patients until the behavior subsides or can be

Table 7–5. Precautions for Non-Hospital Settings

Settings

Psychiatric facilities
Long-term care facilities
Home care
Schools
Occupational settings

Precautions

Universal blood and body fluid precautions
Standard disinfection and cleaning procedures
Care with sharps
Attention to biting and injuries

controlled. The patient may need further evaluation to determine if any additional precautions are indicated. This should be done on an individual basis, with no restrictions placed on any patient unless absolutely necessary.

Long-term Care Facilities/Nursing Homes. Patients with AIDS can be safely cared for in long-term care facilities. No precautions in addition to those already mentioned are needed. Special attention should be paid to the patients with AIDS to prevent decubiti or infection from occurring.

Community Facilities. No additional precautions are needed beyond those described in this chapter (Bryant, 1986; Lusby et al., 1986). It is advisable that any needles or sharp instruments contaminated with blood be disposed of in a safe manner. Laws vary in different states as to needle and sharps disposal and these should be consulted, but in all instances needles and sharps must be placed into a rigid, puncture-proof, non-breakable container. A coffee-can with a lid works well when improvising. The container should be disposed of in a manner consistent with local public health regulations. Additional information on the care of persons with AIDS in community settings can be found in Chapter 10. Chapter 5 presents a detailed account of the nursing management of the adult client with AIDS that is applicable to all settings.

School Settings. It is best that as few people as possible be aware of the child's diagnosis; transmission is not casual and will not occur in the school setting. Therefore, there is no need to inform others. Children with HIV infection can safely attend school. It may be helpful to hold a conference including the child's physician, local public health officer, school nurse, and the child's parents when he or she is returning to school. However, the only purpose of such a conference should be to deal with any special needs the child may have so that the nurse may more readily attend to the child if a problem occurs. It is not necessary to inform teachers, administrators, parents, classmates, and other students of the child's diagnosis, as there is no risk to them of transmission. The child may participate in regular school activities without restriction, unless deemed necessary for medical reasons by the child's physician.

Children with poor hygiene who are unable to control their excretions and secretions may need to be restricted from certain classroom activities but only in the severest of cases should the child be prohibited from attending school. Exclusion from school may also be appropriate for children exhibiting certain unacceptable behaviors, such as biting others. These children must be assessed periodically for changes in mental status which may have impact on their behavior and hygiene.

If a child with HIV infection sustains an injury, the nurse should take the same precautions as other out-patient nurses when in contact with the child's blood and body fluids. Any objects contaminated with blood should be cleaned and disinfected immediately with a germicide. For example, toys should be washed, disinfected, and rinsed well before being given to children. Common sense should prevail when dealing with other, similar objects. Additional information on children and adolescents with AIDS in school settings can be found in Chapter 6.

Occupational Settings. The same precautions as mentioned previously should be followed by occupational health nurses handling a company or industry's industrial emergencies and work-related problems for persons with AIDS or HIV infection. Such employees may continue to work without restriction unless medically indicated otherwise by their physicians. Co-workers should not be informed of the person's diagnosis.

Risk of HIV Infection

Because of the high rate of mortality associated with AIDS, there is concern and fear among nurses working with patients with AIDS and among people living with persons with AIDS about acquiring HIV infection. There is also fear among many employees (especially health care workers) who might have HIV infection or AIDS about the possibility of transmitting the virus to patients or co-workers (Table 7–6). Research on the risk of infection to health care workers and to household contacts is on-going.

Health Care Workers. Several studies, including some currently in progress, demonstrate that the risk of acquiring AIDS or HIV infection from occupational

Table 7–6. Risk of HIV Infection

Risk of HIV Infection *to*   Health care workers,   Household contacts   or *from*   Employees with AIDS/HIV infection   *requires*:
1. actual percutaneous or mucous membrane exposure to blood or body fluids or   2. sexual contact

exposure is extremely low (Anonymous, 1984; Flynn et al., 1987; Gelberding et al., 1986; Henderson et al., 1986; Hirsch et al., 1985; Kuhls et al., 1987; McCray & CNSG, 1986; Neisson-Vernant et al., 1986; Oksenhendler et al., 1986; Stricoff & Morse, 1986; Weiss et al., 1985). By definition, "exposure" involves actual percutaneous or mucous membrane exposure to the blood or body fluids of a patient with HIV infection, whereas "contact" refers to virtually any other activity between the patient with HIV infection and the health care worker. This may involve touching the patient, transporting a patient, performing a bed bath, giving postural drainage or physical therapy and any other type of activity involved in providing routine care to a patient. No risk of acquiring HIV infection from routine contact with a patient who is infected has been demonstrated and a very low risk of infection is associated with percutaneous or mucous membrane exposure to the blood or body fluids of a patient with HIV infection. Hundreds of health care workers with percutaneous exposures to blood or mucous membranes of open wounds contaminated by blood or body fluids have been prospectively followed. Only a handful of these people became infected with HIV as a result of this exposure. Each of these individuals denied risk factors other than the described work exposure. Those with non-needlestick exposures had not observed barrier precautions at the time of the exposure resulting in infection; barrier precautions will have little effect in protecting a health care worker following a needlestick exposure. Despite these unfortunate cases, routine patient contact which does not involve actual exposure cannot result in infection with a virus transmitted blood-to-blood.

The risk of HIV infection to health care workers after exposure remains low. Barrier precautions as stated previously, should prevent actual exposure, and infection cannot occur without exposure.

Much concern has been expressed about the need to identify patients with AIDS or HIV infection for the benefit of protecting health care workers. Although it is generally desirable to know all that is possible about a patient's overall medical condition, knowing a person's HIV antibody status is not necessary for nurses to protect themselves. In many states, HIV antibody testing is illegal without the explicit consent of the patient, and in all instances posting a diagnosis on a patient's door breaches confidentiality and a patient's right to privacy. Observing good hygiene and good infection control and barrier precautions will protect health care workers whether or not they are aware of the diagnosis of the patient.

Patients with HIV infection need the same good quality nursing care provided for all patients. Fear of AIDS does not protect a nurse. Knowledge and understanding of the transmission of HIV helps in dealing rationally with reasonable precautions and offers protection from exposure and subsequent potential infection.

Household Members. There is little increased risk of HIV infection to household contacts of infected patients without sexual contact, and none at all when a few guidelines are followed (Bryant, 1986; Lusby et al., 1986). Good hygiene should be practiced to prevent transmission of all organisms within the home, especially to prevent infecting a person with AIDS with an opportunistic organism. Razors or toothbrushes, which may come into contact with blood or body fluids, or other personal articles of this nature should never be shared.

A person with HIV infection need not eat from any special dishes or with special utensils; routine washing with hot soapy water will remove and destroy the virus. As a matter of routine, however, no household members should ever eat from the same utensils or drink from the same glass or cup.

There is no need for the laundry of a patient with AIDS to be segregated as HIV will be destroyed by hot water and soap in a washing machine. If clothing is soiled with blood or body fluids, bleach should be added to the wash. There have been no documented cases of transmission of HIV due to fomites (inanimate articles) other than contaminated needles; even if clothing is soiled with infected blood, transmission of the disease would not occur with such contact.

Employees with AIDS. Much concern has been expressed about the employee with AIDS or HIV infection, and more specifically, an infected health care worker. The only instance in which an employee could transmit AIDS to another employee or to a patient would be in situations in which there is both a high degree of trauma to the patient that would provide a portal of entry for the virus (e.g., during surgery) and access of blood or serous fluid from the infected health care worker to the open tissue of the patient. The instances in which this would be possible are rare, and the chances of a health care worker infecting a patient or another employee are unlikely, therefore each situation involving HIV infection in an employee needs to be handled individually. Precautions to prevent transmission of HIV infection from health care workers to patients are simple. All health care workers should wear gloves for direct contact with mucous membranes or non-intact skin of all patients. Health care workers who have exudative lesions or weeping dermatitis should refrain from all direct patient care and from handling patient care equipment until the condition resolves. It is not necessary to terminate the worker's employment, and rarely are work restrictions indicated. Protecting the privacy of the employee and his or her diagnosis is important. Numerous companies and corporations have established policies permitting persons with AIDS to continue working as long as they are physically able; the only limitations would be those in which there is an increased risk of infection to the employee. Recent court cases have resulted in rulings protecting a person with an infectious condition from employee discrimination under certain circumstances. This would apply to persons with HIV infection since it is not casually transmitted or airborne.

The CDC does not restrict personal service workers (e.g., hairdressers, manicurists, or others providing services that involve casual contact with their clients) or food workers from work solely because of HIV infection since no documented cases of AIDS have been transmitted in these settings. Employees should not be restricted from using equipment and facilities in the work place, including telephones, toilets, drinking fountains, eating facilities, or office equipment.

There are no work situations which would require or even warrant HIV antibody screening of employees, and this is advised against strongly. The use of this test as a screening device raises serious questions concerning employee privacy rights.

Fear of AIDS may cause employees, including health care workers, to refuse to work beside others infected with HIV. Such situations include health care workers who refuse to work with patients with AIDS, office employees refusing to work with other employees who are infected as well as employees refusing to work with clients who have AIDS. In many of these situations, legal action has been taken against the employee. In those cases which have been challenged by the employee, the standard which has been maintained is that the employer has an obligation to inform and educate the employee about the transmission of HIV if that employee is to work with clients or patients with AIDS. In situations in which employees who do not work directly with persons with AIDS but due to unfounded fears refuse to perform a part of their job, education regarding HIV infection and its transmission should precede any corrective action on the part of the supervisor. If an individual employee refuses to work, he or she will be protected only if the refusal is both reasonable and based on a good faith belief in the existence of an imminent threat of serious injury or death (Bayer, 1986; Matthews & Neslund, 1986; Mills et al., 1986). The most effective way to prevent this from occurring is by education of all employees about the transmission of HIV and methods of prevention in those situations where it is possible (i.e., working with infected patients).

Summary

The importance of education when dealing with AIDS/HIV infection cannot be stressed enough. For the nurse in his or her practice, knowing and understanding how HIV is transmitted and the simple and practical methods to prevent transmission should be emphasized. Observing universal precautions with all patients is important, but even more so is understanding why the precautions have been established and how they halt transmission. Understanding these basic facts helps alleviate unfounded fears and enables people to deal more effectively and compassionately with patients with HIV infection in whatever capacity this may be.

References

Anonymous. (1984). Needlestick transmission of HTLV-III from a patient infected in Africa. *Lancet*, 1, 1376–1377.

Bayer, R. (1986). Notifying workers at risk: The politics of the right-to-know. *American Journal of Public Health*, 76, 1352–1356.

Besner, J., Thiessen, M., Sutherland, R., et al. (1986). Acquired immunodeficiency syndrome (AIDS). *Alberta Association of Registered Nurses*, 42, 25–27.

Bryant, J.K., (1986). Home care of the client with AIDS. *Journal of Community Health Nursing*, 3, 69–74.

Centers for Disease Control. (1987a). Human immunodeficiency virus infection in transfusion recipients and their family members. *Morbidity and Mortality Weekly Report*, 36, 137–140.

Centers for Disease Control. (1987b). Recommendations for preventing HIV transmission in health-care settings. *Morbidity and Mortality Weekly Report Supplement*, 36, 1S–18S.

Centers for Disease Control. (1985). Recommendations for preventing transmission of infection with human T-lymphotropic virus type III/lymphadenopathy-associated virus in the workplace. *Morbidity and Mortality Weekly Report*, 34, 681–695.

Corea, A. (1987). Discussion of departmental policies. UCLA Hospital. Personal communications.

Eickhoff, T.C., Axnick, K.J., Brimhall, D., et al. (1984). A hospitalwide approach to AIDS: Recommendations of the advisory committee on infections within hospitals. *Infection Control*, 5, 242–248.

Flynn, N.M., Pollet, S.M., Van Horne, J.R., et al. (1987). Absence of HIV antibody among dental professionals exposed to infected patients. *Western Journal of Medicine*, 146, 439–442.

Garner, J.S., Simmons, B.P. (1983). CDC guidelines for isolation precautions in hospitals. *Infection Control*, 4, 245–325.

Gerberding, J.L., Bryant, C.E., Moss., A., et al. (1986). Risk of acquired immunodeficiency syndrome (AIDS) virus transmission to health care workers (HCW): Results of a prospective cohort study. Program of the 2nd International Conference on AIDS, Paris, France, p. 124.

Gerberding, J.L., the University of California, San Francisco Task Force on AIDS (1986). Special Report: Recommended infection-control policies for patients with human immunodeficiency virus infection—an update. *New England Journal of Medicine*, 315, 1562–1564.

Harris, L.J. (1986). A safe working environment for hospital nurses. *Quality Assurance Bulletin*, 36, 237–238.

Henderson, D.K., Saah, A.J., Zak, B.J., et al. (1986). Risk of nosocomial infection with human T-cell lymphotropic virus type III/lymphadenopathy-associated virus in a large cohort of intensively exposed health care workers. *Annals of Internal Medicine*, 104, 644–647.

Hirsch, M.S., Wormser, G.P., Schooley, R.T., et al. (1985). Risk of nosocomial infection with human T-cell lymphotropic virus III (HTLV-III). *New England Journal of Medicine*, 312, 1–4.

Holloway, N.M. (1986). AIDS awareness in the Emergency Department. *Critical Care Nurse*, 6, 90–93.

Jackson, M.M., Healy, S.A., Straube, R.C., et al. (1986). The AIDS epidemic: Dilemmas facing nurse managers. *Nursing Economics*, 4, 109–116.

Kuhls, T.L., Viker, S., Parris, N.B., et al. (1987). Occupational risk of HIV, HBV and HSV-2 infections in health care personnel caring for AIDS patients. *American Journal of Public Health*, 77, 1306–1309.

Lusby, G., Martin, J.P., Schietinger, H. (1986). Infection control at home: A guideline for caregivers to follow. *American Journal of Hospice Care*, 3, 24–27.

Martin, L.S., McDougal, S., Loskoski, S.L. (1985). Disinfection and inactivation of the human T lymphotropic virus type III/lymphadenopathy-associated virus. *Journal of Infectious Diseases*, 152, 400–403.

Matthews, G.W., Neslund, V.S. (1986). The initial impact of AIDS on public health law in the United States—1986. *Journal of the American Medical Association*, 257, 344–352.

McCray, E., The Cooperative Needlestick Surveillance Group (1986). Occupational risk of the acquired immunodeficiency syndrome among health care workers. *New England Journal of Medicine*, 314, 1127–1132.

Mills, M., Wofsy, C.B., Mills, J. (1986). Special report: The acquired immunodeficiency syndrome; infection control and public health law. *New England Journal of Medicine*, 314, 931–936.

Neisson-Vernant, C., Afri, S., Mathez, D., et al. (1986). Needlestick HIV seroconversion in a nurse. *Lancet*, 2, 814.

Oksenhendler, E., Harzic, M., LeRoux, J.M., et al. (1986). HIV infection with seroconversion after a superficial needlestick injury to the finger. *New England Journal of Medicine*, 315, 582.

Spire, B., Barre-Sinoussi, F., Montagnier, L., et al. (1984). Inactivation of lymphadenopathy associated virus by chemical disinfectants. *Lancet*, 2, 899–901.

Stricoff, R.L., Morse, D.L. (1986). HTLV-III/LAV seroconversion following a deep intramuscular needlestick injury. *New England Journal of Medicine*, 314, 1115.

Weiss, S.H., Saxinger, W.C., Rechtman, D., et al. (1985). HTLV-III infection among health care workers—association with needlestick injuries. *Journal of the American Medical Association*, 254(15), 2089–2093.

Chapter 8

Psychosocial and Neuropsychiatric Aspects

Jacquelyn Haak Flaskerud

AIDS generates a unique series of stresses for patients, their lovers, spouses and family members, and health care professionals. It creates serious problems for everyone with whom the person has close contacts, including friends and employers. It causes stress in HIV positive healthy people, in those with LAS and ARC, and in the general public (Christ & Wiener, 1985).

Unique Social, Psychological, and Medical Features of the AIDS Epidemic

AIDS/HIV infection and its related conditions have a constellation of unique characteristics which makes them public health problems without contemporary counterpart. AIDS is a relatively new, communicable, sexually transmitted, lethal disease. It was first identified and occurs most frequently in socially stigmatized groups: homosexuals and intravenous (IV) drug users. The diagnosis of AIDS is a catastrophic event because it is known to have a rapid downhill course, no curative treatment and an extremely poor prognosis. The complexity and multiplicity of problems confronting people with AIDS and the psychological terror it engenders affect every aspect of a person's life. Specific features of the AIDS epidemic contribute to the unique psychosocial and medical aspects of the disease (Batchelor, 1984; Christ & Wiener, 1985; Dilley et al., 1986; Holland & Tross,

---

This chapter expands on information in two articles in the *Journal of Psychosocial Nursing*, "AIDS: Psychosocial aspects," 25(12), 8–16 and "AIDS: Neuropsychiatric complications," 25(12), 17–20.

1985; Morin & Batchelor, 1984; Rubinow, 1984; Wells, 1985; Wolcott, 1986; Wolcott et al., 1985):

1. Persons diagnosed with AIDS/HIV infection are generally young. About 21% are in their 20's, 47% in their 30's, and 21% in their 40's (CDC, 1988).

2. The diagnosis may force the person's identification as a likely member of a stigmatized minority.

3. The social stigma and fear associated with the contagious aspect of the disease can cause avoidance of social and physical contact by others, sometimes including the person's family.

4. Because of moral disapproval and negative societal attitudes, there is a tendency to blame the infected person for the disease in the two largest transmission groups.

5. Persons with AIDS/HIV infection are vulnerable to feelings of guilt, self-hatred, rejection, and ostracism as well as to the commonly recognized feelings of fear, anxiety, depression, and anger that accompany life-threatening illnesses.

6. AIDS is associated with the highest incidence of neurologic and neuropsychiatric morbidity of any serious common illness not primary to the nervous system.

7. AIDS is associated with severe chronic physical disability which leaves persons debilitated and disfigured.

8. Health care professionals and the current patient treatment system for PWAs are severely taxed and often overwhelmed by the complexity and multiplicity of problems associated with AIDS. This situation is likely to worsen as the numbers of patients increase. In addition there may be a lack of knowledge and sensitivity among health care workers that is detrimental to patient care.

9. The disease has had a highly visible social and political impact. There is a constant barrage of media attention given to it that is not always accurate, is often stressful, aggravates public fears and leads to attempts at repressive measures such as quarantines.

Because of these characteristics of the disease and the epidemic, the care of PWAs requires special attention to the psychosocial and neuropsychiatric aspects of the disease they are experiencing. Also of concern to health professionals are the stresses experienced by the lovers, spouses and families of PWAs and the stresses they themselves experience in giving care to PWAs.

Psychosocial Assessment of Seriously Medically Ill Patients

Knowledge of the psychosocial problems associated with cancer provides a generally applicable framework for understanding the psychosocial consequences of AIDS and for designing strategies to meet patients' needs. It should be noted,

Table 8–1. Psychosocial Assessment

1. Past psychosocial history
2. Current distress and crisis
3. Past and current coping
4. Social support needed and available
5. Life cycle phase
6. Illness phase
7. Individual identity
8. Experience with loss and grief

however, that unlike cancer patients, PWAs with opportunistic infections have no structured regimen to follow to help them cope with the fear of the progressive effects of their disease. Infections must be treated as they occur. In addition PWAs often do not experience the remissions, improvement, and plateaus that cancer patients do.

Concepts important to the care of seriously medically ill patients have relevance to the care of PWAs (Christ & Wiener, 1985; Dilley et al., 1986; Holland & Tross, 1985; Joseph et al., 1984; Mount, 1986; Wolcott, 1986; Wolcott et al., 1986). Information about persons with HIV infection in various categories of assessment can assist the health care professional in anticipating reactions, needs and vulnerability to psychological dysfunction and in designing an appropriate psychosocial intervention model (Table 8–1).

Past Psychosocial History. The person's past history of interpersonal relationships, education and career can provide insight into vulnerability to psychological dysfunction. Nonprescribed drug and alcohol use and prior psychiatric care are other indicators of psychological function. Psychologically healthy individuals usually have stable jobs and stable interpersonal relationships. Psychologically vulnerable HIV-infected persons may have pre-illness behaviors that include drug use and multiple sexual contacts. Presence of a personality disorder, as in intravenous drug abusers, or of a previous psychiatric disorder is more apt to result in severe psychological symptoms and a maladaptive response to the stresses of illness.

Current Distress and Crisis. What are the specific threats and losses the person is experiencing currently? What aspect of the illness is the most distressing and bothersome to the individual at the present time? The person's level of anxiety, fear, and behavioral disorganization will change from one time to the next and will be related to the duration, intensity, and precipitants of the crisis currently being experienced.

Coping. Previous patterns of understanding problems and methods of resolving problems will be called into action by the person. Knowing which approaches have been successful for this person in the past and which approaches are currently being tried will give an indication of how he or she will attempt to cope with the illness and how successful that attempt might be. It will also give direction for providing support to the person's coping mechanisms.

Social Support. What sources of support are available to the person—family? spouse? lover? friends? social groups? What is the person's social identity? To which cultural or subcultural groups does he or she belong? What are the possibilities for support within that social identity? What types of support and assistance does he or she need—practical assistance? social interaction? emotional support? And how can that assistance be provided?

Life Cycle Phase. People have different goals, resources, skills and social roles that are related to their age. The majority of persons with HIV infection are in their 20's, 30's and 40's. Those in their 20's will have fewer resources and skills than those in their 40's. They will be involved in the psychosocial tasks of establishing independence, autonomy, and adult identity. At times of illness this age group typically becomes intensely reinvolved with the family of origin, emotionally and financially. Older persons (those in their 30's and 40's) will have more resources (money, housing, insurance) and will have established independent adult roles. At times of illness they are more likely to depend on a spouse or lover and friends for support.

Illness Phase. Needs of people for psychosocial support differ according to the phase of illness they are experiencing. Stresses on the person are different at diagnosis, treatment, and after treatment phases. They also differ depending on the clinical syndrome the person is experiencing: an opportunistic infection, a neoplasm, or a central nervous system disease. Emotional reactions and methods of coping will also differ in response to the illness phase.

Individual Identity. An individual's personal identity will also affect his or her reaction to a life threatening illness. The person's sources of self-esteem, his or her valued achievements and future goals all make up a personal identity. These and an individual's orientation to living and search for meaning will all play a role in how this illness is personally perceived and how it will be faced and combatted.

Loss and Grief. The losses the individual has experienced, is experiencing currently, and anticipates experiencing as a result of the illness will affect the kind of psychosocial support that is needed. Persons could be currently grieving a loss and could be going through the grief process. They could have previous experiences with loss and grief and feel some recognition and equanimity toward the process, or they might have no previous experience and be anxious and fearful about anticipated losses and the grieving process.

An assessment of the person with HIV infection in these various areas will provide the health care professional with the information needed to design a psychosocial intervention plan for him or her. This plan can be individualized to meet the specific needs of individuals as they move through the various phases of the disease and the phases of their emotional and social responses to the illness. The common psychosocial crises that occur in PWAs have been identified, and intervention strategies have been designed to support the person during these crises.

Psychosocial Stresses on the PWA

The major psychological stress on PWAs is the knowledge and awareness that they have a lethal disease with the potential for a rapidly declining course to death. Most symptoms are of fear, anxiety and depression. Social stresses on PWAs include exposure, stigma, rejection, abandonment and isolation. Common reactions are guilt, fear, anger and suspicion (Christ & Wiener, 1985; Coates et al., 1984; Cohen & Weisman, 1986; Dilley et al., 1986; Durham & Hatcher, 1984; Fiske, 1986; Holland & Tross, 1985; Macks, 1986; Newmark, 1984; Ostrow & Gayle, 1986; Perry & Markowitz, 1986; Ryan, 1984; Seymour, 1986; Steinbrook et al., 1985; Wolcott, 1985, 1986).

Certain crisis points occur in the course of the disease and the illness that precipitate intense anxiety, fear, and/or depression (Table 8–2). The initial crisis is at diagnosis. The same existential issues that accompany a diagnosis of cancer occur with AIDS. The normal response is characterized by disbelief, numbness and denial followed by anger, acute turmoil, disruptive anxiety and depressive symptoms. High levels of anxiety can exist for two to three months post diagnosis and can take the form of panic attacks, agitation, tachycardia, impulsive behaviors such as sexual acting out, and suicidal ideation.

The treatment phase is often accompanied by weakness, depression, alienation, and dysphoria. Patients fear disfigurement, debilitation, and pain. Treatment is often accompanied by isolation procedures which make patients feel alienated and socially abandoned. The termination of treatment often brings on feelings of increased anxiety and fears of renewed disease progression. Hypervigilance with

Table 8–2. Crisis Points and Emotional Response

Stresses	Emotions/Behaviors	Interventions
Crisis points in the illness		
Diagnosis	Intense anxiety, fear, anger, guilt, impulsive behavior	Crisis intervention, Pharmacotherapy
Treatment	Depression, weakness, alienation, dysphoria, fear of disfigurement, disability, pain	Individual therapy, Education
Treatment termination	Anxiety, fear	Resource provision
New symptoms	Hypochondriasis, demanding and dependent behavior, anxiety	Stress reduction techniques
Recurrence and relapse	Depression, dependence, apathy, isolation, suicidal ideation, dysphoria, fear of abandonment	Support groups
Terminal illness	Deterioration, decline, ambivalence, dependence, disinterest, resolution	Supportive assistance

bodily functions and the appearance of new symptoms can result in hypo-chondriacal concerns, demanding behavior toward medical personnel, and excessive dependence on health care givers.

Recurrence of disease and relapse are often accompanied by feelings of hopelessness, helplessness, sadness, low self-esteem, discouragement, loss of control, dependence, isolation, and suicidal ideation. Patients fear being abandoned by health care givers who might decide that continued treatment is futile. This stage may also be accompanied by cognitive impairment because of central nervous system disease. The terminal phase of illness is marked by deterioration and decline, and can be accompanied by ambivalence, dependence, and disinterest and/or resolution.

During the crisis points in the disease and illness course, PWAs have need of a full range of psychosocial interventions. These include immediate crisis intervention and/or individual therapy to deal with feelings of extreme anxiety, fear, and anger and with impulsive behavior and suicidal thoughts and behaviors. Persons with HIV infection should be encouraged to express their anxiety, fear, sadness, and anger and to grieve with the understanding that grief is a healing process. Pharmacotherapy should be used for intense anxiety, depression, and insomnia. Whenever possible health care givers should support and enhance the person's coping mechanisms and defenses and not work in opposition to these unless they are dangerous or destructive. Patients also need on-going psychosocial support in the form of support groups to dispel self-blame and guilt, provide reassurance, share information and experiences, and reduce feelings of isolation and loneliness. Experience with persons with HIV infection in support groups and research on levels of distress in persons with AIDS, ARC and LAS suggest that three separate support groups be developed for persons with clinical disease: one for persons with LAS and ARC, one for persons with Kaposi's sarcoma, and one for other PWAs. These suggestions are based on the differing levels of anxiety and areas of concern of these people.

In addition, infected people need education regarding the disease and its treatment, liaison with community resources to help them resolve practical problems, instruction in stress and anxiety reduction techniques such as relaxation, and supportive intervention from a social network that includes family, friends, health professionals, volunteers, and clergy in the forms of encouragement, comfort, concern, compassion, affection, and spiritual assistance.

All of these interventions play a role in the treatment of PWAs during crisis stages. Which of these will take priority at any given time depends on individual response and can be determined by completing a psychosocial assessment of the patient at varying crisis points. If at all possible, it is desirable that the patient be assigned a primary care giver, primary care nurse, or a case manager to coordinate service needs and provide a central and familiar person the patient can see to provide continuity of care throughout the course of the illness, hospitalizations, and referrals.

Table 8–3. Internal Conflicts and Emotional Responses

Stresses	Emotions/Behaviors	Interventions
Psychological conflicts		
Transmission	Anxiety, fear, anger,	Education
Protection from infection	Suspicion, guilt	Resource provision
Previous lifestyle	Internalized homophobia or societal prejudices	Support groups
Personal relationships	Loneliness, abandonment	Stress reduction techniques

People with HIV infection are subjected to an unusual number of psychological or internal conflicts (Table 8–3). Some of these revolve around transmission of the disease: who the person got it from or to whom he or she might have passed it on. Emotional responses to these internal conflicts can be directed toward self and others and involve anxiety, fear, anger, suspicion, and guilt.

Similar concerns and conflicts are evident in the person's efforts to protect him- or herself from the risk of infection. Fear of associating with others, anger and suspicion of others who might transmit infection, and guilt and loneliness from abandoning friends to protect self are all involved in this conflict. People may also experience guilt over their previous lifestyles, especially if they have had a number of anonymous sexual partners or have used intravenous or recreational drugs. The extent of this guilt and self-blame can result in an internalization of society's prejudicial attitudes toward the group(s) to which they belong. Among homosexuals this is called internalized homophobia, but it can happen in any group toward which society expresses disapproval, e.g., drug abusers, prostitutes, sexually promiscuous persons.

Finally, many conflicts occur over continuing personal relationships, especially if these have a sexual focus. Fears of social abandonment, of isolation, and of loneliness all accompany giving up intimate sexual relationships. This is especially true if sexual relationships were used to provide interpersonal contacts.

Some of these psychological conflicts can be resolved through education groups which focus on transmission and protection from infection. Some conflicts can be resolved through support groups and finding reassurance and shared experiences among other persons with the same concerns. Support groups can also help prevent loneliness and isolation. Community resources can help people build social networks and develop sustained relationships that are not predicated on sex or drug use and sharing. The use of stress reduction techniques, such as relaxation or other behavioral techniques, can assist an individual in dealing with personal fears and anxieties.

Table 8–4. Social Stress and Emotional Responses

Stresses	Emotions/Behaviors	Interventions
Social conflicts		
Exposure	Fear of abandonment, isolation and rejection	Support groups
Stigma		
Sexual activity		Support assistance
Employment and insurance	Guilt, anger, suspicion	
Social support limitations	Insecurity due to loss of job and health benefits	Resource provision
Distance from family	Loneliness Alienation	Stress reduction techniques

Persons with AIDS/HIV infection are also subject to an unusual number of social conflicts and stresses (Table 8–4). The first of these could involve public identification as a member of a highly stigmatized group. Both of the largest transmission groups for HIV infection are socially stigmatized: male homosexuals and IV drug abusers. Persons who have chosen to treat their sexuality or their drug use as private matters are now subject to exposure and the consequent possibility of rejection by family and friends. Because the diagnosis is AIDS, they are also susceptible to abandonment by friends who know of their sexuality or drug use but are afraid of the disease. At a time when people most need social support, comfort, compassion, and closeness, they might be left alone and isolated. Confiding the diagnosis to family and friends is often not a matter of personal choice. It is frequently difficult to hide a diagnosis of AIDS because of the obvious physical signs that accompany it, such as frequent illness, disfigurement, and debilitation.

Patients with ARC and LAS and persons who are HIV positive are faced with a dilemma as to whether to confide in friends and family because of the highly probable stigma and social rejection that might result from receipt of this information. Persons who are HIV positive and asymptomatic or who have LAS or ARC have a need for counseling on the benefits and risks of sharing information with others. They also need information on behavioral changes that will eliminate the potential of infection of others or re-exposure to the virus. In addition, counseling should include information promoting optimal health and immune functioning that might include attention to diet, habits, sleep, exercise, and reducing occupational and interpersonal stress. Getting HIV positive persons involved in AIDS-related activities such as support groups and peer counseling helps to dispel feelings of impotence and victimization.

Levels of psychologic distress in persons with ARC or who are HIV-infected are often high. Some studies have found that persons with ARC scored higher than persons with AIDS on several self-report measures of distress (Macks, 1986).

In addition among the persons with AIDS, one-third had not discussed their health problems or sexual orientation with their families or employers, but two-thirds of persons with ARC had not done so. While a significant number of persons who test HIV positive appear to change their sexual behavior, concern has been raised over persons who test seronegative. Some try to protect their negative status but on others the news has a disinhibiting effect due to a belief that they are immunologically buffered (Staff, *AIDS Record*, 1987). Data from several reports, however, suggest that gay men in several metropolitan areas have significantly reduced their high risk sexual practices in response to counseling and education (Macks, 1986).

Persons who are HIV-infected are subject to similar social conflicts regarding their sexual activity. Drastically altering sexual activities can have the effect of leaving the person socially isolated and alone. This is especially true of persons who used sexual encounters to establish interpersonal contacts. Even persons with stable relationships will be left with dramatic changes in their sexual behavior that could have an impact on the relationship, on feelings of closeness and on the ability to give and receive love, comfort and affection.

Persons with AIDS have been confronted with a variety of problems in the area of employment and insurance. Some individuals have been fired from their jobs because of employer and co-worker fears of contacting AIDS. In some cases this discrimination has extended to the families of PWAs. Others have had to leave jobs because of physical disability. In many cases health insurance is lost when the job is lost. In addition, some insurance companies have tried to avoid covering PWAs because of the high cost of care. Many PWAs are without financial security, resources, and insurance. Community resources that they might need include social security benefits, Medicaid, and visiting nurse services.

Finally, many persons with AIDS have limited social support networks. Many times families are not involved with the person or they live in geographically distant and separate places. This could be due to alienation from the family because of lifestyle or due to relocation in large urban areas such as New York, San Francisco, or Los Angeles which are far from where their families live. In some cases PWAs are abandoned by their families when they learn of the AIDS diagnosis. This could be the result of a desire to avoid social stigma, an incorrect belief that homosexuality or drug use causes AIDS rather than a virus and that the disease is just retribution, or fear of contagion. This situation leaves the person at a crucial time without a family to assist with basic physical needs and to provide emotional support and forces a greater dependence on spouses, lovers and friends. Community resources can play a role in providing for basic physical needs through services such as shopping, housekeeping, and other practical services to PWAs at home. Some clergy and churches have become involved in assisting visiting parents and siblings to find places to stay when they come from out of town. The gay community and gay service agencies in the large cities have organized a variety of supportive services for persons with limited or distant social support networks. Political and social organizations are less common to drug abusers who have AIDS, women with AIDS and children with AIDS, and specialized services are not as available to these persons.

As can be noted from the foregoing discussion, the psychosocial stresses on persons with AIDS are overwhelming. They call for a range of psychological and social interventions, and at any given time in the course of a person's disease, they can call for all the interventions and services discussed in this section at one time. Complicating the picture of psychosocial stresses and provision of appropriate psychological and social services are the central nervous system dysfunctions that occur with AIDS, leaving patients in critical need of social and physical assistance.

Neuropsychiatric Complications

Estimates of neuropsychiatric dysfunction in persons with HIV infection range from 30% to 70%. Some studies have shown that neurologic dysfunction is the first manifestation of AIDS in 25% of patients (Macks, 1986). Persons with AIDS appear to be susceptible to lymphomas and B cell neoplasms which have a predilection for the central nervous system (CNS). Other causes of CNS complications are nonviral infections, toxic metabolic disturbance and viral syndromes. Disorders such as toxoplasmosis, progressive multifocal leukoencephalopathy, typical or atypical mycobacterial infection, CNS lymphoma, and metastatic Kaposi's are usually detectable from computed tomography (CT) findings. By far the most common neurologic clinical presentation, however, is a viral syndrome, a nonfocal encephalopathy, that has come to be known as AIDS-dementia complex or AIDS encephalopathy. Several reports have provided evidence that the virus that causes AIDS is found in the CNS and cerebrospinal fluid of patients with neurologic syndromes. Therefore, most investigators now believe that AIDS-dementia complex is caused by direct cerebral infection by HIV (Beckham & Rudy, 1986; Clark & Vintners, 1987; Dilley et al., 1986; Hoffman, 1984; Holland & Tross, 1985; Lowenstein & Sharfstein, 1984; Macks, 1986; Navia et al., 1986; Shapira & Schlesinger, 1986). Often laboratory and physical findings are non-specific. Common laboratory findings include mild to moderately dilated ventricles and/or cerebral atrophy on CT scans and generalized slowing or normal results on the electroencephalogram (EEG). Elevated protein and pleocytosis may be evident in the cerebrospinal fluid (CSF) on lumbar puncture.

Symptoms of CNS Complications

Early recognition of neuropsychiatric complications is important as these can be the first indication of toxoplasma, cryptococcal, or cytomegalovirus infection

Table 8–5. Symptoms of CNS Complications in HIV Infection

Initial Complaints	Early Symptoms	Later Symptoms
Forgetfulness	Unsteady gait	Cerebellar ataxia
Recent memory loss	Incoordination	Confusion
Poor concentration	Loss of interest in work	Disorientation
Decreased spontaneity	Loss of libido	Seizures
Poor cognitive flexibility	Blunted affect	Mutism
Psychomotor slowing	Withdrawal	Incontinence
		Hemiparesis, paraparesis
		Blindness
		Delirium
		Coma

Adapted from Holland & Tross, 1985

or of primary lymphoma and can signal the need for treatment. A variety of treatments are available for the various infections and neoplasms.

Initial complaints of persons with AIDS-dementia complex may resemble those associated with depression and anxiety and require differential diagnosis that includes neuropsychologic testing. Early recognition of symptoms is important as many persons have experienced relief from these symptoms from treatment with azidothymidine (AZT). Initial symptoms may resemble those that a person might manifest in response to a diagnosis of AIDS when they are experiencing an acute existential crisis (Table 8–5). These same presentations also resemble an acute exacerbation of a chronic depression or a typical loss-grief response, both of which could occur in persons who are HIV-infected. They have cognitive, affective, behavioral, and somatic components similar to those seen in major affective disorders. However, the most typical differentiating symptoms are failures in cognition. Deficits are noted in the speed of processing new information, memory, and ability to complete several step tasks (Dilly et al., 1985). There have been some case reports of persons with ARC or HIV seropositive tests who have also complained of mild to moderate cognitive impairment. Again these complaints are difficult to differentiate from the anxiety and/or depression that can accompany a diagnosis of ARC or HIV infection.

In contrast, some persons experience symptoms that mimic bipolar affective disorders, schizophrenia, and hysterical disorders. Cyclic symptoms may occur, ranging from apathy to manic behaviors such as hyperactivity, agitation, irritability, pressured speech, flight of ideas, grandiosity, and lack of sleep. Schizophreniform symptoms may be present, including hallucinations and delusions. Untoward expressions of hostility, temper tantrums, and antisocial behavior may occur. The impairment of cognitive function can again be a differentiating sign: defects in memory, retention, and recall; difficulty in dealing with abstract concepts; and problems in grasping, retaining, and following through on instructions. In comparison, although schizophrenic reactions are often confused, they may usually be distinguished by the patient's clear orientation and ability to retain and recall past events. A final possibility for the nurse to consider would be the patient with a dual diagnosis, e.g., a psychiatric diagnosis of schizophrenia or psychotic depression that preexisted or coincides with the diagnosis of AIDS dementia. In this case separating the symptoms of each disease might be necessary to designing an adequate treatment plan.

Soon after the initial symptoms, persons with HIV infection experience other symptoms of neurologic impairment. Some of these also are typical of depression: loss of interest in work, loss of libido, blunted affect, and social withdrawal. Others are more typically neurologic in character and include disturbance of time and place orientation, incoordination, unsteady gait, and defect in a coherent train of expression. Eventually there takes place a deterioration in motor activity with problems in writing, eating and personal grooming; later delusory and hallucinatory experiences and severe impairment of motor control may occur. Late symptoms demonstrate progressive dementia, mutism, seizures, blindness and paresis.

Assessment and Care of CNS Complications

Nurses must be alert to the manifestations of neuropsychiatric symptoms and be able to differentiate them from anxiety or grief reactions, depression, bipolar illness, and schizophrenia. In addition, family members, lovers, and spouses can be made aware of these symptoms and alerted to report them and seek medical attention if they should occur.

Two nursing diagnoses are most typically involved in the various CNS complications of AIDS. These are (1) alteration in thought processes and (2) sensory and perceptual deficits (McDonnell and Sevedge, 1986). For alteration in thought processes, a neurological assessment can be performed with emphasis on cerebral function. Changes may be noted in the following areas:

1. General appearance/behavior
2. Mood and emotions
3. Affect (flat, inappropriate)
4. Intellectual level
5. Orientation and memory (immediate and delayed)
6. Ability to follow simple to complex commands
7. Ability to perform motor tasks when requested to do so
8. Judgment, personality
9. Speech (slurred, dysarthria, aphasia)
10. Thought patterns (incoherence, delusions, hallucinations)
11. Thought content (preoccupation, perseveration, confabulation)
12. Attention and concentration
13. Ability to recognize the form of a solid object by touch (stereognosis)

Folstein et al. (1975) have developed a mini mental state exam that is an extremely useful screening tool for clinicians (see Appendix D). It includes assessment of orientation, registration, attention and calculation, recall, language, and level of consciousness. It is especially useful for persons who might be experiencing AIDS dementia because it assesses various aspects of memory and cognition, such as recall, repetition, following directions, reading, writing, copying, attention, and calculation.

For sensory and perceptual deficits, a neurologic assessment which focuses on the cranial nerve, cerebellar, and sensory systems can be performed. Changes may be noted in the following areas:

1. Pupillary reflexes (reaction to light)
2. Ocular movements (follow finger)
3. Vision acuity (blurred, presence of floaters)
4. Taste (sugar, salt, etc.)
5. Facial movement (frown, wink, etc.)
6. Pharynx and tongue movements
7. Smell (lemon, peppermint, etc.)
8. Hearing
9. Vestibular alterations (vertigo, nystagmus)
10. Arms (finger-nose, finger-finger, pronation-supination, patting or tapping tests)
11. Legs (heel-knee, heel-toe walking)
12. Trunk (gait, station)
13. Touch (cotton wisp)
14. Pain (pin prick)
15. Temperature (heat and cold)
16. Position (position of thumb)

The care of persons who have developed neuropsychiatric complications requires compassionate and supportive psychological, social and environmental assistance. These people need safe and structured environments. Environments should be constant and consistent with familiar objects, routines, and people. Signs can be posted to guide and direct the person with CNS complications. They need to be involved in decisions about their care and encouraged to be independent to the extent they are able. They need to be oriented to person, place, and time on a regular basis. Clocks, calendars, night lights, an orientation chalkboard, note pads, and information on current events can all assist in helping people remain oriented. Explanations of routines and procedures should be made as simply as possible; routines should be carried out in a consistent manner. Directions for tasks should be given one at a time and redirected if attention wavers. The person's need for stimulation should be assessed and provided at an optimal level to counteract apathy and psychomotor retardation. Medications should be closely monitored as CNS depressants and phenothiazines can have negative effects and be contraindicated. Nurses have to adjust their expectations to account for changes in these persons' abilities to adhere to procedures and treatment and, in some cases, changes in their visual acuity (Holland & Tross, 1985; McDonnell & Sevedge, 1986).

Table 8–6. Psychosocial Stresses on Lover/Spouse

Stresses	Interventions
Guilt over transmission	Lover/spouse support groups or couples groups
Fear of contagion	
Anxiety, fear, depression over life-threatening illness	Individual therapy
	Community resources
Disrupted relationship equilibrium	Attorney, clergy, liaison psychiatry
Decisions regarding treatment	Bereavement groups
Conflicts with family/hospital staff	
Anticipatory and postmortem grief	

Some of these individuals will need constant supervision and others will need assistance with all aspects of daily living. If they are discharged from the hospital, they may need a full range of community services to assist them, including housekeeping, shopping, assistance with eating, bathing, and dressing, transportation to and from the hospital, and visiting nurse services. Families, lovers, spouses and friends need instruction in changes in the person's thought processes, mood, memory, and sensory and perceptual deficits. They need help in planning the adjustments to be made in the PWA's daily living activities and home environment. They need referrals to community resources and respite services. Support groups and psychotherapy can be important resources for families, friends, and the person with AIDS. Family teaching involves also the skills needed to assess the progression of neurologic deficits in order to seek medical attention in a timely manner.

Psychosocial Stresses on the Lover/Spouse of the HIV-Infected Person

There are widespread consequences of a diagnosis of AIDS that affect the person's entire social support network. Affected most immediately and extensively are the spouse or lover of the PWA. These people experience both psychological and social effects of having a partner with AIDS (Christ & Wiener, 1985; Lang et al., 1985; Ostrow & Gayle, 1986; Quinn, 1986; Wolcott, 1986; Wolcott et al., 1985, 1986) (Table 8–6). Psychological stresses experienced by the lover or spouse of a PWA might include guilt about possibly having transmitted the disease. It could also include fear over personal vulnerability to AIDS from sexual contact with the PWA. Each of these issues can be discussed in support groups for the spouse/lover of the PWA or in support groups for couples in which one partner has AIDS. Through sharing experiences, support groups help members avoid self-blame and guilt. They also provide information on contagion and transmission as well as a safe setting in which members can discuss frankly needed changes in sexual practices.

The psychological stresses related to a diagnosis of a life-threatening illness and the premature death of a young adult can cause the same existential crisis, anxiety, and depression in the lover/spouse as it does in the PWA. Lovers and spouses should seek individual counseling to assist them in dealing with their acute crisis as well as with the on-going sadness, fear, and anxiety that can accompany the reality of impending death in a young partner. Support groups can also assist in providing emotional support to spouses and lovers.

There are, in addition, various social stresses on the spouse/lover of PWAs. Major stresses occur because of disruption of the equilibrium of the relationship. A relationship based on interdependence, mutual support, autonomy, and egalitarianism may be severely threatened when one partner becomes emotionally and/or physically dependent, unable to contribute financially, limited in his or her ability to provide support, and impaired in cognitive functions. Spouses and lovers can find themselves involved in activities that drain them physically, emotionally, and financially. Caring for the partner with AIDS can involve loss of time from work, constant supervision, and assistance with all aspects of daily living as well as providing emotional support, comfort, compassion and affection. The diagnosis of AIDS also requires a change in sexual activities both to avoid transmission and infection and in response to decreased sexual desires because of illness. All of these changes in the relationship can be intensely stressful and demoralizing to the spouse/lover. Again, support groups for lovers and spouses or for couples can help resolve some of these issues through sharing of experiences. They also provide information on community resources to assist lovers and spouses in the care of the partner.

There are additional stresses associated with frequent and prolonged hospitalization of the partner that can range from the logistics of visiting to making sure that the partner's financial and insurance resources remain adequate, to making decisions about the partner's medical treatment. The lover/spouse is often called on to make decisions when the partner's mental status is compromised or when the partner is extremely ill. Decisions about life support as well as disposition of property often fall to the lover/spouse. These decisions require that the partner and lover/spouse discuss early in the illness the partner's wishes regarding treatment, life support, funeral, burial, and disposition of property. It is necessary that lovers obtain a durable power of attorney in order to carry out these decisions.

Decisions thus arrived at and carried out can create conflicts with hospital staff and with family and can cause additional stress on the lover or spouse. Decisions regarding treatment and life support might conflict with those that hospital staff believe are necessary or indicated. These conflicts can often be resolved with the assistance of the psychiatric consultation-liaison team, hospital chaplain, and hospital attorney. These same persons can assist when conflicts arise with the patient's family. Such conflicts are most common when families are emotionally distant from the patient and do not realize or take into account the extent and depth of the relationship between the patient and lover. Conflicts can arise over treatment issues as well as burial and disposition of property. Again the assistance of hospital liaison psychiatry, clergy, and attorneys can help resolve these situations. They can also be of service in helping the lover or spouse and patient prepare themselves for these situations and take the necessary steps to implement their decisions.

Finally, psychological issues that lovers and spouses of PWAs must face include anticipatory grief over the loss of a partner and postmortem grief when the partner dies. There are AIDS support groups available in large cities that focus specifically on bereavement and the grief process. These groups encourage persons to grieve—to express sadness, fear, loneliness, and anger—with the understanding that grief is a healing process that is important to the recovery of the bereaved.

Psychosocial Stresses on the Family and Friends of the PWA

The families and friends of persons with AIDS are often themselves in need of supportive care (Table 8–7). All of the emotional and social reactions that occur with PWAs, lovers, and spouses also occur with families and friends: shock, denial, anxiety, anger, fear, guilt and depression (Christ & Wiener, 1985; Lang et al., 1985; Ostrow & Gayle, 1986; Quinn, 1986; Wolcott, 1986; Wolcott et al., 1985, 1986). For the family, in addition, there may be pre-existing conflicts between them and the PWA regarding lifestyle and/or sexual preference that may have resulted in emotional and geographic distance from the patient. For others there is only geographic distance due to the person having relocated in a major metropolitan area. Either situation makes the relationship with the PWA difficult and imposes stress on the family. Families who are emotionally distant by choice may feel ambivalent about the PWA or may reject him or her with all the consequent psychological turmoil that this causes them: anger, bitterness, anxiety, embarrassment, and despair. Families who are geographically distant also experience severe situational stresses in attempting to visit with no place to stay and wanting to provide emotional and physical assistance but being unable because of distance.

Some families experience other stresses. For some of them the diagnosis of AIDS is their first knowledge that their child is homosexual, a drug abuser or sexually promiscuous. This news is greeted with shock, anger, bewilderment, rejection, and sometimes guilt. Parents might feel guilty because they believe that they are responsible for the person's lifestyle. This is especially true of mothers,

Table 8–7. Psychosocial Stresses on Families

Stresses	Interventions
Pre-existing conflicts	Supportive interventions of consultation-liaison team, clergy
Revelation of lifestyle	
Guilt over lifestyle	
Fear of social stigma	Support groups
Conflict with patient's lover	Community resources
Physical, emotional, and financial drain	
Loss and grief	

who traditionally have been blamed by society for the actions of their children. Knowledge of a child's homosexuality, drug use, or promiscuity may cause conflict and divided loyalties within a family as well. Sometimes certain family members, usually siblings, have known of the person's lifestyle but have kept it secret from parents. Sometimes a mother has kept it secret from a father. Other times when the person's lifestyle is revealed no one has pre-existing knowledge but some in the family decide to accept it and others to reject it. Fears and suspicions are aroused and loyalties are threatened. In all of these situations families are in need of compassionate, supportive, and constructive assistance from clergy, health care givers, and the psychiatric consultation-liaison team to help them deal with their feelings, work together, help the PWA cope, and assist in his or her care. They can also use practical assistance like housing and transportation and can benefit from sharing feelings and experiences in a support group for families.

As mentioned in the previous section, families sometimes come into conflict with the lovers of PWAs because they perceive them as having too much control in treatment decisions. Families have to adjust to the lover's role as one that is equivalent to that of a spouse. This is especially difficult if they have not met or known each other before. Since the lover's role and responsibilities are socially ambiguous, they often must be clarified in order for families and lovers to work together for the well-being of the PWA.

Other social stresses that families face is whether to disclose the diagnosis of AIDS to friends and then which friends to tell. The fact that their child or sibling has AIDS subjects them to the powerful threat of social stigma and rejection by friends, neighbors, and co-workers. The consequence of this is that they are without the social support that persons would normally receive when a family member is diagnosed with a life threatening illness. This might be true also during their bereavement when some of the emotional support that usually accompanies mourning is not available to them. Whether to tell friends or not can present a major conflict. Because of this situation, support groups become an important part of a family's social network. In addition, clergy can take the lead in establishing an atmosphere of compassion and concern among their parishioners so that the traditional social support of religion is available (see Chapter 12).

Another stress to families is the prolonged debility of the person with AIDS, with great needs for physical, emotional, and financial assistance. These can deplete family resources and drain family members emotionally and physically. The provision of community resources is essential to the supportive care of the family.

Families and friends also face fears of contagion and transmission and will benefit from education regarding the disease. Friends who have been involved in similar behaviors or circumstances as the PWA may feel particularly vulnerable because they might readily identify with the diagnosed person. In addition, they might want to be supportive but not know how. For many the diagnosis that a friend has AIDS leads to difficult reappraisals and evaluations of their own life-styles and behaviors.

Issues of bereavement affect both family and friends. Since PWAs are usually young, lovers, spouses, family, and friends are dealing with loss and grief in the context of an untimely, undeserved, and unjust illness and death. John Kennedy is said to have said at the death of his infant son that "it is an unnatural thing for parents to bury a child." These issues as well as sadness, anger, anxiety, and loss must all be dealt with as part of the grief process. The services of clergy and mental health counselors can greatly facilitate the grief process.

Psychosocial Stresses on Nurses and Other Health Care Givers

Caring for patients with AIDS puts enormous stresses on health care workers (Table 8–8). This is especially true of nurses and interns because they spend the most time with patients and have the most intensive and closest contact with them through the supportive care and procedures they perform. Nurses and other health care workers are subject to a wide range of emotional, social, and work-related stresses, some of which are common to those experienced by patients, lovers, spouses, families, and friends of PWAs and some of which are unique to their position as health care givers (Christ & Wiener, 1985; Holland & Tross, 1985; Macks, 1986; Mount, 1986; Ostrow & Gayle, 1986; Simmons-Alling, 1984; Steinbrook et al., 1985; Wolcott, 1986; Wolcott et al., 1985, 1986).

Initially nurses and other health care workers have anxiety and concerns about contagion and transmission. They are in contact with the patient's body fluids, they administer medications and IV fluids, change beds, bathe patients, and provide toilet care. These concerns include fears of personal exposure (e.g., needle-sticks) and exposure of other staff members. In addition, they have concerns

Table 8–8. Psychosocial Stresses on Nurses/HCWs

Stresses	Interventions
Contagion and transmission	Education
Discomfort with homosexuality and drug abuse	Adequate staff and resources
Intensive complicated care	Psychosocial support groups
Facing own mortality	Crisis intervention and individual support
Repetitive grief	Clear institutional policies and goals on treatment
Conflicts over goals of treatment	Personal stress reduction

about appropriate infection control procedures. This extends to fears of introducing infection to the AIDS patient, of cross infection of other patients, and of teaching infection control procedures to families, friends, lovers, and spouses of patients. Since the introduction through in-service education of adequate and accurate information concerning AIDS and infection control procedures, anxiety has decreased significantly. Willingness to work with patients with AIDS and appropriate precautions and behavior toward PWAs have increased. The fear of transmission has had social consequences for health care workers, some of whom have had spouses or lovers urge them to quit their jobs to avoid infection of themselves and their families. Others have experienced social stigma and avoidance by friends because they work with PWAs.

Other stresses on nurses result from the uncertainty and discomfort they feel in relating to drug abusers, prostitutes, promiscuous persons, homosexuals, and the lover of the gay PWA. Personal values, cultural background, and religious ideals are challenged by the different backgrounds of these patients. Again through education, and with the assistance of the consultation-liaison psychiatric team or mental health consultants, nurses have become more comfortable discussing sexuality openly. This includes knowing enough about bisexuality and homosexuality to understand the issues and problems as they relate to AIDS transmission and being able to discuss sexual precautions and answer questions of lovers and family. Several studies have measured health care workers' attitudes toward homosexuals. On a homophobia scale, both physicians and registered nurses measured in the low-grade homophobic range (Douglas et al., 1985; Macks, 1986).

The intense physical care and emotional needs of hospitalized PWAs can cause health care workers to become overtaxed, stressed, fatigued, and fearful of being overwhelmed by the burden of the intensive complicated care. Enormous demands are made upon their energies by the frequent necessity to meet immediate acute needs and by serious time pressures and overwork. In addition, they feel stressed by their inattention to other responsibilities and other patients necessitated by the seemingly all-encompassing needs of the AIDS population. These stresses increase each day by the mushrooming incidence of the disease and tax institutional resources to the limit. In some institutions, the quality and comprehensiveness of training programs have been questioned because students are taking care of only PWAs and have no experience with patients with other problems.

Nurses have become overwhelmed by caring for PWAs day after day. Infection control procedures often leave them feeling isolated themselves, and they are emotionally and physically drained by the intensive physical and psychologic needs of the patients. AIDS brings to the nurse's attention the constant responsibility for intense, complex monitoring of the sights, sounds, smells and suffering of life and death struggles. Nursing care problems of the patient with AIDS can include, all at the same time, a need for attention to respiratory distress, pain, nausea, vomiting, diarrhea, bleeding, fatigue, motor weakness, breakdown of skin, breakdown of oral mucous membranes, nutritional deficits, fluid volume deficit, alteration in mental status, and acute psychologic distress. Nurses have found it especially difficult to deal with the patient's anger in complex nursing care situations. Interns are often fatigued and overtaxed by the immediate demands of acute situations. Interns are called on to manage acute crises in the illness; they do procedures such as arterial blood gas measurements, blood cultures, lumbar punctures, and bone marrow biopsies. They also feel isolated from the rest of the staff and resentful that residents and attending physicians avoid discussing life-sustaining treatment with patients and families and leave no-code orders up to them.

Dealing with the patient with AIDS has a special impact on health care workers because they and the patients are usually about the same age. Identification and a sense of personal vulnerability to disease and death are elicited by taking care of young, hitherto healthy persons who face rapid physical deterioration and death. Health care workers are forced to recognize the fact of their own death and dying and are faced with the need to re-examine the meaning and quality of their life and living. Physicians have expressed the level of distress they feel when diagnosing pneumocystis pneumonia as "pronouncing a death sentence." The age of the patients has elicited the feeling that it's "like telling your brother that he's going to die." Other especially difficult situations are discussing life sustaining treatments with a patient whom they have just met and who may need immediate intubation.

Nurses often become intensely involved with PWAs because of the time and closeness of the nursing care demanded. To some degree they become a "family" to the patient and in some cases nurses have been asked to hold the durable power of attorney for the patients and make decisions regarding treatment, disposition of property, and burial. This relationship with the patient is highly stressful when the patient dies, and nurses and physicians react much more strongly than they would with patients who have relied more on family and friends for support. Repetitive grief and demoralization occur because of the high mortality of AIDS.

The traditional goals of nursing and medical care impose additional stresses on health care givers. In general these goals are to cure, to prolong life, and to improve the quality of remaining life when its duration is beyond control. Patients with AIDS fall into the second and often the third category. Prolonging life and quality of life interventions become the prime focus of service. However, even this goal cannot be carried out without personal conflict, ambiguity, and conflict among staff. Many of the treatments for AIDS produce debilitating and distressing side effects, so that prolonging life and quality of life can be at odds. Often treatment fails. Health care workers get involved in questions about whether the treatment regimen is justified and become pessimistic and wonder "What's the use?" Their professional identity as persons who improve patients' lives is called into question. These conflicts can result in anxiety and depression among staff. The care of the PWA presents a challenge to the nurse's competency base, to professional and personal values, and to ethical convictions.

In order to meet the psychosocial needs of health care personnel caring for AIDS patients, a multifaceted program of institutional support is required:

1. Regularly scheduled educational and informational updates on HIV and its treatment are needed for all staff. Especially important is instruction on (a) transmission and contagion, (b) bisexuality and homosexuality, (c) assessment of mental status and how to recognize delirium, (d) monitoring cognitive dysfunction and adjusting expectations for patients' independent adherence to procedures and treatment, and (e) hospital and community resources to assist patients and families.

2. Clear, consistent policies and procedures about infection control adhered to by all staff will decrease anxiety about transmission and ensure correct and appropriate behavior toward patients.

3. Clear, consistent, and explicitly stated agreement among all hospital staff on the goals of treatment for PWAs will ensure a common approach and feelings of support for one another among staff. This agreement on goals might address the issues of prolonging life through the use of available treatment, enhancing the quality of life for both patient and family through excellence in symptom control and attention to psychologic, social, spiritual, legal, and financial needs, and providing supportive care until death.

4. Regular and as-needed meetings to provide emotional support for staff specifically related to the care of PWAs and their families will offer a sense of shared experience and social/professional group support to health care workers.

5. Easy access to mental health consultants for patient care support and individual staff member emotional support can provide assistance in crisis situations and on an individual basis. Referrals can be made for staff desiring more long term psychologic support.

6. Adequate institutional resources and support to provide the level of nursing and medical care needed will prevent staff from becoming overwhelmed, fatigued, and overtaxed by the care of PWAs.

On a personal level, nurses and other health care workers can implement several measures that can reduce their stress at work and away from work. At work they can:

1. work regular (consistent) hours or shifts;
2. take lunch and coffee breaks;
3. take brief respite breaks (look out the window, wash hands and face, massage face, isometric exercises); and
4. acknowledge and reward work well done by one another.

Away from work they can:

1. exercise, eat and drink in moderation;
2. create meaningful relationships and commit time to allow this to happen;
3. develop a hobby or diversional activity that is absorbing;
4. not bring work home; and
5. take regular vacations.

Several psychosocial issues that usually arise separately are combined in the treatment of patients with AIDS in such a way that they create unusually difficult problems. These include fears of contagion, disease, and death in young persons; negative social attitudes and personal prejudices; overworked, fatigued and overwhelmed health care workers; and overtaxed institutional resources. Such difficult problems require a set of supportive guidelines for nurses and other health care professionals in the care of patients with AIDS.

Psychosocial Tasks of Health Care Workers Treating Patients with AIDS

In caring for patients with AIDS, nurses and other health care workers engage in a variety of psychological, social, and educational tasks that will ensure that patient needs are met. These provide guidelines for the nurse in meeting the psychosocial-educational needs of the patient (Mount, 1986; Steinbrook et al., 1985; Wolcott, 1986; Wolcott et al., 1985, 1986).

1. Accept, value, and provide longitudinal psychosocial and physical nursing care and medical care to the patient.

2. Support the patient's capacity for hope, determination, and autonomy.

3. Provide accurate medical information concerning treatment alternatives, benefits, and risks.

4. Provide accurate information regarding health enhancing behavioral options in a sensitive, nonjudgmental manner.

5. Understand common psychosocial issues surrounding AIDS and provide assistance or referral for problems.

6. Familiarize herself or himself with community psychological, social, educational, political, and financial resources and make appropriate referrals for patients and families.

7. Recognize and ensure treatment of neuropsychiatric syndromes common to AIDS.

8. Control symptoms, reassure patients that this will be done, and provide supportive care or comfort measures.

9. Carry out patients' decisions concerning life-sustaining treatment and reassure them that they will not be abandoned.

10. Recognize and work to minimize the stress that co-workers experience in caring for patients with AIDS.

Summary

The diagnosis of AIDS presents psychological and social dilemmas, conflicts, and stresses for everyone intimately involved with the PWA, for less intimately involved acquaintances, and ultimately for the entire society. An awareness of these stresses for the people involved, of the psychosocial supports needed and available, and of new developments in the treatment and care of HIV infection will assist the nurse in giving optimal nursing care. In addition, nurses should care for themselves and request from their institutions and one another the support that they need to battle HIV infection and AIDS.

References

Batchelor, W.F. (1984). AIDS: A public health and psychological emergency. *American Psychologist*, 39(1), 1279–1284.

Beckham, M.M., Rudy, E.B. (1986). Acquired immuno-deficiency syndrome: Impact and implication for the neurological system. *Journal of Neuroscience Nursing*, 18(1), 5–10.

Centers for Disease Control. (1988, February 1). *AIDS Weekly Surveillance* Report. AIDS Program, Atlanta, GA.

Christ, G.H., Wiener, L.S. (1985). Psychosocial issues in AIDS. In V.T. DeVita, Jr., *AIDS: Etiology, diagnosis, treatment and prevention* (pp. 275–297). Philadelphia: J.B. Lippincott.

Clark, G.L., Vintners, H.V. (1987). Dementia and ataxia in a patient with AIDS. *Western Journal of Medicine*, 146, 68–72.

Coates, T.J., Temoshok, L., Mandel, J. (1984). Psychosocial research is essential to understanding and treating AIDS. *American Psychologist*, 39(11), 1309–1314.

Cohen, M.A, Weisman, H.W. (1986). A biopsychosocial approach to AIDS. *Psychosomatics*, 27(4), 245–249.

Dilley, J.W., Ochitill, H.N., Perl, M., et al. (1985). Findings in psychiatric consultations with patients with AIDS. *American Journal of Psychiatry*, 142(1), 82–85.

Dilley, J.W., Shelp, E.E., Batki, S.L. (1986). Psychiatric and ethical issues in the care of patients with AIDS. *Psychosomatics*, 27(8), 562–566.

Douglas, C.J., Kalman, C.M., Kalman, T.P. (1985). Homophobia among physicians and nurses: An empirical study. *Hospital Community & Psychiatry*, 36(12), 1309–1311.

Durham, J.D., Hatcher, B. (1984). Reducing psychological complications for the critically ill AIDS patient. *Dimensions of Critical Care Nursing*, 3(5), 300–306.

Fiske, M. (1986). Psychological nursing care of AIDS victims. *Chart*, 83(5), 6, 11.

Folstein, M.H., Folstein, F.L., McHugh, P.R. (1975). Mini Mental State: Practical method for grading the mental state of patients for the clinician. *Journal of Psychological Research*, 12, 189–198.

Hoffman, R.S. (1984). Neuropsychiatric complications of AIDS. *Psychosomatics*, 25(5), 393–400.

Holland, J.C., Tross, S. (1985). The psychosocial and neuropsychiatric sequelae of the acquired immunodeficiency syndrome and related disorders. *Annals of Internal Medicine*, 103, 760–764.

Joseph, J.G., Emmons, CA, Kessler, R.C., et al. (1984). Coping with the threat of AIDS: An approach to psychosocial assessment. *American Psychologist*, 39(11), 1297–1302.

Lang, J.M., Spiegel, J., Strigle, S.M. (1985). *Living with AIDS*. Los Angeles: AIDS Project, Los Angeles.

Lowenstein, R.J., Sharfstein, S.S. (1984). Neuropsychiatric aspects of acquired immune deficiency syndrome. *International Journal of Psychiatry in Medicine*, 13(4), 255–260.

Macks, J. (1986, September). The Paris AIDS conference: Psychosocial research. *Focus: A Review of AIDS Research*, 1(10), 1–2.

McDonnell, M., Sevedge, K. (1986). Acquired immune deficiency syndrome. In M.H. Brown et al., (Eds.): *Standards of Oncology Nursing Practice* (pp. 565–594). New York: John Wiley & Sons.

Morin, S.F., Batchelor, W.F. (1984). Responding to the psychological crisis of AIDS. *Public Health Reports*, 99(1), 4–9.

Mount, B.M. (1986). Dealing with our losses. *Journal of Clinical Oncology*, 4(7), 1127–1134.

Navia, B.A., Jordan, B.D., Price, R.W. (1986). The AIDS dementia complex: Clinical features. *Annals of Neurology*, 19(6):517–524.

Newmark, D.A. (1984). Review of a support group for patients with AIDS. *Topics in Clinical Nursing*, 6(2), 38–41.

Ostrow, D.G., Gayle, T.C. (1986, August). Psychosocial and ethical issues of AIDS health care programs. *Quality Review Bulletin*, 12(8), 284–294.

Perry, S.W., Markowitz, J. (1986). Psychiatric interventions for AIDS-spectrum disorders. *Hospital and Community Psychiatry*, 37(10), 1001–1006.

Quinn, J.R. (1986). The AIDS crisis: A pastoral response. *America*, 154, 504–506.

Rubinow, D.R. (1984). The psychosocial impact of AIDS. *Topics in Clinical Nursing*, 6(2), 26–30.

Ryan, L.J. (1984). AIDS: A threat to physical and psychological integrity. *Topics in Clinical Nursing*, 6(2), 19–24.

Seymour, N. (1986, December). Counseling the patient with a positive antibody test. *AIDS File*. San Francisco: San Francisco General Hospital Medical Center.

Simmons-Alling, S. (1984). AIDS: Psychosocial needs of the health care worker. *Topics in Clinical Nursing*, 6(2), 31–37.

Shapira, J., Schlesinger, R. (1986). Distinguishing dementias. *American Journal of Nursing*, 86,(6), 698–702.

Staff. (1987, March). *AIDS Record*. Washington, D.C.: Bio-data Corporation.

Steinbrook, R., Lo, B., Tirpack, J., et al. (1985). Ethical dilemmas in caring for patients with the acquired immunodeficiency syndrome. *Annals of Internal Medicine*, 103, 787–790.

Wells, R. (1985). AIDS: Express train to death. *Nursing Mirror*, 160(7), 16–18.

Wolcott, D.L. (1986). Psychosocial aspects of acquired immune deficiency syndrome and the primary care physician. *Annals of Allergy*, 57(8), 95–102.

Wolcott, D.L., Fawzy, F.I., Landsverk, J., et al. (1986). AIDS patients' needs of psychosocial services and their use of community service organizations. *Journal of Psychosocial Oncology*, 4(1), 135–146.

Wolcott, D.L., Fawzy, F.I., Pasnau, R.O. (1985). Acquired immune deficiency syndrome (AIDS) and consultation-liaison psychiatry. *General Hospital Psychiatry*, 7, 280–292.

Chapter 9

Risk Factors and HIV Infection

Adeline M. Nyamathi
Jacquelyn Haak Flaskerud

It is commonly recognized that the causal agent in AIDS is a retrovirus formerly known as HTLV-III and recently renamed human immunodeficiency virus (HIV). Groups of persons whose behaviors and circumstances put them most at risk for contracting HIV infection and acquiring AIDS have also been identified: homosexual and bisexual men, intravenous drug abusers, hemophiliacs and blood product recipients, persons who have sexual contact with these groups, and infants born to mothers with HIV infection. However, since AIDS was first recognized, it rapidly became apparent that not all members of these groups became immunodeficient or contracted the complicating diseases when exposed to HIV. Within groups of infected individuals (that is, persons who have antibody to HIV), it is still uncertain who will develop AIDS or related diseases. This variable expression of pathogenic properties is true of all but a few microorganisms infecting humans (Osborn, 1986; Siegel, 1986).

At present it appears that AIDS develops in a relatively small proportion of people with HIV antibody; thus, HIV seropositivity might be viewed as necessary but not sufficient to cause the syndrome. Many seropositive people remain clinically well, with normal immune function or, more commonly, mild depression of immune function (Schechter et al., 1985a).

The important questions thus become, (1) why do so many people not become immunodeficient or contract disease, and (2) what is there about the risk behavior groups that makes them susceptible? The presence of something in addition to HIV exposure seems to be required both to acquire the virus and to become ill from it. One or more co-factors must exist.

Prospective studies are rapidly identifying specific environmental or behavioral components of lifestyle that might prove predictive of positive or nega-

Table 9–1. Risk Factors for HIV Infection

Exposure factors
  Anal receptive sex
  Multiple sexual partners
  Needle and syringe sharing
  Frequency of injection
  Receipt of factor VIII concentrate
  Blood transfusions
  Needlestick
  Parent from risk group

Trigger factors or co-factors

  Non-infectious
  Malnutrition
  Recreational drugs
  Prescribed drugs
  Allogeneic semen and sperm
  Emotional stress
  Age
  Pregnancy

  Infectious
  Antigenic overload
  (e.g., STDs, soft tissue infections, bacterial endocarditis,
  tubercular infections)
  Coincident immune suppression
  (e.g., CMV, HBV, EBV, herpesviruses)

tive outcomes of established HIV infection. Other co-factors being studied are those that would suppress immunity due to either a loss of protective natural defenses or undeveloped protective natural defenses. They include co-infection with pathogens associated with immune depression, malnutrition, allergic disorders, exposure to prescription drugs and recreational drugs, exposure to sperm and semen, a deficient natural resistance system, and genetic parameters (McCombie, 1986; Shearer and Levy, 1984).

Among the groups most at risk for AIDS, those persons with loss of protective natural defenses or induced immunodeficiency would include homosexual and bisexual men, drug abusers, adult recipients of whole blood and blood products, and the sexual partners of these. Persons with undeveloped natural defenses would include infants and possibly older adults (over 50–60 years of age).

Risk Factors and HIV

It appears that several risk factors are involved in determining the pathogenesis of AIDS. These risk factors might be viewed as occurring in two categories: exposure factors and trigger factors or co-factors (Table 9–1). Exposure factors are those risk factors that result in exposure to HIV. Trigger factors or co-factors are those risk factors that either determine a person's likelihood of being infected after exposure to HIV or contribute to disease expression in those who have been infected (Schechter et al., 1985a).

Exposure Factors. Numerous studies in the United States, Canada, Britain, the Netherlands, Denmark, Germany, and France have documented the relationship of specific sexual and lifestyle practices to exposure to HIV infection (Bienzle et al., 1985; Blattner et al., 1985; Evans et al., 1986; Goedert et al., 1985; Groopman et al., 1985; Jeffries et al., 1985; Kingsley et al., 1987; Moss et al., 1987; Newell et al., 1985a; Schechter et al., 1985a; van Griensven et al., 1987; Winkelstein et al., 1987). Receptive anal intercourse, multiple anonymous sexual partners, douching or rectal enemas before receptive anal intercourse, fisting, and the use of anal receptive objects are the main sexual risk factors associated with virus transmission. These risk factors produce exposure to HIV by increasing the probability of sexual contact with an infectious partner, by providing a route for transmission, and by causing trauma to the rectal mucosa, thus potentiating subsequent access of the viral agent to the bloodstream. Moreover, the most recent evidence indicates that the virus infects rectal cells directly rather than entering immune system cells in the bloodstream as was previously thought. Researchers in San Francisco, La Jolla and Bethesda have reported these results (*New York Times*, February 5, 1988).

Other risk factors for exposure to HIV infection have been associated with various aspects of substance abuse (Blattner et al., 1985; Chaisson et al., 1987; Faltz & Madover, 1986; Ginzburg et al., 1985; Siegel, 1986). The disinhibiting effects on behavior caused by alcohol and other drugs are well known and may possibly allow for more frequent and anonymous sexual exposure to the virus. Some drugs also blunt the sensation of pain, thus permitting or extending sexual practices that might not ordinarily be tolerated. The most obvious association of drugs and HIV infection is the direct transmission of the virus through the sharing of hypodermic needles, syringes, and other paraphernalia among parenteral drug users. There is a demonstrated increased risk of seropositivity with increasing numbers of persons with whom needles are regularly shared and with more frequent injections (Blattner et al., 1985). These risk factors produce exposure by increasing the probability of contact with the virus.

Other exposure factors exist for hemophiliacs and blood recipients. The risk of seropositivity for hemophiliacs increases as the number of exposures to factor VIII concentrate increases. Among blood recipients, the number of blood transfusions a person receives is a significant risk factor for HIV seropositivity (Blattner et al., 1985).

Trigger Factors or Co-factors. Co-factors exert an effect on disease expression that is independent of any role in producing exposure to HIV. Co-factors to HIV augment or accelerate immunodeficiency. Co-factors increase the likelihood of being infected after exposure or contribute to the expression of active disease in those who are HIV positive. Co-factors may have additive, deterministic, synergistic, or facilitative roles in the cytopathic effects of HIV on the immune system (Schechter et al., 1985a).

The most prominent immunologic feature of AIDS is a drastic reduction in the number of circulating T helper cells (T4 cells). At the same time, the number of circulating T suppressor cells (T8 cells) often persists at normal levels, thus leading to a reversal of the usual T4/T8 (H:S) ratio of around 2:1 (Wainberg et al., 1987). Co-factors are postulated to contribute to T cell immunodeficiency and immunologic abnormality through a variety of mechanisms.

There are both non-infectious and infectious co-factors involved in the etiology and susceptibility to HIV infection and AIDS. Non-infectious co-factors include dietary factors, use of IV drugs and recreational drugs, exposure to prescription drugs, allergic disorders, stress, age, and pregnancy. The commonest cause of T cell immunodeficiency worldwide is protein-calorie malnutrition. Malnutrition results in defects in macrophage and T cell function accompanied by hypergammaglobulinemia and increased susceptibility to infections (Seligman et al., 1984). Poor nutrition secondary to drug use and the use of drugs to control appetite both can lead to a chronic state of malnutrition which ultimately compromises the body's immune system (Mondanaro, 1987).

The use of alcohol, nitrites (poppers), amphetamines, marijuana, tobacco (cigarettes), and IV drugs (heroin, cocaine and morphine) have all been linked with immunosuppression. Lymphocyte function is suppressed by the presence of clinically observable alcohol (Siegel, 1986). In vitro, nitrites have been shown to suppress various leukocyte functional parameters associated with host defense (Newell et al., 1985b). Nitrite use has been associated with a transient immunosuppression which may weaken the normal defenses against infection (Goedert, 1984; Moss et al., 1987; Newell et al., 1985a). Use of cigarettes and marijuana have been associated with lower helper T cell counts (Newell et al., 1985a; Schechter et al., 1985a). In addition, cigarette smoking, marijuana use, and nitrite inhalation all could predispose the lungs to opportunistic infections. IV drug abusers use substances that have intrinsic immunosuppressive properties and are associated with chromosomal damage. Both IV and non-IV drugs have been associated with a reduction in numbers of T helper cells and an increase in T suppressor cells (Ginzburg et al., 1985; Siegel, 1986).

Frequent use of antibiotics has also been associated with immunosuppression (Ginzburg et al., 1985; McKenna et al., 1986). Chemical immunosuppression, whether from physician-prescribed or self-prescribed antibiotics, has been shown to occur in populations at high risk for sexually transmitted diseases and for soft tissue infections.

Exposure to allogeneic semen and sperm has been suggested as a possible co-factor in AIDS (Shearer & Levy, 1984; Schechter et al., 1985a; Sonnabend et al., 1984). Immunosuppression could occur from exposure to allogeneic cells in passive partners of anogenital sex if sperm and semen can reach the lymphatics and vascular system. This could occur by way of rectal and lower bowel lesions resulting from trauma due to sexual practices and viral infections.

Emotional stress has been persistently associated with reactivation of herpes simplex and with the abrupt onset of malignancy (Osborn, 1986). It has been hypothesized that there is an immunologic component of emotional stress that is a contributor to the progression of symptomatic disease. Stress could play an important role in the progression of disease in HIV-infected persons.

Age is related to immunologic status. Infants are an immunologically abnormal group and the more premature they are, the more immunologically abnormal they will be. Infants have undeveloped natural resistance systems which make them susceptible to multiple infections, including HIV (Osborn, 1986; Shearer & Levy, 1984). In addition, there is an age-related loss of natural resistance in older adults which could make them more susceptible to HIV as well as to other infections (Sandor et al., 1986; Shearer & Levy, 1984).

Pregnancy is another co-factorial mechanism that contributes to immunosuppression. Gestational immunosuppression occurs naturally in the second and third trimesters and can be measured by depressed lymphocyte numbers and functions, which return to normal one month post-partum (Tallon et al., 1984).

Finally, of the possible non-infectious co-factors to HIV, allogeneic blood and blood products may be immunosuppressive, as may factor VIII concentrate. The transfer of allogeneic blood and blood products could compromise the immune system of recipients (e.g., kidney transplants). In persons with hemophilia, immunosuppression may result from infusion of factor VIII replacement therapy (Ablin, 1985; Ablin & Gonder, 1985; Shearer & Levy, 1984).

Infectious co-factors are also involved in the etiology and susceptibility to AIDS. Infectious co-factors can contribute to the progression to AIDS both from antigenic overload and stimulation and from coincident immunosuppression (Osborn, 1986). It has been proposed that if the immune system is chronically overstimulated by a high antigenic load in association with various chronic infections, this overstimulation may interfere with the host's capacity to eliminate infectious agents (Seligmann et al., 1984). A history of multiple infectious diseases, among them syphilis, giardiasis, gonorrhea, chancroid, and parasitic diseases, has been suggested as a co-factor in the acquisition of HIV infection (Moss et al., 1987; Newell et al., 1985a; Osborn, 1986; Sindrup et al., 1986; Sonnabend et al., 1984). Soft tissue infections as well as infections such as viral hepatitis and bacterial endocarditis may result from the IV use of drugs dissolved in non-sterile water mixed with contaminated diluents and impure narcotics, and self-administered through blood- and dirt-contaminated needles and syringes (Ginzburg et al., 1985; Osborn, 1986). These various infections are thought to produce sufficient insult to the immune system to enhance the pathologic effects of HIV on the host.

Another infectious co-factor which might be operative in the progression from asymptomatic infection to overt disease is coincident immunosuppression caused by viruses other than HIV. Chief among those suggested as playing an additive or synergistic role in potentiating the cytopathic effects of HIV are chronic infections with cytomegalovirus (CMV), Epstein-Barr virus (EBV), hepatitis B virus (HBV), and herpesviruses (herpes simplex [HSV] and herpes zoster [HZV]) (Collier et al., 1987; Friedman-Kien et al., 1986; Jeffries et al., 1985; Latchman, 1987; Melbye et al., 1987; Osborn, 1986; Potterat et al., 1986; Schechter et al., 1985a). Infection with these viruses has significant effects on the immune system and may facilitate the progression of HIV infection. The effect of infection with other viruses might be simply immunosuppressive, providing opportunities for reactivation of HIV. Or, they may serve to activate cells that carry HIV, resulting in the full expression of cytopathologic effects (Schechter et al., 1985a).

The various risk factors discussed here play a role in exposure to the virus, transmission of the virus, immunosuppression of the host, and activation or facilitation of the virus. Depending on their combination, they can increase or decrease the risk of HIV infection and the risk of expression of disease.

Risk Factors and Transmission Groups

Risk factors tend to cluster in the different transmission groups for HIV infection, producing groups more or less at risk of infection by the virus. It is important to note here that behaviors and circumstances put people at risk, not the groups with whom they are associated. However, these behaviors and circumstances occur more or less frequently in some groups than others and therefore the term "risk groups" has emerged. This identification has a negative side to it, i.e., the possibility of stigmatization of these groups. A possible positive side is the opportunity to design health education programs that are specific to the lifestyle, practices, and circumstances of specific groups. Each of the groups defined by the Centers for Disease Control (CDC) as transmission groups for HIV infection and AIDS has specific associated risk factors.

Homosexual and Bisexual Men. The majority of studies identifying risk factors have been conducted with samples of homosexual and bisexual men. Many studies have been conducted in all United States cities where AIDS is prevalent and in comparable cities in Europe. These studies are remarkably alike in their identification of risk factors in the homosexual and bisexual male transmission groups.

There is overwhelming agreement among researchers that the greatest risk of exposure to HIV in the homosexual and bisexual male transmission groups comes from anal receptive sexual intercourse and sexual practices (fisting, douching, use of objects) with multiple sexual partners. These risk factors are found to be associated with HIV seropositivity, with generalized lymphadenopathy, with AIDS-related complex (ARC) and with AIDS (Bienzle et al., 1985; Evans et al., 1986; Goedert et al., 1985; Groopman et al., 1985; Jeffries et al., 1985; Kingsley et al., 1987; Moss et al., 1987; Newell et al., 1985a; Schechter et al., 1985a; Schechter et al., 1985b; van Griensven et al., 1987; Winkelstein et al., 1987). These sexual practices are implicated not only in exposure to the virus, but also in transmission of the virus via rectal cells and/or trauma to the rectal mucosa, and in the presence of numerous non-infectious and infectious co-factors of HIV in these host risk groups.

Among the non-infectious co-factors, the use of alcohol, marijuana, and volatile nitrites (poppers) in conjunction with sex has been reported for homosexual men with AIDS (Ginzburg et al., 1985; Goedert, 1984; Newell et al., 1985a,b; Siegel, 1986, van Griensven et al., 1987). These drugs are used to heighten sexual arousal, to relax the anal sphincter during anal receptive inter-course, and to prolong duration of intercourse. The use of these drugs may act also to prolong the duration of exposure to the virus.

In addition, both volatile nitrites and alcohol act as co-factors to HIV infec-tion because of their immunosuppressive effects. The suppression of normal lym-phocyte function in persons using volatile nitrites and alcohol may act as a facilitator of HIV infection or, in the presence of the virus, may be enough to lead to the full-blown syndrome.

Anal receptive sexual practices resulting in trauma to the rectum and bowel provide the route also for exposure to allogeneic semen and sperm. Sperm has been suggested as a possible co-factor in AIDS because of its immunosuppressive char-acteristics (Schechter et al., 1985a; Shearer & Levy, 1984; Sonnabend et al., 1984).

Among the infectious co-factors of HIV for the homosexual/bisexual transmission group, several of the infectious diseases are transmitted sexually and are facilitated by anal receptive sexual activity. Among the many infectious dis-eases associated with HIV infection are gonorrhea, syphilis, and chancroid. These diseases are thought to result in antigenic overstimulation or overload in the host and to act as co-factors which could augment or accelerate the pathogenesis of immunodeficiency (Jeffries et al., 1985; Moss et al., 1987; Osborn, 1986; Schech-ter et al., 1985b; Sindrup et al., 1986; Sonnabend et al., 1984; Weber et al., 1986). The physician-prescribed or self-prescribed use of antibiotics by homosexual and bisexual men in association with multiple infectious diseases has also been as-sociated with immunosuppression (Ginzburg et al., 1985; McKenna et al., 1986).

Other infectious co-factors of HIV for the homosexual/bisexual transmission group are concomitant chronic infections with other viruses: hepatitis B, herpes-viruses, cytomegalovirus, and HTLV-I and HTLV-II. These infections cause coincident immunosuppression with HIV and could be operative in the progres-sion from asymptomatic infection to overt disease (Bentwich et al., 1987; Bienzle et al., 1985; Collier et al., 1987; Friedman-Kien et al., 1986; Getchell et al., 1987; Halbert et al., 1986; Jeffries et al., 1985; Latchman, 1987; Melbye et al., 1987; Osborn, 1986; Potterat et al., 1986; Sandor et al., 1986; Schechter et al., 1985a; Sonnabend et al., 1984).

It is important to note here some of the similarities and differences in homosexual and heterosexual sexual transmission of the virus. Heterosexuals who practice anal receptive sex and who have multiple sexual partners are considered to be at increased risk for HIV infection (Blattner et al., 1985; Cowell, 1986;

Table 9–2. A Comparison of Sociodemographic Characteristics and Risk Factors in Heterosexuals and Homosexuals who are HIV-Infected

Sociodemographic Characteristics and Risk Factors	Sexual Group and Direction of Association with HIV Infection	
	Homosexual	*Heterosexual*
White	↑	↓
Education	↑	↓
Income	↑	↓
Married	↓	↑
IV drugs	↓	↑
Inhaled cocaine	↑	↓
Inhaled nitrites	↑	↓
Number of sexual partners	↑	↓
Rectal trauma	↑	↓
Exposure to feces, semen	↑	↓
Gonorrhea	↑	↓
Syphilis	↑	↓
Cytomegalovirus	↑	↓
Hepatitis	↑	↓
Kaposi's sarcoma	↑	↓
Pneumocystis pneumonia	↓	↑

↑ = Direct relationship; ↓ = Inverse relationship.

Redfield et al., 1985). However, the virus can be transmitted through vaginal receptive sex and has been documented for both male-to-female and female-to-male transmission (Redfield et al., 1985). The question has been raised whether female-to-male transmission is as efficient as male-to-female. Furthermore, questions have been raised about the efficiency of vaginal transmission compared to anal transmission.

Heterosexual sexual activities that are vaginal receptive and vaginal insertive may be less facilitative of transmission of the virus because of the differences in the epithelial lining of the rectum and the vagina (Shearer & Levy, 1984). The susceptibility of the rectum and bowel to trauma and lesions could facilitate not only the transmission of HIV but also other sexually transmitted infectious diseases as well as allogeneic sperm and semen. Both of these have been considered as co-factors in the pathogenesis of AIDS. It should be noted, however, that anal receptive sex is not a requirement for exposure and that bidirectional heterosexual transmission of HIV infection and disease has been documented in studies of female sexual contacts of males with AIDS, of spouses of patients with ARC and AIDS, and in reports from Africa (Redfield et al., 1985).

The similarities and differences mentioned earlier and other similarities and differences in socioeconomic characteristics and risk factors that exist between homosexual and heterosexual groups are given in Table 9–2 (Blattner et al., 1985; Guinan et al., 1984; Redfield et al., 1985).

IV Drug Abusers. The most obvious exposure factor in the IV drug abuser transmission group is the transmission of HIV through sharing hypodermic needles, syringes and equipment. The risk of seropositivity increases as the number of persons with whom needles are regularly shared increases and as the number of injections increases (Blattner et al., 1985; Chaisson et al., 1987; Faltz & Madover, 1986). Chief among the co-factors of HIV in IV drug abusers are the intrinsic immunosuppressive properties of the drugs used. IV drug abusers have many immunologic abnormalities (Ginzburg et al., 1985; Goedert, 1984; Shearer & Levy, 1984; Siegel, 1986). The combined effect of drug use and HIV infection on the immune system may facilitate disease expression.

Other co-factors of HIV among IV drug abusers are the possibility of antigenic overload and consequent immunosuppression due to multiple infections (e.g., cellulitis, abscesses) from the use of nonsterile water, contaminated diluents, impure narcotic, and blood- and dirt-contaminated needles (Ginzburg et al., 1985). Other infections common to IV drug abusers are the viral hepatitides and bacterial endocarditis as well as the traditional sexually transmitted diseases of gonorrhea, syphilis, trichomoniasis, and chlamydia (Mondanaro, 1987; Osborn, 1986). Chemical immunosuppression could also be operating among IV drug abusers because of their physician-prescribed and self-prescribed use of antibiotics for their numerous infections (Ginzburg et al., 1985; McKenna et al., 1986).

Malnutrition may also act as a co-factor of HIV in substance abusers (Mondanaro, 1987; Seligmann et al., 1984; Shearer & Levy, 1984). Drugs have a direct appetite-suppressing effect and alcohol can lead to impaired absorption of food. Malnutrition is further exacerbated by inadequate assimilation of vitamins and amino acids due to damaged liver cells. Ultimately the body's immune system is compromised owing to chronic malnutrition. As noted earlier, the commonest cause of T cell immunodeficiency in the world is malnutrition.

Finally, coincident viral infections such as HBV can act as co-factors of HIV in IV drug users (Conte et al., 1987). Increased HTLV-I and HTLV-II infections, respectively causing an aggressive lymphoma, and hairy cell leukemia, coincident with HIV infection have been observed in intravenous drug users in an AIDS endemic area in New York (Robert-Guroff et al., 1986). A high antibody prevalence for HIV was seen in this group (41%). In addition 9% had antibody to HTLV-I and 18% to HTLV-II. The antibody prevalence for HTLV-I and HTLV-II in the general population is about 1%. These viruses have been shown to adversely influence functioning of the immune system.

Hemophiliacs. The exposure factor for HIV for hemophiliacs in the United States was the blood supply prior to 1983. The virus was introduced into the blood supply by donors who were infected and was transferred to hemophiliacs during transfusion. Hemophiliacs receive blood that is concentrated from the pooled plasma of literally thousands of donors. The virus was evidently able to survive the fractionation procedures then in use, and over 90% of an estimated

20,000 hemophiliacs became seropositive. Severe hemophiliacs receive an average of 122,000 units of clotting factor concentrate annually (Osborn, 1986; Prince et al., 1985).

However, hemophiliacs who were dependent on clotting factor VIII concentrate (hemophilia A) and clotting factor IX concentrate (hemophilia B) might have been measurably immunosuppressed prior to infection (Ablin, 1985; Ablin & Gonder, 1985; Osborn, 1986; Prince et al., 1985; Shearer & Levy, 1984). Immunosuppression resulting from clotting factor concentrate could be a co-factor in susceptibility to infection in hemophiliacs. Likewise, in recipients of multiple blood transfusions, the transfer of allogeneic blood and possibly blood products could cause at least temporary immunosuppression, making them susceptible to HIV infection when present in the blood supply. In hemophiliacs the risk for seropositivity reflects severity of their disease as measured by dosage of concentrate used. In blood transfusion recipients, the number of blood transfusions received is a significant risk factor for HIV seropositivity (Blattner et al., 1985).

Hemophiliacs present the mildest and simplest examples of a co-factor which might augment or accelerate the pathogenesis of immune deficiency (Osborn, 1986). Other than the alloantigens represented in clotting factor concentrate, their other infectious and noninfectious risk factors are not extraordinary. Hemophiliacs are at once the highest transmission group for HIV infection and, among the transmission groups, the lowest for AIDS. Of the 90% of hemophiliacs who are HIV-infected, only 2 1/2% have contracted AIDS (Goedert et al., 1986; Vetrosky et al., 1987).

Women. Exposure factors to HIV infection for women include IV drug abuse (50%) and sexual contact with infected men, principally IV drug abusers (20%) and bisexuals (5%) (Furth, 1987; Mondanaro, 1987; Shearer & Levy, 1984). Women are discussed here separately because of differences in the risk factors for HIV infection operating in women. Among the exposure factors, women who are sexual partners of bisexual men are more likely to engage in anal receptive sex than are other women (Shearer & Levy, 1984). Anal receptive sex has been identified as an exposure and transmission factor of HIV infection in numerous studies. In addition, because of trauma to the rectal mucosa, anal receptive sex also facilitates multiple infections which may act as co-factors to HIV infection.

Among the co-factors of HIV operating in women drug abusers, all of those implicated in IV drug abusers in general would apply in women IV drug abusers as well, including poor nutrition, use of drugs known to suppress the immune system, repeated bouts of infection and high stress. In addition to the concerns raised about nutrition earlier in the discussion of IV drug abusers, women are known to compound their nutritional problems by purposely using drugs to lose weight. In some women, drug dependence coexists with eating disorders. Drugs and starvation are used in combination to control weight (Mondanaro, 1987).

Another co-factor of HIV infection is multiple chronic infections in some transmission groups. Women drug abusers experience more medical problems than their male counterparts (Mondanaro, 1987). Drug dependent women are vulnerable to sexually transmitted diseases and their sequelae, urinary tract infections, soft tissue infections, endocarditis, hepatitis, anemia and diabetes. Furthermore, drug dependent women experience much higher levels of stress than do either male drug abusers or non-drug using women (Mondanaro, 1987). The areas of increased stress include low income, education, and financial resources; living alone and responsibility for children; partners that use drugs; more dysfunction and pathology in the family of origin; and higher levels of anxiety, depression, and recent life change events and lower levels of self-esteem.

Perhaps the co-factor of HIV infection of greatest risk to women is pregnancy. Immunosuppression occurs naturally in the second and third trimesters of pregnancy. Although the information on the adverse effect of pregnancy on HIV infection is limited, what is available is dramatic. Studies have demonstrated that not only do a high percentage of the children of these pregnancies become HIV-infected but that more than 50% of the women became sick with AIDS, and of those more than half died of AIDS within a few months of delivery (Scott et al., 1985; Tallon et al., 1984). This is a pace and rate of exacerbation unknown in the other transmission groups. It is thought to be associated with the synergistic effects of immunosuppression in pregnancy on HIV infection.

Infants. HIV infection is transmitted to infants through transplacental spread from mother to fetus in utero, at delivery, or after delivery, through breast feeding and through blood or platelet transfusions (Klein, 1984; Staff, *AIDS Record*, 1987). For the majority of infants who are HIV-infected, the greatest exposure factor is from an infected mother during pregnancy rather than during birth or afterwards (Staff, *AIDS Record*, 1987).

Chief among the co-factors of HIV infection for infants is that they have undeveloped natural resistance systems which make them susceptible to multiple infections, including HIV. Because their immune system does not develop fully until after birth, infants can be considered immunosuppressed or immunologically abnormal. Infants who are premature have even greater immunologic abnormality (Osborn, 1986; Shearer & Levy, 1984). The significant shortening of average incubation period in infants with AIDS from 2 years or more to less than a year has been explained on that basis (Osborn, 1986; Scott et al., 1985).

Other co-factors of HIV infection that could be operating in infants are the multiple other infectious agents that the mothers of these infants could pass on to them in utero. These include the viruses with which high-risk-group mothers are infected (e.g., HBV, EBV, CMV, HSV); bacteria (e.g., syphilis, tuberculosis); and protozoa. The effects of fetal infection by these agents could result in prematurity, low birth weight, developmental anomalies, congenital disease, and persistent postnatal infection (Klein, 1984). All of these conditions could compromise the ability of the infant to survive. In addition many of these organisms and other organisms can be transmitted at delivery and are associated with neonatal disease (e.g., streptococcus A and B, *E. coli*, *Neisseria gonorrhoeae*, chlamydia).

Aging Population. Another age-related kind of immunologic abnormality worthy of concern is that ascribed to the process of aging (Osborn, 1986). There could be an age-related loss of natural resistance or immunity that would make older adults more susceptible to HIV infection (Shearer & Levy, 1984). This co-factor has been shown to exist for herpes zoster, which has an increased incidence in geriatric populations (Sandor et al., 1986). While this age group is not currently considered at high risk, age-related loss of immunity could operate as a co-factor in HIV-infected asymptomatic persons as they become older. This co-factor could also make older adults more susceptible to other non-infectious co-factors (Shearer & Levy, 1984).

Ethnic/Racial Minorities. Blacks and Hispanics are overrepresented among persons with AIDS (39%) compared to their numbers in the general population (20%). Of the homosexual/bisexual transmission group, 15% are Black and 10% are Hispanic. Among IV drug abusers 50% are Black and 30% are Hispanic. Among women with AIDS, 51% are Black and 20% are Hispanic and among children with AIDS, 58% are Black and 22% Hispanic (Faltz & Madover, 1986; Flaskerud, 1988; Mondanaro, 1987). Blacks and Hispanics are represented in all the transmission groups discussed previously. For reasons largely undetermined thus far, their risk factors appear to differ.

Of the Blacks and Hispanics who are HIV-infected, a greater percentage than Whites were exposed to the virus through practices associated with IV drug abuse. It would seem that the risk factors for HIV infection in IV drug abusers should have the same explanatory value in the occurrence of seropositivity in Blacks and Hispanics as they do in Whites. This does not appear to be true. In a study of heterosexual (male and female) drug abusers in San Francisco, HIV seropositivity was significantly more prevalent in Blacks and Hispanics (14%) than in Whites (6%) (Chaisson et al., 1987). This difference could not be explained by behavioral characteristics (number of persons with whom needles were shared; duration of drug use; number of persons rinsing/cleaning needles) or sociodemographic characteristics (age, sex, history of prostitution, type of drug program). This racial/ethnic difference has also been reported in New York and New Jersey with much higher rates of seropositivity (54% for Blacks and 16% for Whites) (Robert-Guroff et al., 1986; Weiss et al., 1985). In the New York study, Whites and Blacks did not differ significantly with respect to age, sex, frequency of drug taking, or place of origin of drugs. Blacks had used both heroin and cocaine for a longer period than White drug users.

Similarly it would seem that among the homosexual/bisexual transmission groups, established risk behaviors should have similar power in explaining the occurrence of seropositivity and disease for Whites and Blacks. Again this does not appear to be the case. In a large, prospective study of homosexual/bisexual men in San Francisco, the seropositivity of Blacks (65.5%) was significantly greater than that of Whites (48.7%) and the seroconversion over two years was significantly greater for Blacks (20%) than for Whites (6.4%). These differences could not be explained by three established risk factors: i.e., receptive anal intercourse, multiple sexual partners, and needle sharing did not differ significantly between the groups (Samuel & Winkelstein, 1987).

In order to explain the differences in ethnic/racial groups, future studies will need to examine more carefully the other co-factors to HIV infection discussed in this chapter: malnutrition, use of recreational drugs, antigenic overload, and coincident immunosuppression by other viruses. Other useful indicators might be access to health care services, general morbidity and mortality rates, education and income.

One study of coincident viral infection with HTLV-I, HTLV-II and HIV (HTLV-III) in intravenous drug abusers in New York demonstrated that Blacks (46%) were more likely than Whites (11%) to be seropositive for HTLV-I or HTLV-II (Robert-Guroff et al., 1986). Seventy-three percent of Blacks were antibody positive for HTLV-I, II, or III (HIV) compared to 26% of Whites. While probably an artifact of sampling, 100% of persons studied with soft tissue infections (mostly staphylococcus and streptococcus) were Black. Since both multiple infections resulting in antigenic overstimulation and coincident immunosuppression by other viruses have been identified as possible co-factors in HIV infection, these merit more intensive study in determining differences in racial/ethnic groups.

Risk Factors and Risk Reduction

The identification of risk factors can reduce the risk of exposure to HIV infection in the general population and in the transmission groups and can reduce the risk of progression from asymptomatic infection to ARC or AIDS in those infected. Furthermore, defining the risk factors of susceptibility could permit the identification of additional potential transmission groups and allow for the initiation of early preventive steps. Finally, if it can be demonstrated that such risk factors contribute to susceptibility to AIDS, perhaps the degree of concern reaching near-hysteria by the public and health care workers can be reduced.

Identification of the most common exposure and transmission factors in HIV infection has become the focus of public health education programs to prevent HIV infection in all segments of the population, but particularly among transmission groups. Assessment and identification of co-factors is an equally urgent task: 1.5 to 2 million HIV-infected asymptomatic individuals in the United States alone now live under the potential threat of a lethal disease. The likelihood that the disease will occur may be influenced if not actually determined by co-factors specific to a particular group. These co-factors may be fairly easy to control through public health education campaigns. It may be possible through health education to define lifestyles that facilitate continued well-being for many years.

In order to control the spread of HIV infection and AIDS, a multifactorial approach to cause, prevention, and cure is most likely to be effective. A multifactorial approach considers changes in the host, the agent, and the environment in order to combat disease. Public health education programs can be designed with these factors in mind. Host factors are those behaviors that individuals can engage in or change that will prevent exposure to HIV or progression to disease expression. Agent factors include identifying the virus, developing antiviral treatments, and developing a vaccine against the virus. Environmental factors involve HIV infection control in hospital and community settings and decreasing the risk of opportunistic infections. All of these factors should be included in public health education campaigns. Health education should include information for the public on the prevention of infection and disease, the treatments and services available to those infected and diseased, and environmental control of and reduction of infection.

The remainder of this chapter will focus on changes in host behavior to prevent the spread of infection and disease. Identification of the agent and control of the agent are considered more fully in Chapters 3 and 4, respectively. Control of environmental factors is considered in Chapters 5, 7, 10, and Appendix C. Nursing care as it relates to host, agent, and environmental factors is discussed in depth in Chapter 5.

Primary Prevention: Exposure to HIV

Persons who are HIV antibody negative can protect their negative status and prevent infection by avoiding certain behaviors and practices most closely associated with infection. These include behaviors associated with sexual transmission, intravenous transmission and perinatal transmission.

There is no risk of sexual transmission for those who practice sexual abstinence. Likewise, there is no risk of infection if neither partner is infected. This would be true of mutually monogamous couples since the introduction of HIV in the United States (mid-1970s) and for couples who have been shown to be HIV antibody negative in serologic testing (Blattner, 1986; Francis & Chin, 1987).

For couples outside of these situations, the extent of risk can be decreased by limiting the number of sexual partners and by selecting partners from groups at low or no risk of infection. The prevalence of infection varies by sex, geography, and sexual practices. Risk of infection is lower in women, outside the AIDS endemic areas (large urban areas in New York, California, Florida, Texas, New Jersey, Illinois, Pennsylvania, Georgia, Massachusetts, and the District of Columbia), in those not practicing anal receptive intercourse, and in those with few sexual partners (Blattner, 1986; Francis & Chin, 1987).

Finally, the risk of infection is decreased in those who practice protective sex. Protective sex is sexual activity in which no semen, vaginal fluid, or blood is exchanged between partners. Such practices involve kissing, hugging, caressing, genital manipulation (all in the absence of open lesions) and vaginal and anal in-

Table 9–3. Risk of Sexual Transmission of HIV

Absolutely safe
  Abstinence
  Mutually monogamous with noninfected partner

Very safe
  Non-insertive sexual practices

Probably safe
  Insertive sexual practices with the use of condoms and spermicide

Risky
  Everything else

tercourse provided a condom is worn and a spermicide is used. The risk of sexual transmission of HIV for various practices is given in Table 9–3.

There are specific practices that homosexual men can avoid to reduce their risk of infection. These include anal receptive intercourse and multiple sexual partners. In combination these currently produce the highest risk for HIV infection in the United States (Blattner, 1986; Francis & Chin, 1987; Kingsley et al., 1987). Avoidance of anal intercourse is the principal focus of efforts to reduce risk in the male homosexual community.

Among heterosexual men and women, reducing the number of sexual partners and practicing protective sex at all times can reduce the risk of infection. Anal receptive intercourse is also a danger among women with bisexual partners and among prostitutes, both male and female.

Intravenous transmission of HIV can be prevented both in recipients of blood and blood products and in IV drug abusers and experimenters. Infection through donated blood and blood products can be prevented through donor exclusion, serologic testing for HIV antibodies, and heat inactivation of products like factor VIII concentrate. Donor exclusion can be facilitated by education of donors, active interview strategies at blood banks, and confidential post-donation self-exclusion (Ascher & Francis, 1987). Serologic testing of donors for HIV antibody uses both the enzyme-linked immunosorbent assay (ELISA) techniques and the confirmatory Western blot assay. Recently the indirect immunofluorescent antibody (IFA) test has provided an external standard against which ELISA performance can be judged. Furthermore, the recent addition of HBV antibody-core testing of blood donors should further eliminate donors at risk for HIV infection, because a substantial proportion of those at risk for HIV infection are also at risk for HBV (Ascher & Francis, 1987). Finally, preliminary reports of heat inactivation of factor VIII concentrates suggest that this approach can protect hemophiliac factor VIII recipients from acquiring HIV infection (Blattner, 1986; Vetrosky et al., 1987). These precautions should virtually eliminate the risk of HIV infection from transfusion of blood and blood products.

For intravenous drug abusers, exposure to HIV infection can be eliminated by stopping the use of IV drugs. In order for this to occur addicted persons need

Table 9–4. Risk of Transmission Through IV Drug Use

Absolutely safe
  Stop the use of IV drugs

Very safe
  Use sterilized injection paraphernalia

Probably safe
  Clean injection paraphernalia with bleach

Risky
  All other activities

to be referred to rehabilitation programs. To make this possible, health care workers, local and federal governments, and the general public will have to take a greater interest in the welfare of drug abusers. Currently drug abusers arouse little sympathy or interest. Health care workers put little effort into promoting health or preventing illness among this group. Public health education efforts directed at the rehabilitation of drug abusers or at the prevention of AIDS among drug abusers are not extensive. Little encouragement is given drug abusers to enter treatment programs. In addition, the number of rehabilitation programs available is not at all adequate to the need for programs if the goal is to stop drug abuse or if all drug abusers wished to enroll in such a program. A massive infusion of government and public support is necessary for a major rehabilitation effort.

In the absence of stopping the use of IV drugs, exposure to HIV infection could be prevented if unsterilized injection paraphernalia were not shared among individuals. At a minimum, those persons who use IV drugs should clean their equipment with a readily available disinfectant (e.g., bleach). Other possibilities are to provide sterile needles and syringes for IV drug abusers (Table 9–4).

Outside the addicted population are substantial numbers of persons who experiment with drugs. Educational programs for teenagers, for communities in which drug use is high, and for the staff of drug clinics need to emphasize the danger of sharing needles and equipment.

Intravenous drug abusers will likely serve as the major entry of HIV infection and AIDS into the heterosexual community, especially into poor, urban communities. An aggressive prevention effort is required to prevent further spread of HIV into social/ethnic minority communities. Finally, drugs are implicated in a broader sense in the spread of HIV infection. The use of drugs in conjunction with sexual practices is prevalent in many groups, including homosexual males, teenagers, and prostitutes, and has a disinhibiting effect on sexual practices. A public health education campaign similar to the one linking drinking and driving is called for in linking substance abuse to the possibly lethal consequences of sexual activity in the case of AIDS.

Perinatal transmission of HIV can be avoided if infected women do not become pregnant. Pregnancy carries a high risk of infection to infants and accelera-

Table 9–5. Risk of Perinatal Transmission

Absolutely safe
    Abstinence
    Sterilization

Very safe
    Birth control measures and abortion

Probably safe
    Use of condoms

Risky
    Pregnancy

tion of the development of AIDS in HIV-infected mothers. Women who are in high risk behavior groups (IV drug abusers, prostitutes, women with multiple sexual partners, with STDs, and with sexual partners at high risk) should be encouraged to be tested for HIV infection. Those who are infected should be encouraged to postpone pregnancy until more is known about the risks to themselves and their infants. Women who are HIV-infected and become pregnant should be given abortion counseling early in their pregnancy (first trimester) (Francis & Chin, 1987; Guinan & Hardy, 1987; Wofsy, 1987) (Table 9–5).

Secondary Prevention: Prevention of Disease Expression

Persons who are HIV antibody positive and asymptomatic can engage in a number of activities to prevent their progression to lymphadenopathy syndrome (LAS), ARC, and AIDS. These activities center on minimizing or eliminating the effects of co-factors, both infectious and noninfectious. Co-factors were identified earlier in this chapter as risk factors that augment or accelerate immunodeficiency, that is, they contribute another factor besides HIV to immunosuppression of the host. Through public health education, persons who are HIV-infected can become aware of the particular co-factors to HIV that might be operating with them. Through lifestyle changes, persons with HIV infection can also minimize or eliminate immunosuppressant factors and emphasize factors that promote immune functioning.

The non-infectious co-factors identified earlier were malnutrition, use of recreational drugs and alcohol, pregnancy, stress, age, and exposure to allogeneic sperm and semen. First, regular medical evaluations and follow-up are advised. Second, health maintenance efforts, including proper nutrition, abstinence and sobriety, stress management, safer sex practices, and not sharing needles may all decrease the risk of seropositivity developing into LAS, ARC, or AIDS.

Calorie-protein malnutrition is a major cause of immunosuppression. Persons who are HIV-infected can be taught to eat an adequate diet with essential nutrients including protein, carbohydrates, fat, vitamins, and minerals. Persons who are HIV-infected need to ensure that their daily intake of calories and protein is adequate and that their vitamin intake is sufficient. Information on nutrition and meal planning could be an important aspect of public health education for several of the transmission groups. Both homosexual men and heterosexual women may have eating disorders or may diet excessively related to their desire to be exceptionally thin to enhance their physical attractiveness. Information on the dangers of this kind of dieting and conversely on what constitutes adequate nutrition may be needed.

Another group that may need nutrition information is the urban poor. Even when diets are adequate in calories in this group, they are often deficient in protein, vitamins, vegetables, and fruit, and high in fat. Among the urban poor are the IV drug abusers and substance abusers who often are poorly nourished due to the appetite suppressant effects of drugs, toxic effects of alcohol on the gastrointestinal tract, and inadequate assimilation of vitamins and amino acids due to damaged liver cells (Mondanaro, 1987).

The use of alcohol, recreational drugs, and IV drugs is another cause of immunodeficiency (Siegel, 1986). Persons who are HIV-infected should be taught the effects of substance abuse on the immune system and should be encouraged to give up the use of alcohol, nitrites, marijuana, cigarettes and IV drugs. The suggestion is that removal of such potential precursors or determinants may allow for recovery from and/or avoidance of AIDS in individuals who have not yet progressed to the full-blown syndrome (Siegel, 1986).

Women who are HIV-infected must be given information on the effects of pregnancy on the progression of disease. Pregnancy itself has an immunosuppressant effect that can accelerate the pace of exacerbation of AIDS. Seropositive women should not get pregnant; they should use a reliable method of birth control. Other information that women need to know about pregnancy and AIDS is that over 70% of pediatric AIDS is attributed to maternal transmission; that they do not need to be sick to pass on HIV to the fetus; that there is no way to prevent the fetus from becoming infected if the mother is infected; and that the virus may be contracted through breast milk (Mondanaro, 1987; Wofsy, 1987). Counseling on birth control, pregnancy, and abortion should be part of any health education program for women.

Emotional stress has also been shown to affect immunosuppression. The effects of stress can be mitigated or reduced through regular exercise, adequate and regular amounts of rest and sleep, relaxation techniques, and effective coping. Persons in some of the transmission groups have inadequate or inaccurate knowledge of the benefits of exercise, thinking instead that no exercise is more beneficial if a person has the chance of becoming sick. Acceptable and feasible programs of exercise might have to be designed for members of some groups.

Walking is an exercise available to all and is not overtaxing. Similarly, the importance of adequate regular rest and sleep might need to be explained to persons who believe that they can "catch up" on rest and sleep or that being sleep deprived has no effect. Teaching relaxation techniques is probably necessary for all groups as information about these is relatively new.

Finally, coping response may have a role in immunologic function (Locke et al., 1984). Coping responses to stress have been described as occurring in three ways: (1) manipulation of the stress-producing situation; (2) reinterpretation of the situation; and (3) action to control the stress resulting from the situation (Hefferin, 1980). Good copers are those who use all three coping responses. A person's typical coping response can be assessed and alternative or additional responses can be taught to help the person deal with stress. Persons who cope effectively with the stress of HIV infection would be those who are able to (1) change their behaviors in the face of HIV infection, e.g., their nutrition, their use of drugs and alcohol, their sexual activity, their needle sharing activity; (2) reinterpret their HIV status as an opportunity to practice health maintenance rather than as a death sentence; and (3) engage in stress reducing activities such as exercise, relaxation techniques, and rest and sleep.

All persons who are HIV-infected need information on the meaning of infection. They cannot assume that they will or will not develop AIDS. Information should include that they are probably infected for life and that they are probably contagious for life. This information means that they should not engage in unsafe sexual practices and/or needle sharing, nor should they donate blood, plasma, body organs, or other tissue. They can thus help to prevent the spread of HIV to non-infected individuals. However, neither should they engage in unsafe sexual practices or share needles with other seropositive persons. There is a possibility that repeated exposures to the virus may increase the possibility of developing AIDS. Unsafe (unprotected) anal sexual practices also expose the person to allogeneic sperm and semen. As noted earlier repeated exposure to sperm and semen through the rectum can have immunosuppressant effects. Persons who are HIV-infected would want to avoid these effects.

The infectious co-factors of HIV infection also contribute to immune suppression and can be avoided by changes in behavior that could result in more competent immune functioning. Unsafe sexual practices, anal receptive sex in particular, and IV drug use and needle sharing result in many infections besides HIV. These infections are believed to result in antigenic stimulation and overload, causing a burden on the immune system and/or a chronic coincident immunosuppression. In the presence of HIV infection, these other infections act as co-factors in the development of disease expression. Many of the infectious co-factors of HIV infection can be prevented by the same changes in sexual practices that could prevent HIV infection: avoiding anal intercourse and multiple sexual partners. Anal receptive intercourse is associated not only with HIV infection but also with other sexually transmitted diseases that present a health threat to male homosexuals and male and female prostitutes: hepatitis B, cytomegalovirus infection, herpes simplex, amoebiasis, syphilis, and gonorrhea (Kingsley et al., 1987). Whether through the ability of immunosuppression to provide opportunity for activation of HIV, or actual activation of cells carrying HIV, coincident chronic infections have significant effects on the immune system and on the progression of HIV infection. Avoiding anal intercourse should be the principal focus of any public health education program as it reduces the risk of HIV infection, reduces the numbers of repeated exposures to the virus, reduces the risk of other sexually transmitted diseases, and thereby also reduces the effects of infectious co-factors. Short of that, condoms should be used for all insertive sexual practices to reduce the risk of infection.

There is evidence that public health education and the fear of AIDS has resulted in a reduced number of sexual partners in homosexual and bisexual men and a change to safer sexual practices. These changes have coincided with significantly reduced rates of gonorrhea and syphilis between 1982 and 1986, which have been observed in London, Stockholm, Seattle, New York, Denver and San Francisco (Bell, 1986; Carne et al., 1987; Gellan & Ison, 1986; Handsfield, 1985). Reduced rates have been observed in heterosexuals as well, although the decline has not been as dramatic. It seems apparent from these changes in sexual behavior in homosexual men that preventive measures and the fear of AIDS are the major factors in motivating change. It is not quite as apparent what is motivating heterosexuals, but no other obvious reason is evident.

In London as well as in Baltimore, Chicago, Los Angeles, Pittsburgh and Washington, D.C., significantly lower seroconversion rates were noted in men who reduced or stopped receptive anal intercourse than in men who continued the practice with at least two or more partners (Kingsley et al., 1987). Major newspapers have reported even more striking results that HIV seropositive homosexual men who stopped receptive anal intercourse reconverted to a seronegative status. Scientists have not as yet confirmed this report. However, it is clear from several studies that modification of this high-risk behavior can have a substantial impact on risk, both as an exposure factor and as a co-factor of HIV infection.

Among IV drug abusers, the risks of infectious co-factors can be reduced significantly by stopping the use of IV drugs, by using disinfected needles and syringes, by stopping needle and equipment sharing, and by decreasing the number of injections. All of these practices, uncorrected, result not only in HIV infection but also in multiple infections among IV drug abusers. Chief among these infections are frequent and chronic soft tissue infections (cellulitis, abscesses), bacterial endocarditis, and the viral hepatitides. In addition, IV drug abusers who use prostitution to support their drug habits are also frequently infected with all of the sexually transmitted diseases described previously. These chronic multiple infections can play a role as co-factors in the progression of disease in HIV-infected individuals. Stopping the use and sharing of dirty and infected needles and syringes could result in reduced HIV infection, reduced number of exposures to the virus, reduced risk of other infections, and thus reduced effects of infectious co-factors. The focus of public health education for drug abusers should be to stop the use of drugs, to stop sharing dirty needles and syringes, and to practice safer sex (use condoms, stop anal receptive intercourse, and reduce number of sexual partners).

There is initial evidence that IV drug abusers in the United States are beginning to change their needle sharing habits out of fear of AIDS (Staff, *NIDA Notes*, 1987). In Europe (Netherlands, England, Italy), the threat of AIDS combined with the availability of clean equipment through needle exchange programs has reduced the number of addicts using contaminated and dirty needles and syringes (Staff, *NIDA Notes*, 1987). Although there has been a reduction in needle sharing, more drug rehabilitation and AIDS education programs are needed for IV drug abusers in the U.S. There are three groups who should be targeted for AIDS prevention and three different program approaches that are needed. First, drug users wanting to stop the IV use of drugs should be given treatment. Second, drug users not likely to stop should be taught safe injection methods. Finally, persons not yet injecting should be educated about the risks of this behavior.

Tertiary Prevention:
Enhancing Immunocompetence

For persons who have developed clinical LAS, ARC, or AIDS, elimination of all the risk factors, both exposure factors and co-factors, discussed previously is necessary to avoid immunosuppression from sources other than HIV. In addition, various therapies other than drugs for enhancing immunocompetence are being tested.

Nutrition. While the exact contribution nutritional status plays in the progression of AIDS is unclear at this time, there are many aspects of malnutrition which have been shown to affect cellular immunodeficiency (Beach and Laura, 1983; Benkov et al., 1985). In general, nutritional aspects play a critical role in host resistance. This has been evident in studies of an association between nutritional status and development of infectious processes, and the outcome of infectious processes and functioning of major organs such as the heart, liver, and GI tract (Chandra & Scrimshaw, 1980; Chlebowski, 1985; Dossetor et al., 1977; Hughes et al., 1974). Profound muscle wasting is evident in heart and respiratory muscle atrophy, and in impaired digestion secondary to inadequate production of pancreatic enzymes and flattened intestinal villi (Bentler and Stanish, 1987).

In a body composition study of 33 persons with AIDS, where measurements of total body potassium, fat, concentrations of serum proteins and albumin and water volume were recorded, Kotler et al. (1985) found that patients with AIDS were significantly underweight, and depleted of potassium, body fat content, serum protein concentrations, and intracellular water volume. The reasons for the development of malnutrition were related to impaired intestinal absorption, intestinal damage due to bacterial parasites or viral infections, intestinal malfunction as a result of malnutrition itself, or decreased pancreatic secretion and intestinal brush border enzyme activities. Other contributing factors to malnutrition include GI manifestations such as oral and esophageal candidiasis and herpes gingivostomatitis, vomiting, and persistent diarrhea and fever (Da Prato and Rothschild, 1986).

Kotler et al. (1985) report that the later course of AIDS is most likely influenced by malnutrition. In particular, the effect of protein-energy malnutrition is significant on the immune system and the ability to deal with infection (Chandra, 1987). Evidence of impaired immunity has been the absent or reduced delayed cutaneous hypersensitivity response to common microbial antigens, decreased number of thymus-dependent T lymphocytes, reduced capacity of neutrophils to kill ingested bacteria, reduced activity of various complement proteins, decreased concentration of IgA antibody, decreased ability to bind antigen, and decreased total number of T lymphocytes, particularly the T helper lymphocyte population. As a result of such changes in the immune defense, development of infectious diseases such as tuberculosis, bacterial diarrhea, herpes, pneumocystis pneumonia (PCP) and candidiasis are increased.

Therapies directed at reversing or altering the progressive weight loss associated with AIDS may be critical (Chlebowski, 1985). Assessment of nutritional status is a necessary first step in supporting these individuals, particularly in a syndrome whose treatment has yet to be discovered. Assessment and follow-up should include anthropometric measures and evaluation of visceral proteins (serum albumin, total iron-binding capacity, a complete blood count, and serum potassium). Blood urea nitrogen, creatinine, and liver function tests should be taken as indicated. Weight should be reassessed at least weekly, and frequent assessment of appetite also is recommended (Bentler & Stanish, 1987).

Provision of a detailed nutritional plan is important to provide guidance in meal preparation (Klug, 1986). As inadequate nutrition may be affected simply by the emotional state of the individual, Schietinger (1986) recommends arranging for volunteers to buy groceries or bring hot cooked food to the house or for friends to visit during mealtimes. To increase calorie intake, the availability of frequent high-calorie, nutrient-dense snacks is recommended. Particularly when oral lesions are evident, the provision of soft or bland foods such as puddings, ice cream, and non-acidic juices can increase caloric intake. Supplementation with vitamins in amounts not greater than one or two times the Recommended Daily Allowance should be considered to offset deficits. When fever is present, protein allowances should be increased by 10% per degree Celsius of fever or 5.4% per degree Fahrenheit of fever (Bentler & Stanish, 1987).

When diarrhea is problematic, the nurse should first try prescribed anti-diarrheals after each loose or watery stool (Schietinger, 1986). Should the stools exceed the recommended daily dose of the medication, it is best then to proceed with around-the-clock administration.

In the event that oral or tube intake is limited, GI tube feeding may provide an alternate supply of nutrients in the presence of a functioning GI system (Bentler & Stanish, 1987). When diarrhea is present or when there is an inability to tolerate bolus feedings, a continuous drip using an enteral feeding pump is indicated. Finally, if oral or GI tube feedings are inadequate or contraindicated, total parenteral nutrition (TPN) may be considered, but with caution, as there is an increased incidence of infection in immunocompromised individuals; long-term TPN has been associated with both increased risk of infection and liver damage.

To maintain and nourish the existing functioning immune system, the diet should be high in protein and calories. Ungvarski (1985) recommends calorie intake can be increased by using extra peanut butter, honey, and sour cream. To increase protein intake, skimmed milk powder can be added to regular milk, and foods such as canned cream soups, cream, cheese, peanut butter, and eggs can be increased. In addition, strategies can be implemented for dealing with altered sense of taste, nausea, and lactose intolerance (Lang et al., 1985).

Zinc Supplementation. Zinc deficiency has been associated with depressed cellular immunity, particularly T4 function, killer T cell function, and thymic involution (Chandra, 1987; Da Prato & Rothschild, 1986). In addition, as seminal fluid contains a fair amount of zinc, multiple ejaculations may be a significant source of zinc loss in an individual who is marginally depleted as a result of inadequate intake or malabsorption. The administration of oral zinc supplement has been found to improve immune responses by increasing numbers of circulating lymphocytes, intracutaneous delayed hypersensitivity reactions, and specific antibody IgG responses to ingested antigens. In addition, zinc administration has been found to offer significant protection against formed mycotoxins and to heal intestinal mucosal lesions (Chandra, 1987; Da Prato and Rothschild, 1986).

Vitamins. Vitamins have been found to be essential for optimum immune functioning. Deficiencies in vitamins A, B6, and E have reportedly led to reduced lymphocyte response to mitogens and antigens, decreased antibody responses, and impaired cellular immunity (Chandra, 1987).

In a clinical study of six patients given ascorbate, patients reportedly had considerable improvement in their condition (remission of biopsy proven Kaposi's sarcoma) (Cathcart, 1984). The reason proposed for the improvement was that ascorbate is able to suppress the symptoms of disease and reduce the tendency for secondary infection because it functions as the premier free radical scavenger and is better able to saturate every cell of the body, making it superior to any other free radical scavenger. Ascorbate was found to neutralize the suppressor factor in AIDS patients in concentrations of 10 to 20 g of ascorbate a day. While some consider this amount far too toxic to use in humans, other research supports the use of high doses and finds this dose is easily tolerated and not toxic (Kalokerinos, 1981; Klenner, 1971; Stone, 1972).

Persons with LAS, ARC, or AIDS should eliminate the use of alcohol and recreational drugs and IV drugs. These have a negative effect on nutrition. They not only suppress appetite but also irritate the GI tract and lead to impaired absorption of food. Damaged liver cells resulting from substance abuse can be responsible for inadequate assimilation of vitamins and amino acids, and can lead to malnourishment.

Damaged liver cells have other negative effects for persons with clinical disease. Many of the therapeutic drugs used to treat the opportunistic infections have toxic side effects. A well-functioning liver is necessary to metabolize these toxins. Finally, alcohol and drugs have immunosuppressant effects and create even greater difficulties for persons whose immune systems are compromised by HIV.

Preventing Polymicrobial Enteric Infection. Other factors which are recognized as potent immunosuppressants are the polymicrobial enteric infections (Matossian, 1986). Toxins produced by the microbial organisms compromise the individual's immune functioning to the point where the AIDS virus is able to express itself in an opportunistic manner (Da Prato & Rothschild, 1986). The pathogenesis of this outcome has been found to include an increase in mucosal cyclic adenosine monophosphate, depression of mucosal immunity leading to diarrhea and further nutrient and electrolyte loss, and altered macrophage phagocytosis and T cell immunologic unresponsiveness.

Nurses can play a crucial role in prevention of enteric infections. It is essential to teach individuals that a low-microbe diet can be achieved by using canned, bottled, and pasteurized foods, broiling and cooking meat well, scrubbing and washing fruits and vegetables, and avoiding prepared foods such as tuna and egg salads, cold meats, and the like (Ungvarski, 1985).

Reducing the number of microbes in the home can be accomplished by using a dilute solution of household bleach to clean surfaces which may come in contact with food. Damp dish towels and sponges are germ catchers; therefore, the use of paper towels is recommended. For persons with pets, rubber gloves should be worn when emptying pet litter boxes or trays and cleaning bird cages.

In addition, persons with LAS, ARC, or AIDS can avoid infection by eliminating anal receptive intercourse or at least using condoms. This sexual practice in the absence of the use of condoms, is associated with many sexually transmitted diseases (e.g., CMV, HBV, HSV, amoebiasis, gonorrhea, and syphilis). Trauma and lesions of the rectal mucosa provide the route for infection to occur. Anal receptive intercourse may be the source of many of the opportunistic infections that flourish in persons with clinical disease.

Reducing Psychological Stress. Psychological stress can be immunosuppressive and play a role in increasing the individual's vulnerability to disease (Dorian et al., 1982; Locke et al., 1984; Linn et al., 1982; McClelland et al., 1982). In studies indicating evident psychological stress, such as a competitive qualifying examination or death in the family, immunologic impairment was documented (Dorian et al., 1982). Research in this area suggests that how a person reacts to the stressor (ability to cope) has a greater impact on immunologic impairment than how much stress was experienced (Locke et al., 1984). In a study of the correlation of self-reported life stress and distress symptoms with natural killer cell activity in 114 healthy undergraduate volunteers, Locke et al. (1984) found subjects who reported major life stressors but few distress symptoms (good copers) had significantly higher natural killer cell activity than those experiencing high levels of distress and life stresses (poor copers).

There is no question that the diagnosis of AIDS presents the individual with major psychological concerns. Moreover, personal characteristics of the individual, such as depression, can result in altered immunologic responses (Linn et al., 1982). In addition, the absence of social support can play a part in the manifestation of disease as a disease facilitating co-factor (Cobb, 1976). The psychologic and social stress experienced and its impact on immunologic function thus may play a significant role in progression of disease. In addition to the stress management approaches discussed earlier in this chapter (exercise, sleep and rest, relaxation techniques), psychosocial nursing interventions can benefit the person with AIDS and are discussed in Chapter 8.

Summary

Risk factors play a major role not only in exposure to HIV infection but also in disease expression and progression. It is crucial that these risk factors be identified and become a focus of public health education programs. Changes in behaviors related to known risk factors have been demonstrated to improve the health of persons at all stages of HIV infection. This information must be communicated to the transmission groups and to the public at large. As new risk factors are identified, these must become a part of health education in the prevention of AIDS. Since health education is a major nursing intervention, it is imperative that nurses make themselves aware of developments in the area of risk factors and HIV infection.

References

Ablin, R.J. (1985). Transglutaminase: Co-factor in aetiology of AIDS? *Lancet*, 1(8432), 813–814.
Ablin, R.J., Gonder, M.J. (1985). Immunological abnormalities in South African homosexuals—a non-infectious co-factor? *South African Medical Journal*, 67, 40.
Ascher, M.S., Francis, D.P. (1987). Is the blood supply safe from AIDS? *California Physician*, 4(7), 18–19.
Beach, R., Laura, P. (1983). Nutrition and the acquired immune deficiency syndrome. *Annals of Internal Medicine*, 99, 565–566.

Bell, S.H. (1986). Incidence of gonorrhoea and fear of AIDS. *Lancet*, 2(8516), 1159.

Benkov, K., Stawski, C., Sirlin, C., et al. (1985). Atypical presentation of childhood acquired immune deficiency syndrome mimicking Crohn's Disease: Nutritional considerations and management. *The American Journal of Gastroenterology*, 80, 260–265.

Bentler, M., Stanish, M. (1987). Nutrition support of the pediatric patient with AIDS. *Perspectives in Practice*, 87, 488–491.

Bentwich, Z., Saxinger, Z., Ben-Ishay, R., et al. (1987). Immune impairments and antibodies to HTLV III/ LAV in asymptomatic male homosexuals in Israel: Relevance to the risk of AIDS. *AIDS Targeted Information Newsletter*, 1(10), 9.

Bienzle, U., Guggenmoos-Holzmann, I., Zwingenberger, K., et al. (1985). Lymphadenopathy and antibodies to HTLV-III in homosexual men. *Klinische Wochen-schrift*, 63, 597–602.

Blattner, W.A. (1986). Etiology and prevention of acquired immunodeficiency syndrome: The path of interdisciplinary research. *Journal of Chronic Disease*, 39(12), 1125–1144.

Blattner, W.A., Biggar, R.J., Weiss, S.H., et al. (1985). Epidemiology of human T-lymphotropic virus type III and the risk of the acquired immunodeficiency syndrome. *Annals of Internal Medicine*, 103(5), 665–670.

Carne, C.A., Johnson, A.M., Pearce, F., et al. (1987). Prevalence of antibodies to human immunodeficiency virus, gonorrhoea rates, and changed sexual behavior in homosexual men in London. *Lancet*, 1(8534), 656–658.

Cathcart, R. (1984). Vitamin C in the treatment of acquired immune deficiency syndrome (AIDS). *Medical Hypothesis*, 14, 423–433.

Chaisson, R.E., Moss, A.R., Onishi, R., et al. (1987). Human immunodeficiency virus infection in heterosexual intravenous drug users in San Francisco. *American Journal of Public Health*, 77(2), 169–172.

Chandra, R. (1987). Nutrition and immunity: I. Basic considerations. II. Practical applications. *Journal of Dentistry for Children*, 54(3), 193–197.

Chandra, R., Scrimshaw, N. (1980). Immunocompetence in nutritional assessment. *American Journal of Clinical Nutrition*, 33, 2694–2698.

Chlebowski, R. (1985). Significance of altered nutritional status of acquired immune deficiency syndrome. *Nutrition and Cancer*, 7, 85–91.

Cobb, S. (1976). Social support as a moderator of life stress. *Psychosomatic Medicine*, 3, 300–314.

Collier, A.C., Meyers, J.D., Corey, L., et al. (1987). Cytomegalovirus infection in homosexual men. *The American Journal of Medicine*, 82, 593–601.

Conte, D., Ferroni, G.P., Lorini, G.P., et al. (1987). HIV and HBV infection in intravenous drug addicts from Northeastern Italy. *AIDS Targeted Information Newsletter*, 1(10), 9.

Cowell, S. (1986). Emerging risk factors for acquired immune deficiency syndrome and risk reduction education. *Journal of Applied Community Health*, 34, 216–219.

DaPrato, R., Rothschild, J. (1986). The AIDS virus as an opportunistic organism inducing a state of chronic relative cortisol excess: Therapeutic implications. *Medical Hypotheses*, 21(3), 253–266.

Dorian, B., Garfinkel, P., Brown, G., et al. (1982). Aberrations in lymphocyte subpopulations and function during psychological stress. *Clinical and Experimental Immunology*, 50, 132–138.

Dossetor, J., Whittle, J., Greenwood, B. (1977). Persistent measles infection in malnourished children. *British Medical Journal*, 2, 1633–1635.

Evans, B.A., Dawson, S.G., McLean, K.A., et al. (1986). Sexual lifestyle and clinical findings related to HTLV-III/LAV status in homosexual men. *Genitourinary Medicine*, 62, 384–389.

Faltz, B.G., Madover, S. (1986). AIDS and substance abuse: Issues for health care providers. *Focus*, 1(9), 1–2.

Flaskerud, J.H. (1988). Prevention of AIDS in Blacks and Hispanics: Nursing implications. *Journal of Community Health Nursing*, 5(1), 49–58.

Francis, D.P., Chin, J. (1987). The prevention of acquired immunodeficiency syndrome in the United States—an objective strategy for medicine, public health, business, and the community. *Journal of the American Medical Association*, 257(10), 1357–1366.

Friedman-Kien, A.E., Lafleur, F.L., Gendler, E., et al. (1986). Herpes zoster: A possible early clinical sign for development of acquired immunodeficiency syndrome in high-risk individuals. *Journal of American Academy of Dermatology*, 14, 1023–1028.

Furth, P.A. (1987). Heterosexual transmission of AIDS by male drug users. *Nature*, 327, 193.

Gellan, M.C.A., Ison, C.A. (1986). Declining incidence of gonorrhoea in London: A response to fear of AIDS? *Lancet*, 2(8512), 920.

Getchell, J.P., Heath, J.L., Hicks, D.R., et al. (1987). Detection of human T cell leukemia virus type I and human immunodeficiency virus in cultured lymphocytes of a Zairian man with AIDS. *The Journal of Infectious Diseases*, 155(4), 612–616.

Ginzburg, H.M., Weiss, S.H., MacDonald, M.G., et al. (1985). HTLV-III exposure among drug users. *Cancer Research* (suppl.), 45, 4605s–4608s.

Goedert, J.J. (1984). Recreational drugs: Relationship to AIDS. *Annals of the New York Academy of Sciences*, 437, 192–199.

Goedert, J.J., Biggar, R.J., Winn, D.M., et al. (1985). Decreased helper T lymphocytes in homosexual men. *American Journal of Epidemiology*, 121(5), 637–644.

Goedert, J.J., Biggar, R.J., Weiss, S.H., et al. (1986). Three-year incidence of AIDS in five cohorts of HTLV-III infected risk group members. *Science*, 231, 992–995.

Groopman, J.E., Mayer, K.H., Sarngadharan, M.G., et al. (1985). Seroepidemiology of human T-lymphotropic virus type III among homosexual men with the acquired immunodeficiency syndrome or generalized lymphadenopathy and among asymptomatic controls in Boston. *Annals of Internal Medicine*, 102, 334–337.

Guinan, M.E., Hardy, A. (1987). Epidemiology of AIDS in women in the United States—1981 through 1986. *Journal of the American Medical Association*, 257(15), 2039–2042.

Guinan, M.E., Thomas, P.A., Pinsky, P.F., et al. (1984). Heterosexual and homosexual patients with the acquired immunodeficiency syndrome. *Annals of Internal Medicine*, 100, 213–218.

Halbert, S.P., Kiefer, D.J., Friedman-Kien, A.E., et al. (1986). Antibody levels for cytomegalovirus, herpes simplex virus, and rubella in patients with acquired immune deficiency syndrome. *Journal of Clinical Microbiology*, 23(2), 318–321.

Handsfield, H.H. (1985). Decreasing incidence of gonorrhea in homosexually active men—minimal effect on risk of AIDS. *Western Journal of Medicine*, 143, 469–470.

Hefferin, E.A. (1980). Life cycle stressors: An overview of research. *Family and Community Health*, 2, 71–90.

Hersh, E.M., Reuben, J.M., Mansell, P.W.A., et al. (1983). Immunologic studies of the acquired immune deficiency syndrome: Relationship of immunodeficiency to extent of disease. *Annals of the New York Academy of Sciences*, 364–372.

Hughes, W., Price, R., Sisko, F. (1974). Protein-calorie malnutrition: A host determinant for pneumocystis carinii infection. *American Journal of Diseases of Childhood*, 128, 44–52.

Jeffries, E., Willoughby, B., Boyko, W.J., et al. (1985). The Vancouver lymphadenopathy—AIDS study: 2. Seroepidemiology of HTLV-III antibody. *Canadian Medical Association Journal*, 132, 1373–1377.

Kalokerinos, A. (1981). *Every second child*. New Canaan: Keats Publishing.

Kingsley, L.A., Kaslow, R., Rinaldo, C.R., Jr., et al. (1987). Risk factors for seroconversion to human immunodeficiency virus among male homosexuals. *Lancet*, 1(8529), 345–349.

Klein, J.O. (1984). Current concepts of infectious diseases in the newborn infant. In *Infectious Diseases in the Newborn Infant*. Chicago: Year Book Medical Publishers, Inc., pp.405–446.

Klenner, F. (1971). Observations on the dose and administration of ascorbic acid when employed beyond a range of a vitamin in human pathology. *Journal of Applied Nutrition*, 23, 61–88.

Klug, R. (1986). Children with AIDS. *American Journal of Nursing*, 86, 1126–1132.

Kotler, D., Wang, J., Pierson, R. (1985). Body composition studies in patients with the acquired immunodeficiency syndrome. *The American Journal of Clinical Nutrition*, 42, 1255–1265.

Lang, J., Spiegel, J., Strigle, S. (1985). *Living with AIDS: A self-care manual*. AIDS Project Los Angeles.

Latchman, D.S. (1987). Herpes infection and AIDS. *Nature*, 325, 487.

Linn, B., Linn, M., Jensen, J. (1982). Degree of depression and immune responsiveness. *Psychosomatic Medicine*, 44, 128–132.

Locke, S., Kraus, L., Leserman, J. et al. (1984). Life change stress, psychiatric symptoms, and natural killer cell activity. *Psychosomatic Medicine*, 46(5), 441–453.

Matossian, M. (1986). Did mycotoxins play a role in bubonic plague epidemics? *Perspectives in Biology and Medicine*, 29, 244–256.

McClelland, D., Alexander, C., Marks, E. (1982). The need for power, stress, immune function and illness among male prisoners. *Journal of Abnormal Psychology*, 91, 61–70.

McCombie, S.C. (1986). Tonsillectomy as a co-factor in the development of AIDS. *Medical Hypotheses*, 19, 291–293.

McKenna, J.J., Miles, R., Lemen, D., et al. (1986).Unmasking AIDS: Chemical immunosuppression and seronegative syphilis. *Medical Hypotheses*, 21, 421–430.

Melbye, M., Goedert, J.J., Grossman, R.J., et al. (1987). Risk of AIDS after herpes zoster. *Lancet*, 1(8535), 728–731.

Mondanaro, J. (1987). Strategies for AIDS prevention: Motivating health behavior in drug dependent women. *Journal of Psychoactive Drugs*, 19(2), 143–149.

Moss, A.R., Osmond, D., Bacchetti, P., et al. (1987). Risk factors for AIDS and HIV seropositivity in homosexual men. *American Journal of Epidemiology*, 125(6), 1035–1047.

New York Times, February 5, 1988.

Newell, G.R., Mansell, P.W.A., Wilson, M.B., et al. (1985a). Risk factor analysis among men referred for possible acquired immune deficiency syndrome. *Preventive Medicine*, 14, 81–91.

Newell, G.R., Mansell, P.W.A., Spitz, M.R., et al. (1985b). Volatile nitrites—use and adverse effects related to the current epidemic of the acquired immune deficiency syndrome. *The American Journal of Medicine*, 78, 811–816.

Osborn, J.E. (1986). Co-factors and HIV: What determines the pathogenesis of AIDS? *Bio Essays*, 5(6), 287–289.

Potterat, J.J., Muth, J.B., Markewich, G.S. (1986). Serological markers as indicators of sexual orientation in AIDS virus–infected men. *Journal of the American Medical Association*, 256(6), 712.

Prince, H.E., Kreiss, J.K., Kasper, C.K., et al. (1985). Distinctive lymphocyte subpopulation abnormalities in patients with congenital coagulation disorders who exhibit lymph node enlargement. *Blood*, 66(1), 64–68.

Redfield, R.R., Markham, P.D., Salahuddin, S.Z., et al. (1985). Heterosexually acquired HTLV-III/LAV disease (AIDS-related complex and AIDS). *Journal of the American Medical Association*, 254(15), 2094–2096.

Robert-Guroff, M., Weiss, S.H., Giron, J.A., et al. (1986). Prevalence of antibodies to HTLV-I, -II, and -III in intravenous drug abusers from an AIDS endemic region. *Journal of the American Medical Association*, 255(22), 3133–3137.

Samuel, M., Winkelstein, W. (1987). Prevalence of human immunodeficiency virus infection in ethnic minority homosexual/bisexual men. *Journal of the American Medical Association*, 257(14), 1901–1902.

Sandor, E.V., Millman, A., Croxson, T.S., et al. (1986). Herpes zoster ophthalmicus in patients at risk for the acquired immune deficiency syndrome (AIDS). *American Journal of Ophthalmology*, 101, 153–155.

Schechter, M.T., Boyko, W.J., Jeffries, E., et al. (1985a). The Vancouver lymphadenopathy—AIDS study: 4. Effects of exposure factors, cofactors and HTLV-III seropositivity on number of helper T cells. *Canadian Medical Association Journal*, 133, 286–292.

Schechter, M.T., Boyko, W.J., Jeffries, E., et al. (1985b). The Vancouver lymphadenopathy—AIDS study: 1. Persistent generalized lymphadenopathy. *Canadian Medical Association Journal*, 132, 1273–1279.

Schietinger, H. (1986). A home care plan for AIDS. *American Journal of Nursing*, 86(9), 1021–1028.

Scott, G.B., Fischl, M.A., Klimas, N., et al. (1985). Mothers of infants with the acquired immunodeficiency syndrome. *Journal of the American Medical Association*, 252, 363–366.

Seligmann, M., Chess, L., Fahey, J.L., et al. (1984). AIDS—an immunologic reevaluation. *New England Journal of Medicine*, 311(20), 1286–1292.

Shearer, G.M., Levy, R.B. (1984). Noninfectious cofactors in susceptibility to AIDS: Possible contributions of semen, HLA alloantigens, and lack of natural resistance. *Annals of the New York Academy of Sciences*, 437, 49–57.

Siegel, L. (1986). AIDS: Relationship to alcohol and other drugs. *Journal of Substance Abuse Treatment*, 3, 271–274.

Sindrup, J.H., Weismann, K., Wantzin, G.L. (1986). Syphilis in HTLV-III infected male homosexuals. *AIDS Research*, 2(4), 285–288.

Sonnabend, J.A., Witkin, S.S., Purtilo, D.T. (1984). A multifactorial model for the development of AIDS in homosexual men. *Annals of the New York Academy of Sciences*, 437, 177–183.

Staff (1987). Gammaglobulin being used to treat pediatric AIDS cases. *AIDS Record*, 1(7), 6.

Staff (1987). International experts discuss needle sharing and AIDS. *National Institute on Drug Abuse Notes*, 2(3), 1–2.

Stone, I. (1972). *The Healing Factor: Vitamin C Against Disease.* New York: Grosset and Dunlap.

Tallon, D.F., Darach Corcoran, D.J., O'Dwyer, E.M., et al. (1984). Circulating lymphocyte sub-populations in pregnancy: a longitudinal study. *Journal of Immunology,* 132, 1784–1787.

Ungvarski, P. (1985). Learning to live with AIDS. *Nursing Mirror,* 160, 20–22.

van Griensven, G.J.P., Tielman, R.A.P., Goudsmit, J., et al. (1987). Risk factors and prevalence of HIV antibodies in homosexual men in the Netherlands. *American Journal of Epidemiology,* 125(6), 1048–1057.

Vetrosky, D.T., Schmidt, B.A., Sobio, H. (1987). AIDS and the hemophilia patient. *Physician Assistant,* 11, 19–31.

Wainberg, M.A., Portnoy, J., Tsoukas, C., et al. (1987). Specific stimulation of lymphocytes from patients with AIDS by herpes simplex virus antigens. *Immunology,* 60, 275–280.

Weber, J.N., Rogers, L.A., Scott, K., et al. (1986). Three-year prospective study of HTLV-III/LAV infection in homosexual men. *Lancet,* 1(8491), 1179–1182.

Weiss, S.H., Ginzberg, H.M., Goedert, J.J., et al. (1985). Risk of HTLV-III exposure and AIDS among parenteral drug abusers in New Jersey. *The International Conference on the Acquired Immunodeficiency Syndrome: Abstracts.* Philadelphia: American College of Physicians.

Winkelstein, W., Jr., Lyman, D.M., Padian, N., et al. (1987). Sexual practices and risk of infection by the human immunodeficiency virus—the San Francisco men's health study. *Journal of the American Medical Association,* 257(3), 321–325.

Wofsy, C.B. (1987). Human immunodeficiency virus infection in women. *Journal of the American Medical Association,* 257 (15), 2074–2076.

Chapter 10

Community Issues

Adeline M. Nyamathi
Michael Hedderman

The impact of AIDS on the community has been overwhelming. Nurses and other health care professionals along with private and public organizations are now joining together to promote health and prevent the spread of this dreaded disease in the community.

Nurses are involved in the community in the prevention of AIDS through public health education, counseling the public about sexual practices, counseling persons who have human immunodeficiency virus (HIV) infections and AIDS-related complex (ARC), and making referrals to community resources for education, testing, and support. Prevention and education activities take place in health settings, social settings, and occupational or work settings. In addition, nurses provide direct care to clients with AIDS and their families in community settings such as homes, clinics, long-term care facilities, and hospice facilities. Direct care includes case management of the client's physical, emotional, and social needs as well as education on the disease; financial, housing, and health resources; and referrals to community AIDS services, centers, and support groups.

Prevention of AIDS/HIV Infection:
Implications for Education, Counseling and Referrals

Because there is currently no cure or vaccine for AIDS, education relating to its prevention is the only way to curb the epidemic. In order to make an impact, education programs must be targeted for all individuals, regardless of risk classification. Most importantly, the content of programs should be culturally sensitive, tailored to the educational level of the population served, and address aspects such as the etiology and signs and symptoms of HIV infection, risk assessment and reduction, diagnostic strategies, and screening modalities. In addition, as a result of the tremendous social stigma that AIDS has evoked, of significant importance is the provision of psychosocial, legal, and ethical counseling. Lastly, persons in the community should become familiar with the multitude of resources which exist should the need for support be manifested.

The strategy for providing health education for the community at large is an issue that has long been debated by health professionals and community organizations. An existing barrier that has diminished society's realization of the extent of this dreaded disease is explained by the Centers for Disease Control's (CDC) illustration of AIDS as the tip of an iceberg. Society is able to see only the visible tip of the iceberg which represents persons diagnosed with AIDS; few individuals realize that below the tip looms an invisible base that includes persons who are not as yet diagnosed with AIDS, who are asymptomatic or who suffer from symptoms and illnesses which result from HIV infection. As a result, society is unaware of the thousands of asymptomatic individuals who are seropositive for the AIDS antibody. This lack of knowledge consequently plays a key role in the transmission of HIV. Other barriers which present difficulty for effective education include the emotionally laden issues of homosexuality/bisexuality and intravenous (IV) drug abuse and the necessity for health professionals to discuss sensitive and intimate aspects of sexual practice, as well as protective strategies in the use of illegal drugs. Such issues may naturally evoke discomfort for educators and learners alike. Lastly, the absolute need for outreach to groups that are at highest risk for exposure to AIDS, such as prostitutes, drug abusers, homosexuals, and bisexuals, or to groups that are socioculturally diverse, such as the urban poor or racial/ethnic minorities, is difficult because these groups are often the segments of the population hardest to reach.

Education

In order to enhance the hope that the transmission of AIDS can be curbed and promote such a reality, nurses must primarily focus their attention on groups of persons whose behaviors put them at high risk for AIDS. According to July 1987 CDC statistics, over 95% of the population with AIDS belong to one of the following groups: sexually active homosexual or bisexual men, present or past abusers of intravenous drugs, individuals who have had transfusions with blood or blood products, persons with hemophilia or other coagulation disorders, persons who have had sexual contact with someone with AIDS or at risk for AIDS, and infants born to infected mothers. Prevention efforts must provide information on each of the main transmission routes and must be relevant to age, education, economic factors, cultural factors, and sexual orientation. Currently prevention and education programs have been targeted mostly at white homosexual men and white heterosexual women. Plans are under way for a massive public health education program in the schools. Heterosexual and bisexual men and ethnic/racial groups other than whites and IV drug abusers have not had adequate public health education to prevent the spread of HIV infection and AIDS.

Homosexual men are politically and socially organized and more educated than the other transmission groups. These characteristics provide advantages and opportunities for public health education. A highly educated group is more receptive of education; political and social organizations take the lead in education and provide settings, support, and opportunities for education. The educational focus for homosexual and bisexual men is to stop anal receptive sex or at a minimum use condoms and to decrease (preferably to one) the number of sexual partners.

However, education strategies for reaching the public must be targeted for individuals who rarely seek health care as well as the health conscious groups. IV drug abusers exemplify a hard to reach group. Creative strategies aimed at the hard to reach groups must be devised, for instance training accepted and trusted members of the subgroup such as reformed drug dealers and abusers to spread the facts about prevention of transmission of the AIDS virus. Providing advice on cleaning needles and syringes (or works) for individuals refusing to stop using IV drugs or proposing needle exchange programs are yet other strategies which may be considered controversial by some persons in the health professions, but may represent the only means to access certain segments of the population.

Particular focus on educating the female population is essential, as informed women can have a positive impact on curbing perinatal transmission and sexual transmission of AIDS in their present and future partners. Women have traditionally held social and cultural roles and strong family values that make them key figures in the education of the community. The values placed on maintaining and supporting the family network, on mothering, nurturing and care of the sick among women help ensure the spread of health education in the community. These characteristics are evident in ethnic/racial minority communities as well as in white communities. Black women have a strong and independent role in the Black community. Black family networks are extensive and cohesive and provide valuable services that include socialization, care, support, mutual aid, and advice (Staples, 1981). In addition, Black women are frequently involved in social, public, and religious service outside the home. Hispanic women, though often characterized as submissive, play important roles in influencing family members. Furthermore, Hispanic women also play important roles in public service and education. Because of the values placed on motherhood, they have a special influence on husbands and sons (Fitzpatrick, 1981). Hispanics also have cohesive extended family networks and a strong sense of family obligation (Alvirez et al., 1981; Fitzpatrick, 1981).

For themselves, women need to be aware that AIDS is often manifested differently in females than in males, which may result in delayed health care, more severe presentation of the disease, and prolonged hospitalization (Mantell et al., 1987; Shaw, 1986). In addition, women need to know about the risks of pregnancy to women who are HIV positive. Pregnancy is immunosuppressive and accelerates the rate of disease expression. Women should be educated regarding the use of IV drugs, birth control, abortion, and high-risk-group partners. A special emphasis should be placed on the education of women of color, who are becoming a group which deserves intensified attention. Latest statistics clearly demonstrate that while to date only 7% of all AIDS cases are female, 70% of these are Black and Hispanic, and 29% occur in heterosexual relationships. Even more striking is the statistic that heterosexual cases of AIDS have increased at twice the rate of homosexual cases over the past year (CDC, 1987).

For individuals who seek regular or periodic health care, sexually transmitted disease clinics, drug treatment centers, hemophilia treatment centers, and perinatal and family planning clinics are practice settings where the need for prevention activities exist. Education can be enhanced by displaying AIDS educational literature in waiting rooms and examining rooms and by having the literature available in languages spoken by the population being served (Shaw, 1986). Increased awareness of AIDS and facts relating to transmission of the virus can be displayed by educational graphics on the walls and by means of the medical intake questionnaire that is administered to all new clients. Finally, nurses providing direct patient care are in a unique position to deliver risk reduction information. In most settings, it is the nurse who spends a considerable amount of time with clients and who is most suited to accurately assess a client's awareness of risk reduction and provide the most valued information.

The CDC and the Surgeon General have recommended that AIDS prevention be taught in schools and some states have mandated this specific instruction. Any student who is sexually active, using drugs, or sexually abused is at risk for contracting AIDS; however, the adolescent is generally considered most vulnerable. The most efficient means of disseminating information to young people is through the schools and beginning no later than the seventh grade. AIDS prevention curricula should include etiology, methods of transmission, precautions and techniques for prevention, need for abstinence, conditions and infections seen in the disease, a comparison of AIDS to other sexually transmitted diseases, and necessary changes in behavior, such as use of condoms and reducing the number of sexual partners. Information on the risks of IV drug use should include resources and counseling services. If the school provides a family life or sex education program, the AIDS material can be incorporated into that curriculum.

Counseling

Psychosocial Support. Due to the devastating nature of the disease and the fear and isolation which accompany it, an awareness of the need for psychosocial support is critically important to reinforce. While psychosocial adjustment to illness is dependent upon the individual's previous level of psychosocial adjustment and social support, persons at greatest risk for AIDS—homosexuals, drug abusers, and prostitutes—may be at increased risk for maladaptive psychological and social adjustment as a result of limited social networks and estranged family ties.

The provision of psychosocial support is essential in motivating these PWAs to accept the limitations of their illness, which includes facing the fear of death, possible disfigurement, and debilitation. Persons with HIV infection and AIDS must maintain a sense of control over their lives and promote a quality of life which is rewarding and worth living. Nurses can best assist individuals in achieving these goals by adequately preparing persons with HIV infection and AIDS regarding health promotion, lifestyle factors, and treatment options and assisting them in decision-making processes.

The threat of AIDS has reportedly affected the quality of life of many healthy homosexual individuals as well. Presenting complaints oftentimes include insomnia, anxiety, and severe somatic symptoms. Affirming the practice of safer sex, supporting the practice of getting involved with other people on other than sexual terms, and spending time discussing fears can often help to distinguish between realistic concerns and imagined risks or fears. In addition, the use of relaxation exercises, positive visualization techniques, self-hypnosis, and professional therapeutic relationships oftentimes enhances coping effectiveness.

In order for psychosocial interventions to be based upon documented need, it is essential that the nurse obtain a brief psychosocial assessment. During the interview process, a sense of dignity can be fostered by portraying a positive regard by verbal and nonverbal behaviors, by therapeutic communication skills, and by the maintenance of a private and confidential environment. The assessment should include information about the nature and stability of the patient's residential and occupational arrangements, the quality of his or her relationships with family, partners and significant others, and the amount of socioemotional support these individuals can provide. In addition, information regarding the person's reactions to and knowledge of his or her disease, beliefs, attitudes, and expectations regarding treatment and outcome, and some preliminary information about usual coping ability would assist nurses in providing the most appropriate resources available (Christ & Wiener, 1985).

Community resources worth investigating include self-help groups for persons with HIV infection and AIDS and their families and partners. By providing access to individuals who experience similar situations, self-help groups can help dispel feelings of isolation and loneliness, enhance quality of life, and give a sense of dignity and hope. Reportedly, many of these self-help groups have been successful in helping members remain sexual and enjoy life to the fullest. Strategies employed by self-help groups include discussions of specific physical and sexual behaviors which serve to reduce anxiety and strengthen new or existing relationships. Self-help affiliations have also responded to the special needs of people with AIDS by providing housing, help with daily chores, and surrogate emotional families when necessary. (Additional information on the psychosocial care of persons with AIDS can be found in Chapter 8.)

Sexual History Taking and Sexual Counseling. Since AIDS is often a sexually transmitted disease, assessing the client's awareness and practice of sexually risky behaviors is an imperative first step in prevention. (Additional information on sexual history taking can be found in Chapter 5.) It is essential, therefore, for nurses to discuss sex with their clients in detail and with great sensitivity. Particularly since the topics of sexuality and sexual practices are of utmost privacy and intimacy, it is especially important for the nurse to be as comfortable as possible when providing counseling or questioning about sexual behaviors. An optimal comfort level in nurses will promote a sense of comfort and enhance a nonthreatening relationship with their clients.

Wells and colleagues (1986, 1987), contend that it is best to alert clients of the need to discuss their sexual practices. Providing an explanation for why it is important to talk about sex, acknowledging the difficulty of discussing sexuality, and reassuring the individual that it is OK to be embarrassed are strategies to help ensure a trusting and comforting relationship between health professional and client. In addition, a sense of control can be enhanced by assuring clients that while honesty is of high regard, they may refrain from answering questions that are too difficult or embarrassing to answer at the present time. Nurses should be able to recognize signs of discomfort in the client by manifestations such as vague answers, silence or signs of embarrassment and promptly defer questioning until a future time.

Suggested strategies which may ensure valued communication between nurse and client include active listening whereby nonverbal indicators of listening such as nodding, leaning forward, and maintaining eye contact are manifested; providing periodic facilitative comments such as "please go on" and using open-ended questions. Talking with clients about sex requires effective use of language. Nurses who speak in anatomic terms such as "penis" and "vagina" may be less able to portray their meaning to less educated or culturally diverse individuals, who may be more comfortable with slang. This issue is particularly important when talking to teenagers about sex. An effective strategy nurses can employ to validate their ability in getting across information on sexual practices is to ask the individual to explain what has been discussed. Nurses may be surprised by the new terminology that can be learned and utilized.

Wells (1987) stipulates that in order for nurses to be effective counselors, a nonjudgmental attitude is imperative, since rejection of a person's sexuality may often be viewed as a rejection of the client as a person. If nurses are not in a position to be nonjudgmental, an explanation should be given to the client with an offer to find another health care provider.

The basic information which should be obtained by the nurse in taking a sexual history is displayed in Table 10–1. Sensitive questioning is of critical importance in obtaining this information. In providing insightful strategies for effective history taking, Wells (1987) recommends that the interviewer should not assume that people are generally sexually active. In addition, normalizing the behavior to

Table 10–1. Basic Sexual Information

Marital status
Current sexual status (active or nonactive)
Number of current partners and extramarital affairs
Sexual preference(s)
Frequency of sexual intercourse
Number of sexual partners in the last year
Number of anonymous sexual partners
Level of satisfaction with sexual activity
Specification of sexual practices
Regularity of using contraceptives
Use of condoms (practices and attitudes)
History of specific venereal disease(s)
Knowledge of venereal diseases and how they are acquired
Participation in sexual activities which increase the risk of AIDS

Adapted from Wells (1987).

be discussed is helpful in enhancing honest communication. For example, the question, "Many people your age are sexually active. Are you sexually active?" connotes to the client an accepting and open environment to discuss sexual practices. In addition, the replacement of pronouns of gender and such terms as "husband" and "wife" with the term "partner" may alleviate many awkward moments and promote therapeutic discussion (Irish, 1983). Well-constructed questions which will assist interviewers in ascertaining extremely sensitive yet critically important sexual issues are given in Table 10–2.

Counseling people about safer sex practices and reducing high-risk activities is an essential part of the sexual counseling process (Carr & Gee, 1986). By accurately assessing an individual's sexual practices and his or her attitudes, beliefs, and feelings about lifestyle, nurses are best able to determine the individual's present and potential risk of exposure as a basis for designing appropriate counseling.

Table 10–2. Clinically Sensitive Sexual Questions

Many people your age are sexually active. Are you sexually active?
Are you married or in a regular sexual relationship?
Many people are sexually active with more than one person. How many persons are you sexually active with?
Are you sexually active with men? with women? or with men and women?
The next question might offend you, but it is important for me to know in some detail about your sexual preferences. As you know some people have sexual relationships with persons of the same sex, others with persons of the opposite sex. What is your sexual preference?
How often are you having sex these days?
It is particularly important for me to know if you have had any venereal diseases and the kinds you have had.
Now I would like to know some information about the sexual practices you engage in to help me determine with you whether any of these activities may increase your chance of acquiring diseases.
Can you describe the types of foreplay and intercourse activities that you use most often?
Have you ever engaged in any of the following activities: Anal sex? Oral sex? How long ago did you engage in these activities? Were you using a condom at the time? How would you feel about using condoms, or having your partner use condoms, during intercourse?

Adapted from Wells (1987).

Table 10–3. Risk Reduction Through Safer Sex Practices

Absolutely Safe
Abstinence
Mutually monogamous with noninfected
  partner

Safe	*Possibly Safe*
Mutual masturbation	French kissing (wet)
Social kissing (dry)	Anal intercourse (with condom)
Body massage, hugging	Vaginal intercourse (with condom)
Body to body rubbing (frottage)	Fellatio interruptus (oral-genital;
Light S&M activities (without	stop before climax)
bleeding)	Urine contact (water sports)
Using one's own sex toys	Cunnilingus (oral-vaginal contact)
Fantasy, voyeurism	

Risky
Anal intercourse without condom
  (especially for receptive partner)
Manual-anal intercourse (fisting)
Fellatio (especially with semen ingestion)
Oral-anal contact (rimming)
Blood contact
Urine or semen ingestion
Vaginal intercourse without condom

Adapted from Carr & Gee (1986).

In order to be effective, nurses must provide counseling which is not only sensitive and supportive but also presented in a realistic and nonjudgmental manner, since abrupt, unrealistic lifestyle changes produce only short-term results (Carr & McGee, 1986). For example, providing advice for individuals to reduce their number of sex partners and practicing safer sex rather than preaching abstinence from sexual activity are realistic and nonjudgmental ways whereby nurses can effectively curb the spread of AIDS.

Aside from being instructed in safer sex practices, individuals need to be aware of how HIV is spread and how to protect themselves from the transmission of the AIDS virus in other ways (Table 10–3). This includes reducing the number of sexual partners, especially anonymous contacts and persons who have had multiple partners, refraining from injecting self with illicit drugs or sharing needles, and not having sexual contact with people who inject drugs. In addition, individuals should be counseled that condoms and spermicides, in particular, nonoxynol-9, can reduce the risk of transmission of infection. However, individuals should be well informed that improper use of the condom or mishaps (such as tearing and leakage) may account for as much as a 17% failure rate of the condom as an effective barrier.

HIV Antibody Test Counseling. People in the community need to know that antibody testing is available at a variety of test sites in most states and through private doctors and clinics. Information about where to get tested can be provided by state and local health departments, local American Red Cross chapters, and community blood services. However, before planning to take the test, counseling

Table 10–4. Client Counseling About HIV Antibody Test Results

The HIV antibody is a protein naturally produced in the body in response to HIV. The test is highly but not completely accurate.

A Positive Test Result DOES Mean

Antibodies to HIV are present in your blood
You have been infected and your body has produced antibodies
You probably have active virus in your body and should assume you are contagious and capable of passing virus on to others

A Positive Test DOES NOT Mean

You necessarily have AIDS, ARC or LAS
You will necessarily get AIDS, ARC or LAS later on
You are immune to AIDS

A Negative Test Result DOES Mean

Antibodies to HIV are not present in your blood at this time. Three possible reasons for this are:

You have not been infected with the virus, OR
You have had contact with the virus but have not become infected and therefore have not produced antibodies, OR
You have been infected with the virus but have not yet produced antibodies (which usually takes from two weeks to six months, but can be even longer)

A Negative Test DOES NOT Mean

You have nothing to worry about; AIDS is still at epidemic proportions
You are immune to this virus
You have not yet been infected with the virus: you may have been infected and not yet produced antibodies

Adapted from Carr & Gee (1986).

before and after testing is imperative. The implications of HIV antibody testing have been discussed in detail (Bayer et al., 1986). As portrayed by Carr and Gee (1986), the critical issues to be discussed include the significance of positive and negative test results (Table 10–4).

For individuals who are confirmed positive for HIV antibody, it is essential to let them know that once antibody positive they are considered potentially infectious to others by any of the routes that AIDS is transmitted, such as by exchange of bodily fluids, perinatally, breastfeeding, sharing needles or donating blood. In addition, they also should be counseled in the use of condoms and spermicides, which can reduce the risk of transmission of infection.

All antibody positive individuals need counseling to help them cope with the implications of a positive antibody test, as well as to educate them as to what they can and cannot do to protect themselves and others around them. A person who tests positive should be encouraged to see a physician for a thorough checkup and follow-up care. Antibody positive individuals should be instructed to:

1. Inform their sexual partners. Persons who need help in doing this should be referred for counseling. The HIV antibody positive individual and the partner should be made aware of the risks of continued sexual activity and instructed in safer sex techniques.

2. Not share toothbrushes, razors, tweezers, or other items that may become contaminated with blood.

3. Not donate blood, organs, sperm, or other body tissues.

4. Not use drugs, but if they do continue, to be sure not to share needles or syringes, and to enroll in a drug treatment program.

5. Clean spills of blood or other body fluids with household bleach diluted with water (one part bleach to 10 parts water).

6. Inform their doctors, dentists, or other health care workers who provide care about their antibody status.

7. Inform past sexual partners or persons with whom they have shared needles or syringes about the positive test.

8. Avoid pregnancy.

The antibody positive individual should also be instructed in healthy living. Appropriate nutrition, adequate sleep and rest, physical exercise, stress reduction, and avoiding infections all take on an extra dimension of importance. The promotion of a healthy lifestyle is believed to have positive effects on the immune system (Lang, 1985). Every effort possible should be made to protect the confidentiality of persons who are HIV-infected. Counseling, support, and referrals should be provided.

Referrals

Ensure Adequate Financial, Housing and Health Resources. As a result of the mass media sensationalism given to the AIDS epidemic over the past two years, hysterical public reaction has at times led to the ostracism of persons with AIDS based on fear. Social stigma has often led to the loss of employment and resultant loss of medical insurance. In addition, as landlords have became cognizant of the AIDS diagnosis, a fear of exposure or unstable financial condition has led to the loss of housing as well.

Self-care manuals such as *Living with AIDS* (1985) and *Surviving and Thriving with AIDS* (1987) outline strategies which can assist persons with AIDS or other AIDS-related conditions to apply for social services, discuss the concerns individuals may have regarding disability, life, and health insurance plans, and provide worksheets to assist individuals in this process. Important considerations which have implications for eligibility for social services or job continuation include whether the diagnosis is CDC defined and what decisive factors were documented in the diagnosis of AIDS. As the application process for social services can become trying, soliciting the assistance of social workers before hospital discharge regarding matters of financial, housing, and health resources is recommended. In addition, the assistance of friends or representatives from local AIDS-related agencies is beneficial.

Community Resources. Knowledge of community resources is probably one of the most significant assistive strategies that nurses can offer to their clients.

While the AIDS epidemic has had a devastating effect on the community, Christ and Wiener (1985) maintain that a positive aspect has been demonstrated in many communities where collaboration and consolidation of services and resources from traditional and non-traditional agencies, government groups, and organizations for gay and non-gay people have assisted persons with AIDS, their caregivers, lovers, spouses, and family members. Services which have proven helpful can be categorized as Health Services, Human Service Agencies, and Social Support Resources. (Specific community, health education, and health service resources are listed in Chapter 13.)

Health care agencies in the community provide a variety of services. Health care agencies can be public or private, profit or non-profit. Health care agencies can provide HIV antibody testing and counseling. They can provide episodic care for persons with lymphadenopathy-associated syndrome (LAS), ARC, and AIDS. They can provide monitoring and follow-up services. Hospitals in the community offer emergency, acute care and chronic care services. They also sometimes offer hospice services. Home nursing care is available in most communities. In some communities hospice services are out-patient based. Mental health services and psychiatric services are available in both community agencies and hospitals. These services are useful for diagnosing and treating the neuropsychiatric problems associated with HIV infection as well as with the emotional turmoil associated with HIV infection and AIDS.

Human service agencies are often composed of a combination of medical, social, and allied disciplines that are organized in a community activity designed to protect and advance the health of persons with HIV infection and AIDS, their friends, lovers, spouses, caregivers, and family members. The members of these organizations, which may include gay coalitions, patient care groups, family groups, social and health care workers, and AIDS task forces, play an essential role in bringing critically important care issues into focus for political groups. These issues may include timely Medicaid reimbursement for patients, rapidly confronting situations of discrimination, and having AIDS designated as a vital diagnosis for Social Security Disability. In particular, when the scientific, medical, diagnostic, and community organizations coordinate forces, public health concerns such as prevention, education of groups at high risk, expert medical and nursing care, housing, financial resources, insurance, employment, and home, community and hospice care can be dealt with efficiently and expeditiously (Foster & Hall, 1986; Sedaka & O'Reilly, 1986).

Aside from the services of medical institutions where psychiatric-liaison personnel are specially trained in providing crisis intervention for persons with AIDS, community organizations are critical in providing additional support services. In many communities, AIDS task forces have a professional and volunteer staff who assist with financial, legal, and housing concerns. The volunteers are especially helpful as they provide a "buddy system" for persons with AIDS and perform services such as assisting in transportation to hospitals, food shopping, taking care of pets, and providing the emotional presence which is often lacking with individuals inflicted with AIDS. Community groups have also joined in forming self-help support groups for persons with AIDS, friends, lovers, spouses and family as well as the "worried well." These groups provide education, a freedom to discuss reactions in a safe environment, and a forum for discussion of medical treatment, decision-making, financial planning, disability applications, and discriminatory treatment.

Control of the AIDS epidemic will require responses on the part of the entire community. Through professional and community activities, nurses have the ability to affect the outcome of the epidemic.

Community Care

Home Care. The key to home care is a case management approach wherein personal dignity, informed right of choice, and safe care are the hallmarks, and home, hospital, and community resources are linked and integrated (Bryant, 1986). Nurses are often case managers of home care or provide such care.

Case management in the community is concerned with infection control. The key issues of concern are (1) how to prevent the spread of infection to sexual partners, family members, and caregivers and (2) how to control opportunistic infections in the immunosuppressed individual. Klug (1986) highlights the need for nurses to make a careful assessment of the home and identify risk factors in the environment that can predispose to opportunistic infections. These may include poor hygiene, nutrition, or sanitation.

While specific infection control measures for the hospital are discussed in Chapter 7, the following issues are highlighted here (Lusby & Schietinger, 1984):

1. Body secretions, particularly blood and semen, are not to be exchanged.

2. Maintaining a state of personal cleanliness, which includes regular bathing and washing hands before preparing foods and after toileting, is essential.

3. Normal sanitary practices to prevent the growth of bacteria and fungi are critical, especially to the immunosuppressed individual. Bleach in 1:10 dilution (1 part bleach to 10 parts water) is an effective disinfectant.

4. Dishes can be used by all family members if cleaned with hot soapy water.

5. Towels and wash cloths should not be shared without laundering; toothbrushes, razors, enema equipment, and sexual toys should not be shared.

6. The environment should be well ventilated, and the patient should be instructed to cover the mouth when coughing (McCarthy, 1986).

The most important barrier to prevention of infection for caretakers is handwashing for 10 seconds using soap, water and friction. Gloves are useful barriers when handling substances such as feces, urine, sputum, oral secretions, blood, and wound drainage. Universal infection precautions are included in Appendix C.

Another aspect of case management is maintaining nutrition and fluid status. Recognized co-factors which weaken the immune system and place an individual at risk for HIV infection include use of alcohol and recreational drugs and improper nutrition (Schietinger, 1986). Poor nutrition may also contribute further to suppression of cell-mediated immunity and reduce the number and effectiveness of circulating lymphocytes (Johnson & Nance, 1985). Persons with AIDS oftentimes experience nutritional deficiencies secondary to anorexia, intractable diarrhea, oral or esophageal Kaposi's sarcoma, candidiasis, or herpes simplex, which can interfere with the ingestion of foods. In addition, nutritional intake may be altered due to depression, which can affect the planning, shopping, and selection of food. When physical or mental inability to prepare foods is apparent, community resources in the form of buddies or volunteers to buy groceries or visit during meal time or home health aides to prepare meals can be sought (Schietinger, 1986).

During an illness such as AIDS, in which increased metabolic rate due to fevers and infections, loss of appetite, and diarrhea predominate, the requirement for calories may be as high as 5000 per day. Lang (1985) provides specifics regarding dealing with problems of eating, such as altered taste sensation, depression, and fatigue in order to increase calorie content.

For persons with infections of the mouth which restrict swallowing of food, soft foods, blender foods, or a topical anesthetic solution may make swallowing easier. McCarthy (1986) recommends that assessing foods and beverages that do not cause discomfort is worthwhile. In particular, consideration of cultural and social compatibility as well as adequacy of maintaining nutritional and fluid intake are primary considerations. Insertion of a nasogastric tube or total parenteral nutrition may be required as a last resort measure. Lastly, it is essential to advise the individual when to seek health care assistance before major problems of adequate hydration and nutrition take hold.

Pain management is another aspect of community case management. As a distressing sensation, pain is a symptom which nurses should assess and treat in an aggressive and comprehensive manner. The factors which diminish an individual's threshold of pain include insomnia, fatigue, anxiety, fear, anger, and depression while the factors which can raise the threshold include sleep, rest, sympathy, understanding, diversion and analgesic agents (Brody, 1986).

To understand the nature of the pain and intervene properly, nurses must carefully assess the quality, onset, duration and intensity of the pain. Of importance is assessment of the psychologic status of the individual, the emotions experienced, and the factors which seem to accentuate or diminish the pain. An understanding of these factors will assist nurses in intervening appropriately.

In a succinct but clinically helpful review, Brody (1986) outlines the causes of pain experienced by persons with AIDS. The author discusses existing medical treatments that can be instituted before narcotic therapy is utilized and dispels many misconceptions held about the use of narcotic therapy as a last resort. Some of these treatments are:

1. Local therapy such as irradiation of bony metastases for pain control.

2. Aspirin, acetaminophen, and other non-steroidal medications should be tried first since they have lower side effects.

3. All analgesics should be administered on an around-the-clock basis to prevent heightening the pain threshold.

4. Attempt behavioral therapy for pain, such as hypnosis, biofeedback, psychotherapy, acupuncture, physical therapy, ice, heat massage and transcutaneous electrical nerve stimulation.

The ultimate aim of pain management is to allow the patient to function as normally as possible and with the greatest ease for the caregiver.

Fatigue is commonly seen in persons with AIDS and constitutes a major symptom which affects quality of life of these individuals. Fatigue is commonly caused by pulmonary insufficiency as a result of interstitial damage from an opportunistic infection, pneumonia, or pulmonary Kaposi's sarcoma (Schietinger, 1986). Nurses should assist the individual in promoting a safe environment in which optimum levels of activity could be performed. In addition, community resources should be made available when the need for managing changing levels of mobility exists (Foster & Hall, 1986).

As a life-threatening symptom, diarrhea not only is an inconvenience but also can play a major role in electrolyte imbalance, skin breakdown, and nutritional depletion. Particularly when frequent watery stools are evacuated daily and symptoms of anorexia, nausea, and vomiting are present, patients and caregivers should be alert to the signs of dehydration and electrolyte imbalance and have easy access to a physician for evaluation testing. Nursing interventions would certainly call for encouraging fluids and administration of antidiarrheal medications as often as necessary. A bland, low fiber diet or removal of milk products from the diet may be of some help (Schietinger, 1986).

One of the most critical aspects of home care is teaching patients and families to identify when to seek health care assistance. Teaching families to recognize the signs and symptoms of infection, fluid and electrolyte depletion, malnutrition, and neuropsychiatric dysfunction are crucial aspects of home care. Equally important is teaching them the health care resources available should any of these complications occur and urging them to seek assistance appropriately and in a timely manner. Support and teaching by the nurse are especially useful in helping families assist persons with neuropsychiatric dysfunctions who are living at home, in preventing infection, and in preventing fluid and nutrition depletion.

Hospice Care. The hospice concept originated as a commitment to provide supportive, residential hospice services in a humane, cost effective and appropriate setting for people with terminal illness (Martin, 1986). Many of the residents of in-patient hospice facilities are people without homes or primary caregivers who do not require the intensity of care provided by a hospital or skilled nursing care facility. A hospice is designed for people who need 24 hour supervision to ensure personal safety and help with the basic activities of daily living: cooking, cleaning, shopping, bathing, laundry, and transportation. Hospice services are also available on an out-patient basis in the home and provide the same services (see Chapter 12).

Martin (1986) has described four essential components of a hospice program. These are a multidisciplinary team, staff education, staff support and reimbursement considerations. The multidisciplinary team should be composed of the following persons:

Nurses assume the case manager role and are primarily responsible for (a) the assessment of the person's condition, (b) communicating changes in condition to the appropriate team members, (c) intervening when necessary, and (d) educating in the principles of infection control. Nurses are vital members of any hospice program and are required on 24 hour call.

Home Health Aides are essential in providing the clients with specific aspects of care, which range from feeding and bathing to around-the-clock supervision of the confused individual.

Social Workers in addition to nurses are effective in providing counseling services for loss, bereavement, fear of contagion, dysfunctional family situations, guilt/shame, or change in role. They also facilitate the acquisition of public support, e.g., Medicare, Medicaid, or other available public assistance.

Physician Consultants provide up-to-date clinical information, are available for emergency consultation, and assist with the development of a care plan for each patient.

Community Liaisons provide a link to complementary services in the community, such as banks, transportation agencies, and AIDS service organizations.

Physical, Occupational, and Speech Therapists assist with the client's independence, perform strengthening exercises, and assist with modifying the home environment.

Volunteers or buddies provide a multitude of valuable functions from running errands to delivering physical and emotional care when specially trained.

The critical elements for a well-functioning hospice are cohesiveness of team members and frequent education sessions, which deal with the facts about AIDS as well as discussing psychosocial and bereavement issues. With a multidisciplinary focus, the person diagnosed with AIDS can be cared for comfortably in the familiar surroundings of a home environment or in an inpatient hospice setting.

Death and dying counseling and support are a major component of hospice care. Kubler-Ross's (1969) five-stage model provides nurses with an understanding of the experience of death and dying. The stages, all or only some of which may occur in any order, include: (1) shock and denial, (2) anger and rage, (3) bargaining, (4) depression, and (5) acceptance. An understanding of these stages will provide the foundation for instituting effective interventions for assisting individuals throughout the grieving process. When in contact with persons of different cultures, nurses should be aware that widely differing beliefs and stages accompany dying. Nurses should educate themselves as to how the dying process is manifested in other cultures so that clients may benefit from their support and interventions.

Although denial may assist individuals in preventing significant disturbances in equilibrium, the implications of a situation oftentimes result in delayed health care and noncompliance to a therapeutic regimen. Especially with AIDS, some persons have denied the diagnosis of the disease or the implications it has with respect to their lifestyles. When denial is excessive, nurses should be patient and wait for the client to feel the time for awareness is present. In particular, when there is nothing hopeful with which to replace denial, stripping individuals of this defense mechanism can be dangerous (Wolcott et al., 1985, 1986).

During the anger or "why me, why not him!" phase, anger may be often focused on nurses and other health caregivers. While this is a trying time for nurses, it is important for the staff to try to understand the anger, listen and accept, and encourage full verbal expression of the patient's feelings.

Bargaining represents the stage wherein individuals attempt to problem solve about the illness and its terminal outcome. It is important for the nurse to demonstrate care and concern, listen carefully to the client's ideas and assist him or her in evaluating alternative therapies.

As the realization of death is close at hand, depression may constitute a major concern, to the point where suicidal ideations are prominent. It is essential for nurses to allow the patient to grieve and not give false reassurances. Frequent, brief visits, verbal and nonverbal expressions of caring, expression of emotions and fears, and assisting in the "life review" may be helpful strategies for persons experiencing the grieving process (Wolcott, 1986).

Summary

The care of persons with HIV infection/AIDS occurs at all levels of prevention in the community. Promotion of health is an important aspect of community education, counseling, and referral that nurses provide. It is important for persons who are not yet infected. It is equally important, if not more so, for people who are HIV-infected or who have clinical disease (LAS, ARC, or AIDS). Diagnosis and treatment of disease and tertiary care are also components of community care. These services can be delivered through home care and hospice care in the community.

References

Alvirez, D., Bean, F.D., Williams, D. (1981). The Mexican American family. In Mindel, C.H., Habenstein, R.W. (Eds.): *Ethnic Families in America* (pp. 269–292). New York: Elsevier.

Bayer, R., Levine, C., Wolf, S. (1986). HIV antibody screening. *Journal of the American Medical Association*, 256(13), 1768–1774.

Brody, R. (1986). Pain management in terminal disease. *Focus*, 1(6), 1–2.

Bryant, J. (1986). Home care of the client with AIDS. *Journal of Community Health Nursing*, 3(2), 69–74.

Callen, M. (Ed.) (1987). *Surviving and Thriving with AIDS*. New York: People with AIDS Coalition.

Carr, G., Gee, G. (1986). AIDS and AIDS-related conditions: Screening for populations at risk. *Nurse Practitioner*, 11(10), 25–46.

Centers for Disease Control. (1987, July). *AIDS Weekly Surveillance Report*—United States AIDS Program, Atlanta, GA.

Christ, G., Wiener, L. (1985). Psychosocial issues in AIDS. In V.T. DeVita, Jr., *AIDS: Etiology, diagnosis, treatment and prevention.* (pp. 275–297). Philadelphia: Lippincott.

Fitzpatrick, J.P. (1981). The Puerto Rican family. In Mindel, C.H., Habenstein, R.W. (Eds.): *Ethnic Families in America* (pp. 189–214). New York: Elsevier.

Foster, J., Hall, H. (1986). Public health and AIDS. *Caring*, 5(6), 4–11, 73, 76–78.

Irish, A. (1983). Straight talk about gay patients. *American Journal of Nursing*, 83, 1168–1170.

Johnson, C., Nance, B. (1985). Getting your house in order. In J. Lang, J. Spiegel & S. Strigle (Eds). *Living with AIDS, a self care manual*, pp. 55–80. AIDS Project, Los Angeles.

Klug, R. (1986). Children with AIDS. *American Journal of Nursing*, 86, 1126–1132.

Kubler-Ross, E. (1969). *On death and dying*. New York: Macmillan.

Lang, J., Spiegel, J., Strigle, S. (Eds.). (1985). *Living with AIDS, a self care manual*. AIDS Project, Los Angeles.

Lang, J. (1985). Nutrition and Exercise. In J. Lang, J. Spiegel, & S. Strigle (Eds.): *Living with AIDS, a self care manual*, pp. 25–27. AIDS Project, Los Angeles.

Lusby, G., Schietinger, H. (1984). Infection precautions for people with AIDS living in the community. (Unpublished manuscript.)

Mantell, J., Belmont, M., Spivak, H. (1987). *Women with AIDS*. 2nd International Conference on AIDS, Paris, France.

Martin, J. (1986). The AIDS home care and hospice program. *American Journal of Hospice Care*, 3(2), 35–37.

McCarthy, P. (1986). Guidelines for AIDS/ARC patient care. (Unpublished manuscript.)

Schietinger, H. (1986). A home care plan for AIDS. *American Journal of Nursing*, 86(9), 1021–1028.

Sedeka, S., O'Reilly, M. (1986). The financial implications of AIDS. *Caring*, 5(6), 38–39, 42–46.

Shaw, N. (1986). Serving your patients in the age of AIDS. *Contemporary OB/GYN*, 28(4), 141–149.

Staples, R. (1981). The Black American family. In C.H. Mindel, R.W. Habenstein (Eds.): *Ethnic Families in America* (pp. 217–244). New York: Elsevier.

Wolcott, D. (1986). Psychosocial aspects of acquired immune deficiency syndrome (AIDS) and the primary care physician. *Annals of Allergy*, 57(8), 95–102.

Wolcott, D., Fawzy, F., Landsverk, J., et al. (1986). AIDS patients' needs of psychosocial services and their use of community service organizations. *Journal of Psychosocial Oncology*, 4(1), 135–146.

Wolcott, D., Fawzy, F., Pasnau, R. (1985). Acquired immune deficiency syndrome (AIDS) and consultation-liaison psychiatry. *General Hospital Psychiatry*, 7, 280–292.

Wells, K., Linn, L., Bensen, M., et al. (1986). Interviewing. Medical Development Guides. UCLA Department of Medicine, pp. 87–95.

Wells, K. (1987). Sexual history taking. Training for health care providers to address acquired immunodeficiency syndrome. (Unpublished document.)

Chapter 11

Ethical and Legal Issues

Marsha D. M. Fowler
Elizabeth A. Chaney

Acquired immunodeficiency syndrome (AIDS), as a disease which is communicable, devastating, fatal, and socially stigmatized, raises an almost overwhelming number of ethical and legal questions. These questions can be subsumed under several ethical principles and their legal correlates. Though not limited to these, they include:

1. Justice: the allocation of limited nursing resources to care of patients with AIDS and nurses' refusal to participate.

2. Autonomy: withholding and withdrawing treatment.

3. Non-infliction of harm—doing good: mandatory testing, labeling and stigmatization.

While it is beyond the scope of this chapter to discuss any of these at length—and each is worthy of lengthy discussion in itself—each area will be given brief attention with particular concern to pointing nurses toward additional ethical and legal resources for further exploration. For clarity and convenience of discussion, ethical aspects will be discussed first and legal aspects second.

Justice: Nurses' Participation in the Care of Persons with AIDS

The principle of justice deals with the allocation of resources (in this case nursing resources) in a manner that fairly distributes burdens and benefits among patients (Fowler, 1984). Though there are many issues that could be addressed here, the question that will be singled out is that of nurse refusal to participate in the care of persons with HIV infection.

Since the identification of AIDS in 1981, there have been several incidents in which nurses have refused to care for patients with AIDS. In some instances, a real or imagined fear of this led physicians to an indefensible practice of masking the diagnosis on the patient's chart to forestall such situations. The grounds that the nurses gave were stated in terms of the fear of communicability of the disease. However, it was clear that the issue of communicability was a cloak for the real objection—which was to the patient's lifestyle.

Nonetheless, a few comments are in order on the concept of communicability. By the very nature of their work, nurses must accept a level of risk of exposure to disease which exceeds that expected of the general population. As Jameton (1984) notes, "exposing oneself to risks in order to protect patients and to provide care is a well-established conventional obligation of the health professions." Nurses are not obligated, however, to accept more than a "fair share" of risk in maintaining the health of society. Yet, it is not easy to determine what constitutes a reasonable level of risk. In general, there have been four conjoint principles which have been used in determining when acceptance of a risk is a duty and when it is optional or supererogatory. Of the four, one is the most pivotal for discussion here: the benefit that the patient receives outweighs the harm that will accrue to the nurse, and that harm is no more than minimal (Beauchamp & Childress, 1979). Does the benefit that the patient will receive, by virtue of the care which nursing can provide, outweigh the harm to the nurse? And, is the harm to the nurse more than a minimal one?

If the situation were such that the institution could not protect, or offered no protection to, the nurse in instances of infectious or communicable diseases, then the harm to the nurse would both outweigh the benefit to the patient and would be more than minimal. However, clinical institutions customarily have policies and procedures which render the risk minimal when followed in practice. Two points must be made here. The nursing administration of any institution has an obligation to provide the necessary policies, procedures, and equipment for infection control and to protect the well-being of the nurse. Administration has a further obligation to see that those procedures are employed. Second, nurses themselves have an obligation to implement the policies and to use the measures and equipment provided in order to protect themselves. Risk should not be undertaken needlessly. When proper precautions are available and followed, the risk of communicability that AIDS poses to the nurse does not exceed the risk posed by other infectious or communicable diseases; it can be minimized.

Is moral or religious disapproval of a patient's lifestyle sufficient grounds for refusal to care for a patient? No. The *Code for Nurses* (ANA, 1985) is very clear on this point:

> The need for health care is universal, transcending all national, ethnic, racial, religious, cultural, political, educational, economic, developmental, personality, role and sexual differences. Nursing care is delivered without prejudicial behavior.

Although AIDS is not a "homosexual disease," as some have labeled it, many of those who have the disease are homosexual, bisexual, intravenous drug users, prostitutes, known to be promiscuous, or known to have had contact with prostitutes. The lifestyle of the patient and the nature of the health problem, whether approved or disapproved of by either society or the nurse, is not an acceptable moral ground for refusing to care for the patient. Lifestyle is considered a patient attribute which is to be used to individualize the nursing care plan, not to deny it.

The *Code* does allow nurses to refuse assignments. It states, "If ethically opposed to interventions in a particular case because of the procedures to be used, the nurse is justified in refusing to participate" (ANA *Code*, 1985). It is important to note, however, that it is the interventions to which the nurse may object—not the patient. Justice demands a fair allocation of nursing resources, one which is impartial and non-prejudicial.

Autonomy: Withholding and Withdrawing Treatment

One of the characteristics of AIDS is its protracted and debilitating downhill course. It is also characterized by an uneven clinical course with intermittent crises interspersed with more quiescent periods. There are times when individual patients, though "salvageable," will say that "enough is enough." Is it permissible for a patient to exercise his or her autonomy by refusing treatment, even if it is life-sustaining?

The *Code* (ANA, 1985) again provides guidelines for the nurse. It states that:

Truth telling and the process of reaching informed choice underlie the exercise of self-determination, which is basic to respect for persons. Clients should be as fully involved as possible in the planning and implementation of their own health care. Clients have the moral right to determine what will be done with their own person; to be given accurate information, and all the information necessary for making informed judgments; to be assisted with weighing the benefits and burdens of options in their treatment; to accept, refuse, or terminate treatment without coercion; and to be given the necessary emotional support.

The *Code* (1985) alludes to the fact that the way in which the principle of respect for autonomy is generally operationalized in clinical practice is through the doctrine of informed consent. (Informed consent is both an ethical and a legal rule, with some differences between the two forms.) Under conditions of informed consent, patients may indeed refuse treatment, selectively refuse treatment, or terminate treatment once begun. This includes both mundane as well as sophisticated treatments. The *Code* is also correct to point out that a patient who decides not to undergo treatment, or to withdraw from it, must not be abandoned emotionally; when medicine has nothing more to offer the individual patient, nursing has everything to offer, and must do so. That is the nature of the duty to care.

Additional support for the notion that patients may refuse even life-sustaining treatment is found in the report prepared by the President's Commission for the Study of Ethical Problems in Medicine and Biomedical and Biobehavioral Research, entitled Deciding to Forego Life-Sustaining Treatment (President's Commission, 1983). The report states that

. . . nothing in current law precludes ethically sound decision making. Neither criminal nor civil law—if properly interpreted and applied by lawyers, judges, health care providers, and the general public—forces patients to undergo procedures that will increase their suffering when they wish to avoid this by foregoing life-sustaining treatment.

Although there is a general duty to preserve life, there is no duty to preserve it beyond the point of human dignity; doing so violates the sanctity of life principle. The sanctity of life principle states that life is a relative (not absolute) value and that we have a relative (not absolute) obligation to preserve it. To preserve life absolutely, simply because it is human biological life, constitutes vitalism, and is a violation of the human dignity nurses seek to preserve.

In order to avoid engaging in vitalism, the sanctity of life principle must be modified by the quality of life principle. That principle holds that there are some lives of a quality not worth living. But, what constitutes a quality of life not worth living?

For nursing, that determination is not made by any consideration of the social worth or social contribution of the individual. Such decisions are anathema to nursing. Instead, a quality of life not worth living is to be determined from the perspective of the patient himself or herself. It is the patient's value system which identifies the boundaries of an acceptable quality of life. Those values may be expressed directly by the patient, or indirectly through a legal instrument or through family members or loved ones. Care must be taken that second parties who provide statements of the patient's wishes or values, when the patient cannot do so personally, are in fact expressing those of the patient and not their own.

In issues of withholding and withdrawing treatment, it is often easier to withhold than to withdraw it. However, this distinction between the two is an emotional or psychological difference, not a moral or legal one. As the President's Commission (1983) notes:

The distinction between failing to initiate and stopping treatment—that is, withholding versus withdrawing treatment—is not itself of moral importance. A justification that is adequate for not commencing a treatment is also sufficient for ceasing it.

Not to belittle the emotional impact of such decisions, it is nevertheless morally (and legally) permissible to withdraw treatment if the patient does not wish it or if it will not benefit the patient, however difficult that may be psychologically.

In terms of the nurse's participation in withholding or withdrawing treatment, the *Code* (ANA, 1985) states:

Nursing care is directed toward the prevention and relief of suffering commonly associated with the dying process. The nurse may provide interventions to relieve symptoms in the dying client even when the interventions entail substantial risks of hastening death.

Nevertheless, "the nurse does not act deliberately to terminate the life of any person."

Active voluntary euthanasia is receiving a great deal of attention because of the court-condoned actions of physicians in the Netherlands, and because of the advocacy of a number of groups in the United States. Nursing's moral tradition in this country is very clear, from the Nightingale pledge forward; nurses may not actively and deliberately take the life of another, even when socially sanctioned (Fowler, 1984). Assisted suicide, "medical killing," or "euthanasia on demand," terms that have been used recently, fall outside the scope of nursing practice, violate the profession's moral norms, and potentially violate the trust that society must have in members of the profession. If active voluntary euthanasia is made legal in this country, non-nurses (and according to recent decisions by the American Medical Association, non-physicians) will have to be prepared to carry out that function.

Avoiding Harm and Doing Good: Mandatory Testing, Labeling, and Stigmatization

Mandatory Testing. Avoiding harm (nonmaleficence) and doing good (beneficence) are two additional principles used to specify nurses' ethical obligations. Nonmaleficence involves the noninfliction of harm, whereas beneficence involves the prevention or removal of harmful conditions, and positively benefiting another. Sometimes, the two are viewed as the single principle, beneficence. Mandatory testing is an issue which arises in any discussion of beneficence.

There has been a great deal of clamor, from many quarters, calling for mandatory testing, even universal mandatory testing, for HIV antibodies. Others have asked that only selected populations have testing imposed, including prisoners, pregnant women, those applying for marriage licenses, hemophiliacs, known drug abusers, patients admitted to hospitals, health care workers, and all homosexuals. Not all of these categories are composed of persons at risk for either infection or developing the disease.

Apart from the pragmatic arguments that universal mandatory testing would not stop the spread of HIV infection and would be costly and wasteful, ineffective, subject to false positives as well as false negatives, impossible to achieve, and unjustifiable in terms of the principles of public health, it is generally seen as an illegitimate intrusion upon an individual's autonomy and its subrules of informed consent and privacy. Although not all intrusions upon an individual's privacy are ethically unwarranted, required universal mandatory testing for HIV antibodies would be an unprecedented move. It would needlessly subject those at no risk to an unnecessary violation of the right of consent and to an invasion of privacy.

Mass screenings are customarily justified on the grounds of beneficence (and alternatively on grounds of justice and utility)—that is, the purpose of screening would be to stop the spread of HIV infection in order to protect those who are not but might become infected with the virus. However, HIV is not spread by casual contact. Neither is it significantly treatable at this point in time. Thus, it is difficult to calculate any significant benefit or good that might be gained, or harm prevented, by mass screening, sufficient to warrant the violation of autonomy that universal mandatory screening would necessitate. There may, however, be some contexts in which non-universal, group-specific mandatory testing could be justified. Given space limitations, it is possible to give only the briefest of commentaries on mandatory testing of particular groups here.

Certainly, in the interests of protecting others (the principle of beneficence), it could be considered justifiable to test donated blood, semen, or organs. The donor's liberty is not infringed upon as the donation of organs, blood, or semen is a choice the donor makes. In addition, it could be considered justifiable to test those whose work-related tasks make them specifically at risk for infection and transmission, as in the case of prostitutes. However, testing as a prerequisite to obtaining a marriage license or testing of pregnant women is less justifiable; a significant proportion of sex and childbearing takes place outside of marriage in this society.

Mandatory screening has also been proposed for prisoners. The arguments usually given are that many prisoners are intravenous drug abusers, who continue drug abuse within the prison, and that a fair number of rapes take place within prisons. Screening, however, will not stop the spread of HIV infection within a prison; behavioral change will. The solution is not to screen, but rather to exert better control over drug abuse and rape and to provide education. Other groups have been considered for mandatory screening, though it is not possible to debate the merits of those proposals here. It should be noted, nevertheless, that not all mandatory testing is disallowed, but that that which is to be done must have substantive ethical justification.

Labeling and Stigmatizing. Throughout this text it has been noted that AIDS is heavily socially stigmatized. In the public mind, it is usually linked to socially disapproved sexual orientations or behaviors or drug use. But even where there is no nursing disapproval of the person's sexual orientation or behavior, there is a tendency to apply labels that potentially harm the patient. To refer to a person with AIDS as an "AIDS victim" may prove as harmful, in the long run, as more overtly prejudicial labels. Terms such as victim have the potential to generate certain attitudes toward the patient which are not particularly beneficial. As with most labels, there is also a risk of treating the patient as a victim rather than as a person with individual characteristics and needs.

Potter (1977) has identified three essential characteristics of labels which must be satisfied in order for the label to be ethically justifiable. First, the label must treat the person as a person, with specific needs. It should not create expectancy disadvantages. Second, an acceptable label is not indelible, but rather removable and able to account for the contingency of the future. Third, labels must expand opportunities, increasing a person's access to services or assistance that could not be had without that label. Labels must not contract opportunities.

Labels which are applied to persons with HIV infection, whether diagnostic labels or informal ones, must meet these three criteria for the label to be warranted ethically. It is often the case that "socially unacceptable diseases" carry overtly harmful labels. Care must be taken that even those labels applied with compassion do not also harm the patient.

Legal Issues

Any discussion of HIV infection and the law requires a cautionary beginning. A strong case can be made for the argument that sufficient legislated public policy and judge-made legal precedent already exist to protect all parties to any transaction that includes the element of AIDS/HIV infection. For example, the United States Supreme Court has ruled that communicable diseases are handicapping conditions and that persons so afflicted are protected from employment discrimination under situations covered by Section 504 of the Rehabilitation Act of 1974. Confidentiality of medical information laws exists to protect against improper disclosure of information concerning a patient's illness and treatment. Occupational health laws require the employer to maintain a work environment that is free of recognized hazards that cause or are likely to cause death or serious physical damage. Both contract and personal injury law offer a variety of potential remedies for persons who believe they have been injured in an AIDS-related transaction. Nonetheless, despite these existing laws, the political process of determining whether new public policy is needed, and the judicial process of applying existing public policy and legal precedent to AIDS/HIV infection–connected cases, is in an early stage of predictably fervid and erratic development.

Public policy debates presently focus on the desirable scope, if any, of mandatory testing; on the necessity, if any, of specific anti-discrimination statutes to protect persons who have positive antibody tests, AIDS-related complex (ARC), or acquired immunodeficiency syndrome; and on the rights, if any, of nurses to know whether their patients have positive antibody tests, ARC, or AIDS. Lawsuits have been filed to establish the applicability of existing legal theory to an exhausting array of questions: May afflicted children be excluded from school? Is a person presumed damaged if a false statement is made that he or she has AIDS? Is a person liable for damages if he or she fails to disclose an AIDS-related diagnosis and transmits AIDS to a sexual partner? Is it attempted murder to intentionally act to infect another with AIDS? Is it intentional infliction of emotional distress to refuse treatment or services to a person with AIDS, or to a close relative who has sought the services on behalf of the person with AIDS?

What is well-settled law today may be unsettled tomorrow, temporarily or permanently, by a new ruling or a new piece of legislation. The more unsettling changes are more likely to occur in the public policy arena. Judges are inclined to make small, incremental adjustments through application of existing precedent to different sets of facts. Public policy and legal precedent in one jurisdiction may be contrary to public policy and legal precedent in another jurisdiction.

Despite the uncertainties created by transitional phases in public policy and case law development, it remains possible to address some of the AIDS-related legal issues confronted by nurses and, within the caveat set forth earlier, to discuss the implication of existing public policy and legal precedent for those issues. It is also possible, and certainly crucial, to begin to identify the questions that need to be asked by nurses who have to make decisions about their participation as professionals in the medical and social treatment of persons infected with HIV.

Legal Rights and Duties of Nurses toward Patients

The nurse's legal duty with respect to persons who are HIV-infected is no different from the nurse's duty to any patient. When the nurse takes on the responsibility to provide nursing care to a patient, the nurse becomes legally obligated to possess and use that degree of knowledge and skill that would be possessed and used under similar circumstances by a reasonably competent nurse. To find out what that "degree of knowledge and skill" may be in a given circumstance, the nurse must look not only to local or community nursing care standards, but also to state-wide and national nursing standards. State-wide standards are established by licensing boards and state-level professional associations and organizations. National standards are developed by groups who offer certification in a field of nursing, or who develop standards for practice which are published for the benefit of nurses practicing in the particular field. The nursing practice licensure acts may also set forth definitions of nursing practice which, to greater and lesser degrees, describe the scope of the nurse's duty to her patient. For example, the California Business & Professions Code, Section 2725, provides in part:

The practice of nursing . . . means those functions . . . which require a substantial amount of scientific knowledge or technical skill, and includes all of the following: a) direct and indirect patient care services that insure the safety, comfort, personal hygiene and protection of patients; and the performance of disease prevention and restorative measures . . . .

Thus, registered nurses practicing in California have, as a matter of legislated public policy, a duty to provide care and to provide for the safety and protection of their patients.

Even if a particular state legislature has not included an express obligation to provide for patient care and safety, judges have consistently found nurses legally responsible for protecting their patients from harm which a nurse knew or should have known would result from the nurse's action or inaction. The nurse's legal duty to protect patients from harm is central to any analysis of questions concerning the nurse's right to refuse to provide nursing care to an AIDS patient.

The general rule of law holds that nurses are to carry out work assignments and medical orders. There are two widely recognized exceptions to the general rule. First, the nurse is not required to act illegally or to otherwise act contrary to "public policy." In some jurisdictions, more conservative courts may require that the nurse be expressly obligated to adhere to a given "public policy" through legislative enactments. In other jurisdictions, the more active, liberal courts may reason by analogy to find that a nurse must be obligated to act or refuse to act in a particular way in order to give expression to existing public policy.

Second, the nurse is not required to carry out medical orders that the nurse knows or reasonably believes will cause harm to a patient. In fact, an affirmative duty arises to not carry out medical orders which would cause harm, and the nurse is expected to possess the knowledge and skill to fulfill the duty.

The legal requirement that nurses carry out their work assignments derives from the typically broad-brush character of the nurse's oral and written contract of employment with the hiring hospital. Usually, such contracts provide that the nurse will be paid a certain sum for working certain hours as assigned by the institution. While some contracts specify the clinical area to which the nurse is regularly assigned, the non-union employment contract seldom includes restrictions or exemptions. Courts recognize that employers cannot operate a complex service-intensive business if employees who have agreed to accept work as assigned are free to accept and reject individual assignments on a subjective, personal, and unpredictable basis.

Nurses who privately contract with individual patients to provide direct and indirect nursing services may, of course, refuse to enter a contract to care for a known patient with HIV infection. It is legally possible to negotiate a contract with an employer in which the nurse's work duties expressly exclude the nursing care of patients with HIV infection. Whether such a contract could be actually negotiated would depend on many variables, including the specific position the nurse would be employed to fill, the likelihood the employer could control the nurse's contact with patients having HIV infection, and how desperately the employer was seeking an employee with the nurse's particular knowledge and skills. Whether such a contract "ought" to be negotiated is a question the answer to which must be derived from professional nursing ethics.

Despite the limitations just described, nurses may refuse assignments if they are against public policy or unlawful. The exception is recognized in part because the employer is presumed to have notice that such an assignment would be improper and therefore has an opportunity to avoid the situation entirely. In theory, nurses may also refuse assignment if the assignment would pose an unreasonable risk of harm to the patient because the nurse lacks the requisite degree of knowledge and skill to safely care for the patient. As a practical matter, the nurse needs to carefully evaluate the comparative "risk of harm" operating in the situation before refusing an assignment. The nurse should determine whether the "assignment" can be modified to incorporate the nurse's limitations in knowledge and skill, and provide help from a knowledgeable, skillful nurse. Second, the nurse needs to evaluate whether refusing the assignment would constitute "abandonment" of the patient to an even greater risk of harm. Third, the nurse needs to decide upon a course of action to ensure that there is not a chronic recurrence of the "competence"–"abandonment" dilemma in that setting. However, before determining that the employer is requiring the nurse to take action that is against public policy, the nurse needs to carefully evaluate the facts and to weigh the relative risks and benefits to the patient, to the nurse, and to third parties of refusing the assignment.

For example, a common problem has to do with the adequacy of infection control practices with regard to the patient with AIDS. In jurisdictions where the nurse is not informed of the diagnosis, or in circumstances under which the physician or administration does not want to "embarrass" the patient through the use of barrier devices, the nurse is placed in an untenable position. Occupational health and safety laws typically provide that employers maintain safe and healthful working environments for employees and for third parties who may be in the environment. Nurses may be tempted to refuse to care for patients known or suspected of having AIDS unless the hospital implements national guidelines (CDC guidelines) for infection control methods for patients with AIDS, arguing that such an assignment would be against public policy. If the hospital then fires the nurse for refusing the work assignment, the nurse would seek to defend the refusal on the public policy ground that to carry out such an assignment would endanger the nurse and even third parties who would be at risk of acquiring HIV if the nurse became infected.

Before embarking on such a course, a nurse should first obtain legal and professional consultation regarding the precise facts involved and the current state of the law in the nurse's jurisdiction, and should continue such consultation at every step of the nurse's refusal to carry out the assignment. Among the questions which would need to be addressed before a nurse elects to refuse to care for a patient with HIV infection are: What is the probability that the nurse would acquire the disease from the patient, given the nursing procedures to be performed? What measures are accessible to the nurse to reduce the risk? What harm is the patient likely to suffer if the nurse does not provide the care? Is the probable harm to the patient more immediate or remote, more reversible or irreversible, than the probable harm to the nurse? Are there less drastic solutions available other than outright withholding of the nurse's services, pending resolution of the infection control policy problem? Does the nurse's opinion comport with the Centers for Disease Control's guidelines and recommendations? What opportunity has the hospital been given to correct the problem? What are the elements of the legal and ethical foundation for the nurse's action?

Legal Rights and Duties of the Nurse with HIV Infection

In the legal profession, AIDS/HIV infection is viewed as one of the most serious threats to Constitutional rights to appear in the last century. Reflexive reaction to this particular threat of personal destruction—a reaction disproportionate, it seems, to the threat posed by so many other, also fatal, and also presently irreversible conditions—is signaled by unexamined cries for severe curtailment of freedom for those "others" afflicted with HIV.

It is a truism within the legal profession, too, that one's perspective on what ought to be "the law" is directly and invariably affected by one's perspective, i.e., on whose ox is being gored. And so it seems appropriate to give consideration to the legal issues affecting nurses who themselves are infected with HIV—whether work related, lifestyle related, or medically induced through exposure to blood or blood products.

Nurses often ask if they may sue their employer if they acquire HIV infection through employment. The standard answer is two-pronged. First, the nurse must be able to prove that the disease was acquired through work and not through lifestyle activities or medical treatment. Second, if the disease is acquired through work-related activities, the employee has recourse to worker's compensation laws for remedies. Ordinarily, worker's compensation is the only remedy available to an employee who sustains a work-related injury. Such injuries are broadly conceived to be part and parcel of the employer's risk of doing business, no fault is assigned, and the objective is to compensate the employee for the injury and attendant losses. Other actions may be brought against the employer if a complaint can be properly stated for intentionally wrongful acts by the employer which caused the injury.

Nurses who acquire, or are at risk of acquiring, HIV through work and non-work-related circumstances need to be further concerned about the status of the employer's policies and procedures governing the personnel management of employees and prospective employees who have positive antibody tests, ARC, or AIDS. Should the nurse who is HIV-infected be excluded from clinical, hands-on, direct contact with patients? Is a positive HIV antibody test grounds for terminating or refusing to hire a nurse? Is a diagnosis of ARC or a diagnosis of AIDS grounds for terminating or refusing to hire a nurse? Would the licensing board have grounds to discipline nurses by revoking the license if the nurse with HIV infection continued to work in the clinical setting with patients? Although application of law to AIDS/HIV infection questions is still developing, both legislative and case law suggest the nurse would have legal recourse if denied employment. And, the analysis which supports the nurse's right to employment would provide a basis for responding to a licensing board's accusation against the nurse's license.

Action to exclude a nurse from employment or to bring an accusation against the nurse's license should be based on defensible application of information from the Centers for Disease Control. Under present guidelines, the question to be asked is whether the nature of the nurse's contact with patients would be so intimate as to risk exposing the patient to the nurse's body fluids (e.g., semen, blood, vaginal secretions). Under basic personnel management guidelines, the question to be asked is whether the nurse is physically and mentally capable of performing the requisite duties in the assigned position. If not, then the follow-up question would be whether the nurse would be physically and mentally capable of performing other duties in an equal position. If not, then the nurse with HIV infection needs to be managed in the presumably enlightened manner that is used with all physically and/or mentally ill employees.

This line of reasoning is similar to that adopted by the United States Supreme Court in the recent *School Board of Nassau County, Florida, vs. Arline* decision (55 U.S.L.W. 4225, March 1987). In the *Arline* decision, the Court held that contagious diseases are handicapping conditions under Section 504 of the Rehabilitation Act. The Court said that persons with contagious diseases, such as tuberculosis, may not be deprived of employment or other benefits in federally funded programs if they are "otherwise qualified" to participate in such programs or could be qualified to participate if reasonable accommodations were made. Two principal criteria for determining that a person is qualified are: (1) the actual medical risk of contagion; and (2) the person's ability to participate in the protected activity given his or her medical inability. When employers receive federal assistance, the *Arline* decision will most likely be employed to protect nurses with AIDS from discriminatory employment practices.

Furthermore, federal law and many state laws prohibit employers from asking prospective employees about their physical condition unless the questions are directly related to the individual's ability to perform the job duties or would pose a significant hazard to the health and safety of others in the workplace. The burden of showing the direct relationship between questions about HIV infection and the proposed job duties would fall on the employer. A few states, including California, Wisconsin, and Florida, prohibit mandatory HIV-antibody testing of prospective employees.

Mandatory Testing: When, Whom, What Purpose?

Most concerns about mandatory testing focus on the unreliability of antibody screening tests, the misuse of unreliable results, and the potential for overreaching abridgment of fundamental human rights in response to fear, ignorance, and bigotry. Imagine, for example, that a federal law has been enacted which requires that all persons must carry on their persons an identification card which includes the current results of their HIV-antibody test. Imagine, too, that the state of the art of antibody testing has not progressed beyond its current position. What questions come to mind?

What is a "current" result? How often must one be tested to ensure that a "negative" has not coverted to "positive"? What will the test cost? Who will pay for the test? If I am wealthy, can I buy the most sophisticated confirmation tests to overrule a "false positive" screening test? If I am poor, must I be labeled an "AIDS/ HIV carrier" because neither I nor the government can afford the confirmation test to unseat my false positive? If I have a printing press in my basement, can I retire to New Zealand from the profits earned in the counterfeit HIV antibody identification card business?

If the confirmation test is also positive, or if I cannot afford to challenge the screening test, what will be the consequences? Do I have to leave my home and family, to live in a quarantine facility? Do I have to be "marked" in some manner on my person to ensure that potential sexual partners know I am a possible HIV carrier? Or, do I have to be "marked" in some manner on my person so that everyone can determine I am a possible AIDS carrier? Should such marking differentiate between HIV antibody positive tests, ARC, and AIDS? If HIV is transmitted through blood and semen, and not by casual contact, is such intrusion into my privacy and constraints on my liberty "rationally related" to a "legitimate public purpose" and therefore a justified deprivation of my fundamental constitutional right to liberty and pursuit of happiness?

Should persons be required to test negative in order to engage in sexual relationships? How would such a law to be enforced? And, even if it were perfectly enforceable, would it be effective given the possibility of false negative testing and conversion to positive between test dates?

Are there situations in which a person's HIV antibody status should be known? Most persons, including outspoken critics of mandatory testing, agree such situations do exist. Blood, semen, and organ donor programs are three commonly cited examples. There is a difference, however, between mandating that programs obtain such tests before accepting or using the material and mandating that all persons be tested regardless of their involvement in the program.

Should persons whose work requires direct contact with blood, semen, and body organs require information about antibody test results before coming into contact with the patient, specimen, or body? At first reading, the answer might seem a clear "Yes." On the other hand, is such disclosure necessary or could such persons protect themselves by regarding every person, every specimen, every body as a potential carrier of infectious disease? And, perhaps more important, should not such automatic protection be part and parcel of the approach to infectious disease control? Today, the concern is AIDS. But AIDS is not the only infectious disease which is transmitted by blood, semen, and body organs, and tomorrow may bring new pathogens. The protection sought by mandatory disclosure of HIV status seems more reliably purchased through public policy that mandates automatic use of infection control methods in every high-risk encounter.

Mandatory disclosure of information about HIV infection is also subject to criticism because health care professionals do not have an impeccable track record of keeping such information truly confidential. In addition, enforcement of rights to confidential treatment of information fails when the person damaged is unable to pursue the civil law remedies as a result of financial or health restraints.

Few persons injured through improper disclosure of confidential information would think of reporting the unprofessional conduct to the appropriate licensing board for investigation and disciplinary action.

The Right to Refuse Life Support Treatment

It appears well-settled law in the United States that persons who are terminally ill or who have chronic, irreversible, and progressively fatal illness may choose to refuse even life-sustaining treatments. The legal requirements for effective refusal follow closely the ethical criteria, set forth earlier in this chapter, for informed decision-making in health care.

To ensure that such a choice may be implemented even if the patient, through illness, has lost capacity, the patient needs a surrogate decision-maker. Family members usually serve as the patient's surrogate unless the patient is an adult and has already designated an agent under a durable power of attorney for health care, or unless there is a court-appointed conservator or guardian with medical decision-making powers. The durable power of attorney for health care provides an adult an opportunity to designate the person he or she wishes to entrust with major health care decisions, and to inform the designated agent about the kinds of choices the patient would make under various circumstances.

Although much of the media attention has fallen on the incidence of AIDS among middle and upper middle class Caucasian homosexual men, other minority designations are represented in significant numbers:

- 80% of all children with AIDS are children of color;
- 70% of all women with AIDS are non-white;
- 50% of persons with AIDS in major eastern cities are non-white and heterosexual;
- 40% of all persons with AIDS in the United States are members of minority groups (CDC, 1986; 1988).

Opportunities to choose and reject treatment, to designate health care agents, to be protected by conservatorship, or to have decisions made by family members can be severely affected by the poverty and disorganization common to persons who lead lives on the streets as IV drug users, prostitutes, or criminals. The absence of family or other spokespersons does not relieve the health team from a duty to determine the patient's desires concerning treatment, so long as the patient has sufficient capacity to express his or her wishes. The growing trend in law to recognize the nurse's duty to serve as a patient advocate goes hand-in-hand with the responsibility to use every opportunity to elicit information concerning the patient's wishes and desires. Such a responsibility would be particularly important in clinical settings where patients are less likely to have access to lawyers and the court system to protect their rights.

Summary

This chapter addressed the ethical and legal issues of obligation to treat, withholding and withdrawing treatment, and mandatory testing. From both an ethical and legal perspective, nurses have an obligation to provide care for persons who are HIV-infected. Nurses who are HIV-infected have the legal right to workers' compensation if they were infected in the course of their work, and to continue their employment or to be employed. Both legal and ethical rules demand informed consent and allow for the withholding and withdrawing of treatment.

Ethically and legally there is currently no persuasive argument for widespread mandatory testing. Autonomy and the right to privacy are stronger arguments against widespread mandatory testing. It is important for nurses to keep themselves up-to-date on developments in policy and the law. Important resources for nurses in this regard are their state nurses' associations and the American Nurses' Association's "legislative alerts" and "updates," the AIDS Action Council's *Action Alert* (Washington, D.C.) and the AIDS Action Foundation's *News Briefs* (Washington, D.C.).

References

American Nurses' Association (1985). *Code for nurses with interpretive statements.* Kansas City, MO: ANA.

Beauchamp, T., Childress, J. (1979). *Principles of biomedical ethics.* New York: Oxford University Press.

Centers for Disease Control (1986). Acquired immunodeficiency syndrome (AIDS) among blacks and Hispanics—United States. *Morbidity and Mortality Weekly Reports*, 35(42), 655–666.

Centers for Disease Control (1988, February). *AIDS Weekly Surveillance Report*—United States AIDS Program, Atlanta, GA.

Fowler, M.D.M. (1984). *Ethics and nursing, 1893–1984: The ideal of service, the reality of history.* Los Angeles: University of Southern California.

Jameton, A. (1984). *Nursing practice: The ethical issues.* Englewood Cliffs, NJ: Prentice-Hall.

Potter, R. (1977). Labeling the mentally retarded: The just allocation of therapy. In S. Reiser, A. Dyck, W. Curran (Eds.), *Ethics in medicine* (pp. 626–630). Cambridge, MA: MIT Press.

President's Commission for the Study of Ethical Problems in Medicine and Biomedical and Biobehavioral Research (1983, March). *Deciding to forego life-sustaining treatment.* Washington, DC: U.S. Government Printing Office.

Chapter 12

A Family's Experience with AIDS

Rose Haque

In Memory of John

Life is like the seasons...
- *Summer is long and sustaining; growing, living*
- *Fall brings a slowing down; peaceful, flowers dying, leaves falling*
- *Winter brings the end; the death of some plants, but the sleeping of others, hibernation*
- *Spring brings a new start; new life, an energy to new beginnings.*

John died on a sunny clear day in summer, July 2, 1986. Death happens at any season. Summer should be filled with fun and activities, but we had the interruption of death. As I close my eyes and try to think of other summers with John—family trips to the cottage, supper on my porch—they are clouded with memories of last year as we watched John worsen in late spring and die in early summer.

I think of what happened with memories of landmarks of the seasons.

Spring/Easter, two years ago, 1985, was the beginning of our journey with John through the days of his illness to the day he died.

John called one evening and calmly told me, "Rose, I have been to the doctor and had a biopsy of a lesion on my leg. I have Kaposi's sarcoma."

"What are you telling me?"

"I have AIDS."

I couldn't swallow; I could hardly talk. This couldn't be happening. I spoke softly. I began to cry quietly. "Oh, John, it can't be true."

So our journey began.

What can I tell you that will help you to give humane care to patients or to one of your loved ones?

I will tell you our story. I am John's sister and a nurse. Maybe there is a part that applies to your situation so that you can support your relative or your patient, as well as his or her family and friends through this dread disease.

Summer 1984

There were earlier concerns about John having AIDS during the summer of 1984.

He was very fatigued and had a respiratory infection which cleared after treatment with antibiotics. Even though his physician assured him that he did not have AIDS, John's anxieties and fears persisted. We spoke of his concern one summer afternoon, and I remember giving assistance and supporting the doctor's findings. The fear remained for both of us even though we didn't talk again about the illness until he called that evening of April 1985, to tell me his diagnosis.

John came to terms with the possibility of his illness after the episode that summer, and lived his life fully—enjoying his friends and family. It was as though he was preparing himself for this eventuality.

The day after his death we found a letter among his papers that he wrote in reflection during the summer of 1984. He wrote of anticipating the possibility of illness, and hoping that family and friends would stay supportive of him. It was a beautiful letter, which was read by the minister at John's funeral service.

Spring 1985

In April, John told me his diagnosis. At the same time, I was given the diagnosis of early breast cancer, which meant I needed a mastectomy. Our family had to deal with two major crises. Although I was dealing with a multitude of upsetting feelings about my own surgery and my diagnosis, I found myself more worried about John. Although I was fearful, I felt more hopeful for my own outcome.

Life seemed so unfair. I wondered if we would ever get through this.

That Easter our family went to church together. Although knowing what we had to face, we attended services that day with hope. Easter is always filled with hope, and we clung to each other with hope for cures and miracles. The day was celebrated almost as if it were Christmas, with an exchange of small gifts, in case Christmas didn't come for John. This was the beginning of making every minute more precious because there was a deadline now for John's time with us. John was hospitalized for two weeks right after Easter for treatment of pneumonia. He needed intravenous antibiotics and oxygen.

Seeing him so sick conjured up fears of immediate death, although the doctor assured us he would recover from this episode. He told us they would continue to treat John aggressively as long as there was a favorable response, thus giving him more time for quality living.

John was frightened. Although he had accepted the illness, he wasn't yet prepared for death. Nor were we.

The hospitalization brought both the opportunity and the necessity to tell others of John's illness. Often we had heard stories that family and friends abandon and isolate persons with AIDS when they hear the diagnosis. Telling others was a painful task because it reinforced our reality, and there also was the fear of judgment, stigma, and rejection. Once those significant to us knew and accepted his illness, one burden was lifted, which decreased some of our anxiety.

Among our friends and relatives there was a response of shock, disbelief, sadness, and some questioning about the disease and risks for contagion for themselves. The questions stemmed from lack of knowledge and the need for self-protection/preservation, not from curiosity about John's lifestyle or how he had contracted the disease. John's friends, our family, and my friends remained supportive, concerned, and a source of strength through his illness.

Although John's illness was not a secret, I realized I was not entirely open with everyone. I did not initially tell my ten-year-old daughter because I thought she might be afraid of closeness with her uncle. I told her of his cancer and decided to tell her he had AIDS only if she asked for more information.

She approached me one day and said, "Mom, why didn't you tell me Uncle John had AIDS?"

She had seen money being collected at a parade for persons with AIDS and one of our friends told her it was to help people who had the same illness as her uncle.

After I explained my reason of not wanting her to be overly worried, she responded, "Mom, I still love Uncle John. That doesn't matter. I don't have to tell everybody if it would bother them."

She accepted, but she already realized there might be consequences depending on whom she told.

There were other people I did not tell. I chose not to tell people whom I knew casually, because their acceptance was not as important, and I did not want to expend more energy dealing with a possible negative response.

Yet our situation was so different from one that I read in an anonymously authored article titled "Obituary for an Unnamed Man." A man who died of AIDS could not have a proper obituary because of the secret the family wanted kept. So much energy used to deal with the stigma of this illness could be used instead to support the person and his or her family.

John was discharged a few days before my breast surgery so he was able to offer support to me and be at the hospital. As I went home to recover, he was able to return to work. Our family began to reestablish some balance.

He was started on chemotherapy treatment for his Kaposi's sarcoma, with hair loss as the initial side effect. The lesions were responsive to the treatment and we were all hopeful. We felt almost as if life were again normal. We needed to sometimes deny the existence of this disease.

We found that denial was a helpful coping mechanism because it allowed us some relief from the anxiety of approaching death and the anticipatory feelings of grief. It permitted us to direct our energy toward going on with our lives. It is not possible to deal with death and sorrow every day.

Summer 1985

We tried to live in the present and enjoy each day, although we envisioned the future, which had death as its finality. While doing this, we felt the urgency to keep memories which would be with us after John was gone. Those memories were captured in our own minds rather than in any tangible way. We had to deal with all of these thoughts while still having to function with day-to-day responsibilities. The goal was to keep a balance.

The summer had many good memories, such as the 4th of July barbecue, Sunday brunch in the city, visits with family and friends, buying a VCR, and times to laugh.

Fall 1985

John went to the Howard Brown clinic to try out the support group sessions for people with AIDS. Although the sessions were designed as a support system, John chose not to utilize the meetings.

His disease was in a more advanced stage compared with that of others at the meetings, and he did not want to be reminded of the finality of his life. He acknowledged the value of the meetings but found his support from friends, family, and prayer.

Howard Brown Clinic provided services which we utilized at other times during our journey. Volunteers offered companionship and help with errands and household tasks. They also assisted us with some financial support.

September was still upbeat! John was still feeling good, and friends gave him a birthday party. It again took more energy to enjoy the celebration and not focus on next year when John might not be here for his birthday.

By October, John's energy level was decreasing, and he lost a few pounds. He was still working, but it was becoming a struggle. He and his boss discussed a less demanding job but he wasn't ready to make a change since he had such pride in his work. Some people with AIDS are ostracized at work or even lose their jobs. This did not happen with John. His employer and colleagues offered extraordinary support to him.

Late that month he had another crisis of more respiratory problems and ex-treme fatigue. The episode began the night he stayed at my house because he didn't feel well enough to travel to his apartment. That night extended to one week. He needed people nearby to assist with comfort needs and meals; and he was too anxious to be alone.

John was better by the end of the week and returned home, but in the next few weeks he continued declining. Treatment with more antibiotics did not im-prove the symptoms, and important decisions had to be made.

He was not able to continue working, which was a major loss for him and for us because it represented giving up part of his life. His employer and colleagues kept in touch with him and invited him to their Christmas party—offering to pick him up in the company's car.

Thanksgiving marked yet another crisis. John called me that morning, crying and telling me he thought he was dying. He had difficulty breathing all night and was very anxious. Instead of sleeping, he had written a note telling us the type of funeral services he wanted and to whom his possessions should be given. I remember the panicky feeling I had as the reality of death was getting closer.

Our friend Ken, who is also a nurse, lived in a nearby building. John was able to call him for instances such as this. John was having increased shortness of breath but his anxiety was also a contributing factor. It became clear at this point that Ken and I were not only support systems but nurses, and that role was evolv-ing more clearly now.

We suggested that portable oxygen could assist him to breathe easier. John agreed to the plan and our first nursing care measure was taken.

The shortness of breath subsided and John joined us for the planned Thanksgiving dinner.

The second major loss which was occurring for John now was his increasing dependency on others. He enjoyed his privacy and took pride in managing his own affairs. Even though he knew his needs were changing, he was ambivalent about acceptance of this dependency.

Winter 1985

The course of his illness was very erratic. One day John would have better energy and feel able to do more. The next day he had to push himself to do any-thing. He was afraid to count on two good days—and so were we. The good days brought hope and the bad day following would erase that. It was like being on a see-saw, with all of us struggling for balance.

A few days before Christmas John called and said he was having fun making cookies with friends. He sounded "normal," energized, and happy.

Then Christmas Eve came, and John was in great discomfort. His fatigue made it impossible to attend church services. So instead we said prayers at the supper table. Vivid in my memory is the scene of friends and family joining hands for prayer, still hoping for miracles and cures.

The holiday was difficult for all of us.

A week later, just prior to the New Year's holiday, there was a family gathering at an aunt and uncle's home. Our small extended family gathered to celebrate. It was another good day for John. As we watched his higher level of energy and better mood, it was easy to deny this illness—at least for a while.

He joked with everyone and we all laughed. John brought out the fun and "kid" in people. He reminded us to enjoy life and to play.

It was a beautiful afternoon. At one point John offered a toast to the family and said, "Thank you all for being such a support to me. I love you all." In response, my cousin's husband—in his deep, gruff voice—said, "We love you too, John." My older uncle added, "We're all in this together. We still hope." We all swallowed back some tears.

The family support continued in many other ways throughout our journey. Cards, phone calls, small gifts, homemade cookies, and messages of love and concern reached John. One cousin sent him the book *When Bad Things Happen to Good People*, by Harold Kushner. Another friend gave him a copy of Carl Simonton's book *Getting Well Again*. Everyone offered support in their own way.

John spent New Year's Eve at my house. Once again he was fatigued and uncomfortable.

On New Year's Day John and I had a sad but rich experience as we talked for the first time about his eventual death. He was trying to get ready for a dinner at my sister's house, but was plagued with tiredness. He spoke of the continual effort of pushing himself every day to live, and of being tired of fighting the battle of sickness. He was preparing to die and trying to find peace within himself. I cried and shared my sadness as I thought of never seeing him again. I assured him that I, my sister, and our children would manage, but we would miss him terribly. It was the beginning of our saying good-bye.

Facing the death of a close loved one also forces us to face our own deaths. "The dying person is a symbol of what every person fears and knows he must someday face" (Anonymous, 1970). If we can confront and understand our feelings about death, our lives can be enriched by the experience of talking with a dying friend, relative, or patient.

Throughout the journey, other people took different opportunities to say good-bye and reminisce about their relationship with John. One of John's friends whom he had known for 20 years made an audiotape of music about love and friendship. I still cry when I listen to the tape.

Winter 1986

A week later John was told he had another opportunistic infection of tuberculosis. His physician started him on medication which would decrease some of his respiratory symptoms. He called me at work with the news and was excited, and again hopeful. If the quality of life improves, the desire to live is stronger. We were hopeful again, put aside the good-byes, and invested ourselves in the day-to-day living. The roller-coaster effect on one's emotions is incredible!

John's symptoms did decrease. He had somewhat better energy and his cough subsided. The only trade-off was that he could no longer get chemotherapy for the Kaposi's sarcoma due to concern that the chemotherapy would cause suppression of his blood count. This would make his risk greater for more respiratory complications. The lesions continued growing.

The next few months John had good and bad days, but not with the extremes of the fall and early winter. We saw the slow decline, but John persevered. The conversation of New Year's Day was put aside and he pushed himself as much as he could every day.

Friends had a Super Bowl party which was like a New Year's Eve party! There was victory for the Chicago Bears, but also for John. He had looked forward to the party and celebrated with all of his friends.

Because it was a mild winter, he could still get out of his apartment and use public transportation some days. He was as active as possible—visiting people and performing his routine daily activities.

Spring 1986

I decided to have my breast reconstruction surgery the first of April since John's illness was stable. There was no interruption of the plan, and John came to see me afterwards at home. He was able to offer me support and love.

The increase in the Kaposi's sarcoma lesions was the current problem causing John emotional and physical pain. Initially he was able to hide the lesions with clothing. But now they were everywhere on his body. His self-concept of a handsome and physically fit man was changing to someone feeble and ugly. He struggled with acceptance of the changes, but sometimes felt depressed. Because the lesions were causing fluid retention in his legs, walking became more painful and would eventually become impossible.

In spite of his deterioration, he decided to move from his studio apartment to a one-bedroom apartment across the courtyard on May 1. It was financially feasible and he wanted a nicer environment and more space.

We helped him clean the apartment, put things away, and he was quickly resettled. He was so excited about his new space, yet I wondered if the decision to move was realistic since we knew he would not be there for long.

Then I realized it was a good decision because John was still living and had needs which could be met by a change in his environment. He wanted to see sunshine and the outdoors from his windows, and walk around in a larger area. Later, when John was confined to bed, it was easier to have a separate bedroom so we could use the living room to rest and sleep when we stayed with him.

In early May he still was able to do household tasks such as washing dishes and preparing simple meals, but it took more time and energy to accomplish.

It was on Mother's Day when he could not walk up stairs any more; so he was carried up to the small gathering we planned for the holiday. Although it was a Mother's Day party for my sister and me, it was another occasion to celebrate more time with John, as well as to say good-bye. There were exchanges of love and affection, and John thanked us for our love and support of being with him. My daughter cross-stitched a heart which said, "I Love You," and she wrote a note telling him what a good uncle he had been to her. We were all saying good-bye in our own way.

Even though we were preparing for John's death, we still hoped there would be more time. John was not ready to give up life. That process of accepting death and giving up life is complex and gradual.

John never left his apartment again after that family gathering.

As he got weaker, he needed more assistance in getting up from a chair. So I purchased a wing-back chair which provided the support he needed to stand and mobilize himself. We always looked for ways to help him maintain his independence.

He spent most of the day in that chair: resting, watching TV, eating his meals, and receiving visitors. Soon, walking to the bathroom was his biggest accomplishment.

June 1986

He could not be left alone now because of his weakness and inability to walk without assistance.

We were confronted with having to provide 24-hour care for John, so we needed to establish a plan.

The plan evolved with a discussion among John's network of family and friends. We scheduled ourselves to have someone with him around the clock. Since our work schedules were all different, we were able to cover the days and nights. John needed assistance with all of his activities of daily living now, and he was in bed most of the time. The plan was working, but we wondered how we would manage when he needed more nursing care, because John did not want to go to the hospital.

Hospice was suggested by his physician, and John was open to the idea. An initial evaluation was done by a physician and nurse who reviewed John's physical and psychosocial needs. A hospital bed, commode, and walker were ordered and new pain medications were prescribed.

Two volunteers were assigned to work with us several hours a week. They sat with John, and did errands, household chores, or whatever else was needed. Aside from providing this help, they offered compassion and support to us.

The nurse visited weekly and we continued scheduling people from our support network to be with John on a 24-hour basis. Since everyone in our support network had jobs and other responsibilities, it was stressful trying to balance everything.

We soon realized that we had to hire someone to give part of the nursing care. The hospice nurse referred us to home care agencies, and we hired a nursing assistant who cared for John Monday through Friday during the daytime hours. We continued covering the evenings, nights, and weekends.

As time passed, we tired, and hope was changing to acceptance and separation.

The anxiety of contagion was brought back to the forefront again as we provided John's physical care of toileting and changing decubitus dressings. We took the necessary precautions, but we were again reminded of the other issues surrounding this disease.

The hospice staff instructed us to use good handwashing techniques and suggested the use of disposable gloves when in contact with body secretions. They also told us to soak linens soiled with body secretions in a solution of bleach and water prior to laundering. The nurse's aide who cared for John cared for other AIDS patients and was not afraid. She was supportive to him and to us.

Despite the assurance that these were the only precautions necessary to prevent contagion, there was still some anxiety and periodic thought of whether we were absolutely safe. It did not prevent or change John's care, but it took more of our emotional energy to deal with these feelings. This is an issue that must be dealt with in order for care to be given. I found that talking with people in our support network decreased my fears and anxieties, and validated our approach to John's nursing care.

The emotional and physical exhaustion we all felt as we continued caring for John would have been unbearable had it not been for the network of supportive people with whom we could talk, cry, or vent anger.

I remember arriving one day at John's apartment after I finished work to stay with him and relieve another friend. I had had a busy work day. I had to arrange for my daughter's care and now I had to watch my brother die. I cried and vented my anger and frustration to my friend so that John would not be subjected to these feelings. Part of me was wanting the journey to end, for it all to be over, but the other part didn't want to say good-bye. As a nurse who cared for dying patients, I had often told families it was normal to experience this. I had validated their feelings, yet it was difficult for me to accept those feelings within myself.

Work colleagues offered to help with John's care or with whatever tasks would lighten our burden. I know this is not always the case. In speaking of her experience with a relative dying of AIDS, a nurse wrote: "Sometimes nurse colleagues fail to support one another when there is illness in their families. They become overly involved in evaluating the nursing care and forget how to listen and support their colleagues" (Doe, 1986). This was not our experience, however.

Our support network felt like a circle of love surrounding John, which was a lifeline to us as well as to John. Severing that line to John was now the task.

As the weeks of June passed and we saw John's lesions spread and his periodic disorientation, we were involved in anticipatory grieving.

I tried to celebrate my birthday on June 25, envisioning how it would be without him next year, and assuming he would not remember the date. Yet late that evening he had a friend phone me, and John wished me a Happy Birthday. We spoke briefly, but he wanted me to know he had not forgotten.

Some grief preparation can be done before our loved one dies, but only after death can we experience the intensity and depth of those feelings to fully grieve the loss. Anticipatory grief does not diminish the pain, emptiness, and loneliness of post-mortem grief, but it does allow us to prepare for death and to say our good-byes.

John wanted to stay in his apartment, but he was running out of money for rent and nursing care. Although the home care agency's daily costs were reasonable, the accumulation of the expenses was becoming a burden. John had been receiving Social Security disability checks, and public assistance provided for food stamps. Some of the medical expenses were covered by public assistance, but our family still had to use some of our own money and our resources were limited.

We decided we would move him to my home, knowing the change in hospice staff and other routines would be distressing to John and a major adjustment to everyone. We had no other choices, and the tentative plans were made. We decided to tell John closer to the time of the move to decrease his anticipation.

John never knew about this plan because he died on July 2 in his own apartment with his friend, Ken, near his bedside.

The journey had ended.

The network of family and friends came to say good-bye to John at the funeral services and his burial. One of John's friends wrote a song for him and played the music at the service. The minister reinforced our faith in God and spoke of the love between John and his family and friends. He acknowledged the terrible toll that AIDS was taking on many people.

We wrote an obituary for the Chicago *Windy City Times*.

Reflection: First Anniversary of John's Death

A year has passed since John's death, and our lives are in a different place. The initial transition from caring for John to the re-establishment of our own routines and activities was difficult. We have all grieved in different ways, but the support network continued to be a resource for us. It has been a painful process, but healing takes place with time and effort. I now see that there were positive outcomes as a result of our experience with John.

We learned the meaning of courage as we watched John persevere. Our capabilities were tested beyond what we thought we could endure, and we found strength we didn't know existed. Our team efforts realized good care for John, and enabled him to die with dignity. Relationships were strengthened with honest expression of feelings. We gained a different perspective on death and were reminded of our choices in making our lives meaningful.

My personal experience with this illness helped me as a nurse to give better and more sensitive care to patients with AIDS, and to assist their families. I expected John to receive competent care from nurses who were kind and non-judgmental, just as I would provide that care to patients.

Nurses must be willing to explore their own feelings and values related to issues of AIDS. Education, peer exchange, and a willingness to share personal experiences can help us reach our goal of providing humane care to AIDS patients and their families. In sharing my experience with other nurses and friends, I have found many people who are worried about the health of relatives and the threat of AIDS to their families. My experiences have given them courage and helped them deal with their fears and their feelings of embarrassment or of being stigmatized. My experiences have helped other nurses and friends realize that AIDS is a disease that happens to peoples we know and love, not just to strangers.

References

Anonymous. (1970). Death in the first person. *American Journal of Nursing, 70*(2), 338.

Cousins, N. (1983). *Healing heart: Antidotes to panic and helplessness.* New York: Norton.

Doe, J. (1986, August). Just be a friend. *Nursing '86, 16*(8), 71.

Duda, D. (1982). *Guide to dying at home.* Santa Fe, NM: John Muir Publications.

Hafen, B.Q. (1983). *Faces of death: Grief, dying, euthanasia and suicide.* Englewood, CO: Morton Publishing Co.

Kushner, H. (1981). *When bad things happen to good people.* New York: Avon.

O'Conner, N. (1984). *Letting go with love: The grieving process.* Apache Junction, AZ: Mariposa Press.

Sarnoff-Schiff, H. (1986). *Living through mourning.* New York: Viking-Penguin.

Simonton, O.C., Simonton, S.M., Creighton, J. (1978). *Getting well again.* New York: Bantam Books.

Chapter 13

Regional and Educational AIDS Resources

Jacquelyn Haak Flaskerud

Persons with HIV infection have need of a wide range of social, educational, and psychological resources both in the hospital and in the community. Patient education is a nursing intervention that includes providing information on community resources. Instructing patients on the resources available to them is part of discharge planning and frequently is the function of nurses in the hospital. Nurses are called on for information about AIDS in a variety of other settings as well as in the hospital. In schools, occupational settings, community mental health centers, public health, visiting nurse, and home health services, nurses are often the most likely persons to be asked for information by patients, families, and the public.

This section provides information on various resources available to persons with HIV infection and their families, members of the public who are concerned about AIDS, and health care workers caring for persons with AIDS. It is divided into the following sections: AIDS hotlines, national, state, and local resources, and educational materials: computer and audiovisual resources; and books, pamphlets, directories, and newsletters.*

These are provided to assist nurses in their health education and health caring roles. However, lists of resources of this sort may be current only up until the time of publication. Information on HIV infection and new resources to assist in prevention of AIDS and the care of persons with HIV infection and AIDS are constantly developing. Local resources will continue to develop in response to the AIDS crisis. Nurses who are involved with the AIDS epidemic will be interested in keeping themselves up-to-date on information about AIDS and HIV infection. As new resources develop, these can be added to this section of the text to keep it current and a useful reference for nurses.

---

*Adapted from the 2nd edition, AIDS Reference Guide for Medical Professionals, edited by Cindi Dale and JoAnne Avers. Copyright 1986, The Regents of the University of California. Adapted with permission.

AIDS HOTLINES

Several hotlines have been set up across the country to answer questions about the disease and its treatment, as well as other information on local resources.

National

(800) 342-AIDS
National AIDS Hotline
Sponsored by the CDC,
Atlanta, Georgia

(800) 843-9388
AZT Information Hotline

(800) 662-HELP
National Institute of Drug
Abuse Hotline

(202) 245-0471
Gary R. Noble, M.D.,
AIDS Coordinator for the
Public Health Service,
Washington, DC

(800) 221-7044
National Gay & Lesbian Task Force,
New York

(800) 227-8922
National Sexually Transmitted
Diseases Hotline
American Social Health Association

(404) 639-3534
CDC Printed Materials
Atlanta, Georgia

(415) 821-7984
Women's AIDS Network
California

State

Alabama

(205) 261-5017
Alabama State Dept. of Health
Department of STD

Alaska

(907) 276-4880
(800) 478-AIDS (Alaska only)

Arizona

(602) 230-5843
(602) 230-5849
Arizona State Dept. of Health

Arkansas

(800) 445-7720
Arkansas State Dept. of Health

California

(800) 367-AIDS (in northern CA)
(800) 922-AIDS (in southern CA)

(213) 876-AIDS
AIDS Hotline of the AIDS
Project/Los Angeles

(619) 260-1304
San Diego AIDS Project

(800) FOR-AIDS
(415) 864-4376
San Francisco AIDS Foundation

(415) 863-AIDS
San Francisco AIDS Activity
  Office

Colorado

(303) 331-8305
Colorado State Dept. of Health

Connecticut

(203) 556-6593
Connecticut State Dept. of Health

(203) 566-1157
9 am–4:30 pm, Mon–Fri

Delaware

(302) 995-8422
Delaware State Dept. of Health

(800) 422-0429
Gay Health Advocates

District of Columbia

(202) 332-AIDS
Washington, DC

Florida

(800) 352-AIDS
(904) 487-2478
Florida State Dept. of Health

Georgia

(800) 342-3427
(800) 551-2728
Georgia State Dept. of Health

(404) 876-9944
AIDS Atlanta

Hawaii

(808) 922-1313
Hawaii State Dept. of Health

Idaho

(208) 334-5944
Idaho State Dept. of Health

Illinois

(800) AID-AIDS
Chicago, IL

(800) 243-2437
(217) 782-2016
Illinois State Dept. of Health

Indiana

(317) 633-8406
Indiana State Dept. of Health

(317) 542-6200
Indianapolis

Iowa

(515) 281-3031
(800) 532-3301
Iowa State Dept. of Health

Kansas

(800) 232-0040
Kansas State Dept. of Health

Kentucky

(502) 564-4478
(800) 654-AIDS
Kentucky State Dept. of Health

Louisiana

(800) 992-4379
(504) 342-6711
Louisiana State Dept. of Health

Maine

(800) 851-AIDS
Maine State Dept. of Health

Maryland

(301) 945-AIDS
(800) 638-6252

Massachusetts

(617) 727-0368
Massachusetts State Dept. of Health

(617) 536-7733
AIDS Action

Michigan

(517) 335-8371
(800) 872-AIDS
Michigan State Dept. of Health

Minnesota

(800) 752-4281
(612) 623-5414
Minnesota State Dept. of Health

(612) 870-0700
(800) 248-AIDS
Minnesota AIDS Project

Mississippi

(800) 826-2961
Mississippi State Dept. of Health

Missouri

(816) 231-8895
Kansas City Health Clinic

(314) 421-AIDS

Montana

(406) 444-4740
Montana State Dept. of Health

Nebraska

(800) 782-2437
Nebraska State Dept. of Health

Nevada

(702) 885-4800
Nevada State Dept. of Health

New Hampshire

(800) 872-8909
New Hampshire State Dept. of Health

New Jersey

(800) 624-2377
New Jersey State Dept. of Health

New Mexico

(505) 266-0911
New Mexico State Dept. of Health

New York

(800) 221-7044
National Gay & Lesbian Task Force,
New York

(212) 420-2779
IV Substance Abuse–AIDS Hotline,
Beth Israel Medical Center,
New York, NY

(518) 473-0641
(519) 457-7152
New York State Dept. of Health

(212) 682-5510
Hemophilia Foundation,
New York, NY

(212) 807-6655
Gay Men's Health Crisis, Inc.,
New York, NY

(718) 485-8111
New York City Health Dept.
HIV Hotline

North Carolina

(919) 733-7301
North Carolina State Dept. of Health

North Dakota

(800) 472-2180
North Dakota State Dept. of Health

Ohio

(614) 466-4643
Ohio State Dept. of Health

Oklahoma

(405) 271-4061
Oklahoma State Dept. of Health

Oregon

(503) 229-5792
Oregon State Dept. of Health

Pennsylvania

(717) 787-3350
Pennsylvania State Dept. of Health

Rhode Island

(401) 277-6502
Rhode Island Project–AIDS

(800) 592-1861 (in Rhode Island)

South Carolina

(803) 734-5482
(800) 322-2437
South Carolina State Dept. of Health

South Dakota

(605) 773-3364
South Dakota State Dept. of Health

Tennessee

(615) 741-7247
Tennessee State Dept. of Health

Texas

(214) 351-4335
Dallas AIDS Project

(512) 458-7405
Texas State Dept. of Health

Utah

(303) 837-0166
Utah AIDS Project

Vermont

(800) 882-AIDS
(8 am–8 pm, Mon–Fri)
Vermont State Dept. of Health

Virginia

(800) 533-4148
Virginia State Dept. of Health

Washington

(800) 272-AIDS
Washington State Dept. of Health

West Virginia

(800) 642-8244
West Virginia State Dept. of Health

Wisconsin

(800) 334-AIDS
(608) 267-3583
Wisconsin State Dept. of Health

Wyoming

(307) 777-7953
Wyoming State Dept. of Health
AIDS Education Risk Reduction
Program

NATIONAL RESOURCES

AIDS PROJECT LOS ANGELES
7362 Santa Monica Blvd.
West Hollywood, CA 90046
(213) 876-8951
Services:
...manual: Living with AIDS
...self-care newsletter
...referrals
...services for persons with AIDS

AMERICAN CANCER SOCIETY
—NATIONAL
Service & Rehabilitation
4 W. 35 St.
New York, NY 10016
(212) 736-3030
Services:
...information referrals to division
offices

AMERICAN FOUNDATION FOR
AIDS RESEARCH (AMFAR)
40 West 57th, Suite 406
New York, NY 10019
(212) 333-3118
-or-
19601 Wilshire Blvd.
Mezzanine Level
Beverly Hills, CA 90210
(213) 273-5547
Services:
...community education
...professional education
...supports laboratory and clinical
   research projects
...aids research funding
...publishes AMFAR Treatment
   Directory

AMERICAN HOSPITAL
ASSOCIATION
840 North Lake Shore Dr.
Chicago, IL 60611
(312) 280-6000
Services:
...education
...referrals

AMERICAN PSYCHOLOGICAL
ASSOCIATION
1200 17th St., N.W.
Washington, DC 20036
(202) 955-7600
...pamphlet: "coping with AIDS"

AMERICAN RED CROSS
—NATIONAL
AIDS Public Education Program
1730 D St., N.W.
Washington DC 20006
(202) 737-8300
Services:
...printed materials
...referrals to local chapters

CENTERS FOR DISEASE CONTROL
AIDS Activity
Building 6, Room 274
1600 Clifton Rd., N.E.
Atlanta, GA 30333
(404) 639-2891
Services:
...national surveillance
...printed materials
...listing of HIV test sites
...publishers of *Morbidity & Mortality
Weekly Report*

CENTER FOR INTERDISCIPLINARY
RESEARCH IN IMMUNOLOGY
AND DISEASE (CIRID) AT UCLA
c/o Dept. Microbiology & Immunology,
UCLA School of Medicine
Los Angeles, CA 90024
(213) 825-1510
Services:
...publishers of:
  newsletters-
    AIDS Medical Update
    AIDS Nursing Update
  manuals-
    *AIDS Reference Guide for Medical
    Professionals*
...clarification on medical research
  findings

FUND FOR HUMAN DIGNITY
666 Broadway, Room 410
New York, NY 10012
(212) 529-1600
(800) 221-7044 (crisis line:
counseling, information, referrals)
Services:
...manual: *National Directory of
AIDS-Related Services*
...printed material for persons with
AIDS
...AIDS service agencies

GAY MEN'S HEALTH CRISES
P.O. Box 274
132 West 24th St.
New York, NY 10011
(212) 807-6655 hotline
Services:
...referrals
...legal aid
...financial aid
...buddies
...housing
...counseling
...educational information
...literature, videos, speakers

HEALTH WORKERS NEEDLE
STICK SURVEY
Centers for Disease Control
1600 Clifton Rd., N.E.
Atlanta, GA 30333
(404) 639-3406
Services:
...federal studies of health workers
  possibly exposed to AIDS; input
  from hospital infection control
  coordinators is being sought

HEMOPHILIA FOUNDATION
—NATIONAL
AIDS Activity Coordinator
Soho Building, Room 406
110 Greene St.
New York, NY 10012
(212) 219-8180
Services:
...printed material—NRCC publications
...referrals
...workshops for providers

NATIONAL AIDS NETWORK
729 Eighth St., S.E., Suite 300
Washington, DC 20003
(202) 347-0390
Services:
...community education
...professional education

NATIONAL ASSOCIATION OF
PEOPLE WITH AIDS (NAPWA)
519 Castro
San Francisco, CA 94114
(415) 553-2509
Services:
...community education
...publish national quarterly newsletter

NATIONAL COUNCIL OF
CHURCHES/AIDS TASK FORCE
475 Riverside Dr., Rm. 572
New York, NY 10115
(212) 870-2421

NATIONAL INSTITUTE OF ALLERGY AND
INFECTIOUS DISEASES (NIAID)
National Institutes of Health
9000 Rockville Pike
Bethesda, MD 20892
(301) 496-0545

NATIONAL INSTITUTE ON
DRUG ABUSE (NIDA)
5600 Fishers Lane
Rockville, MD 20857
(301) 443-6697

NATIONAL INSTITUTE OF MENTAL
HEALTH (NIMH)
Building 10
9000 Rockville Pike
Bethesda, MD 20892
(301) 496-5608

OFFICE OF PUBLIC AFFAIRS
U.S. Public Health Service,
Hubert H. Humphrey Bldg. Rm. 725-H
200 Independence Ave., S.W.
Washington, DC 20201
(202) 648-8182 (Washington, DC)
(800) 342-AIDS (recorded message)
(202) 245-6867 (Alaska and Hawaii
  call collect)
(202) 245-7702 (Surgeon General's
  office)
Services:
...printed material

SAN FRANCISCO AIDS
FOUNDATION
333 Valencia St., 4th floor
San Francisco, CA 94103
(415) 864-4376
Services:
...newsletter
...printed material
...referrals

STATE AND TERRITORIAL DEPARTMENTS OF HEALTH
(By State or Territory)

Alabama

State Health Officer
Alabama State Dept. of Public Health
381 State Office Bldg.
Montgomery, AL 36130
(205) 261-5052

Alaska

Director, Division of Public Health
Alaska Dept. of Health
P. O. Box H06
Juneau, AK 99811
(907) 465-3090

American Samoa

Director, Dept. of Health
Government of American Samoa
LBJ Tropical Medical Center
Pago Pago, American Samoa 96799
(011-684) 633-4590 (overseas)

Arizona

Director of Health
Arizona Dept. of Health Services
1740 West Adams St.
Phoenix, AZ 85007
(602) 255-1024

Arkansas

Director of Health
Arkansas Dept. of Health
4815 West Markham St.
Little Rock, AR 72205
(501) 661-2111

California

Director,
Dept. of Health Services
714 P St., Room 1253
Sacramento, CA 95814
(916) 445-1248

AIDS Section
Public Health Advisor
(916) 445-0553

Colorado

Executive Director
Colorado Dept. of Health
4210 East 11th Ave.
Denver, CO 80220
(303) 320-8333 ext 6315

Connecticut

Commissioner of Health Services
Connecticut State Dept. of
    Health Services
150 Washington St.
Hartford, CT 06106
(203) 566-4800

Delaware

Director,
Dept. of Health and Social Services
Robbins Bldg.
802 Silver Lake Blvd.
Dover, DE 19901
(302) 736-4701

District of Columbia

Director, Dept. of Human Services
801 North Capitol St., NE
7th Floor
Washington, DC 20002
(202) 727-0518

Florida

Staff Director Health Program
  and State Health Officer
Dept. of Health and Rehabilitative
  Services
Bldg. 1, Room 115
1323 Winewood Blvd.
Tallahassee, FL 32339
(904) 487-2705

Georgia

Director,
Georgia Dept. of Human Resources
Division of Public Health
878 Peachtree St., Room 201
Atlanta, GA 30309
(404) 894-7505

Guam

Director, Dept. of Public Health
  and Social Services
Government of Guam
P. O. Box 2816
Agana, Guam 96910
(011-671) 734-2944 (overseas)

Hawaii

Director of Health
Hawaii Dept. of Health
P. O. Box 3378
Honolulu, HI 96801
(808) 548-6505

Idaho

State Health Officer
Dept. of Health and Welfare
Division of Health
Statehouse
Boise, ID 83720
(208) 334-5945

Illinois

Director of Public Health
Illinois Dept. Public Health
535 West Jefferson St.
Springfield, IL 62761
(217) 782-4977

Indiana

State Health Commissioner
Indiana State Board of Health
1330 West Michigan St.
P. O. Box 1964
Indianapolis, IN 46206
(317) 633-8400

Iowa

Commissioner of Public Health
State Dept. of Health
Lucas State Office Bldg.
Des Moines, IA 50319
(515) 281-5605

Kansas

Secretary of Health and Environment
Kansas Dept. of Health
  and Environment
Forbes Field, Bldg. 740
Topeka, KS 66620
(913) 862-9360 ext 522

Kentucky

Commissioner
Cabinet for Human Resources
Dept. of Health Services
275 East Main St.
Frankfort, KY 40601
(502) 564-3970

Louisiana

State Health Officer
Office of Health Services
  and Environmental Quality
Dept. of Health and Human
  Resources
325 Loyola Ave.
P. O. Box 60630
New Orleans, LA 70160
(504) 568-5052

Maine

Director,
  Maine Dept. of Human Services
Bureau of Health
Statehouse Station 11
157 Capitol St.
Augusta, MN 04333
(207) 289-3201

Mariana Islands

Director, Dept. of Health Services
Commonwealth of the
  Northern Mariana Islands
Office of the Governor
Saipan, Mariana Islands 96950
(011-670) 6111, 6112 (overseas)

Maryland

Secretary, Maryland State Dept.
  of Health and Mental Hygiene
201 West Preston St.
Baltimore, MD 21201
(301) 225-6860

Massachusetts

Commissioner of Public Health
Massachusetts Dept. of Public Health
150 Tremont St.
Boston, MA 02111
(617) 727-2700

Michigan

Director,
Michigan Dept. of Public Health
3500 North Logan St.
P. O. Box 30053
Lansing, MI 48909
(517) 335-8022

Minnesota

Sister Mary Madonna Ashton
Commissioner of Health
Minnesota Dept. of Health
717 Delaware St., S.E.
Minneapolis, MN 55440
(612) 623-5414

Missouri

State Dept. of Social Services
Division of Health
Broadway State Office Bldg.
P. O. Box 570
Jefferson City, MO 65102
(314) 751-4330

Mississippi

Mississippi State Dept. of Health
P. O. Box 1700
Jackson, MS 39215
(601) 960-7725

Montana

Director, State Dept. of Health and
    Environmental Sciences
Cogswell Bldg.
Helena, MT 59620
(406) 444-2544

Nebraska

Director of Health
State Dept. of Health
301 Centennial Mall South
P. O. Box 95007
Lincoln, NE 68509
(402) 471-2133

Nevada

State Health Officer
State Dept. of Human Resources
Division of Health
505 East King St., Rm. 201
Carson City, NV 89710
(702) 885-4740

New Hampshire

Director,
Division of Public Health Services
State Dept. of Health and Welfare
Health and Welfare Bldg.
6 Hazen Dr.
Concord, NH 03301
(603) 271-4501

New Jersey

State Commissioner of Health
State Dept. of Health
CN 360
Trenton, NJ 08625
(609) 292-7837

New Mexico

Director, Health Services Division
New Mexico Health and
    Environment Dept.
P. O. Box 968
1190 St. Francis Dr.
Santa Fe, NM 87504
(505) 827-2389

New York

Commissioner of Health
State Dept. of Health
Empire State Plaza
Tower Bldg., 14th Floor
Albany, NY 12237
(518) 474-2011

North Carolina

State Health Director
Division of Health Services
Dept. of Human Resources
225 North McDowell St.
P. O. Box 2091
Raleigh, NC 27602
(919) 733-3446

North Dakota

State Health Officer
State Dept. of Health
State Capital Bldg.
Bismark, ND 58505
(701) 224-2372

Ohio

Director of Health
Ohio Dept. of Health
246 North High St.
Columbus, OH 43266
(614) 466-2253

Oklahoma

Commissioner of Health
State Dept. of Health
1000 Northeast Tenth St.
P. O. Box 53551
Oklahoma City, OK 73152
(405) 271-4200

Oregon

Administrator, State Health Division
Dept. of Human Resources
1400 South West Fifth Ave.,
Room 811
Portland, OR 97201
(503) 229-5032

Pennsylvania

Secretary of Health
Pennsylvania Dept. of Health
P. O. Box 90
Harrisburg, PA 17108
(717) 783-8770

Puerto Rico

Secretary of Health
Puerto Rico Dept. of Health
Edificio A Hospital de Psiquiatria
Rio Piedras, Puerto Rico 02908
(401) 277-2231

Rhode Island

Rhode Island State Dept. of Health
75 Davis St.
Providence, RI 02908
(401) 277-2362

South Carolina

Commissioner, South Carolina
Dept. of Health and Environmental
  Control
2600 Bull St.
Columbia, SC 29201
(803) 758-5445

South Dakota

Secretary of Health
State Dept. of Health
Joe Foss Bldg.
325 East Capitol Ave.
Pierre, SD 57501
(605) 773-3361

Tennessee

Commissioner of Health
  and Environment
Tennessee Dept. of Health
  and Environment
Cordell Hull Bldg,
Room 344
Fifth Ave., North
Nashville, TN 37219
(615) 741-3111

Trust Territory of the Pacific Islands

Chief, Officer of Health Services
Bureau of Health Services
Office of the High Commissioner
Trust Territory of the
    Pacific Islands
Saipan, Mariana Islands 96950
Cable Address: HICOTT Saipan
(011 670) 9854 (overseas)

Texas

Commissioner of Health
Texas Dept. of Health
1100 West 49th St.
Austin, TX 78756
(512) 458-7375

Utah

Executive Director
Utah Dept. of Health
288 N., 1460 W.
Salt Lake City, UT 84116
(801) 538-6101

Vermont

Commissioner of Health
Vermont Dept. of Health
60 Main St., P. O. Box 70
Burlington, VT 05402
(802) 863-7200

Virginia

State Health Commissioner
State Dept. of Health
The James Madison Bldg.
109 Governor St., Room 400
Richmond, VA 23219
(804) 786-3561

Virgin Islands

Commissioner of Health
Virgin Islands Dept. of Health
P. O. Box 7309
St. Thomas,
U.S. Virgin Islands 00801
(809) 774-6097

Washington

Division Director
Division of Health
Dept. of Social and Health Services
1112 South Quince St.
Mail Stop ET-21
Olympia, WA 98504
(206) 753-5871

West Virginia

State Director of Health
West Virginia Dept. of Health
1800 Washington St., E., Rm 206
Charleston, WV 25305
(304) 348-2971

Wisconsin

Administrator, Division of Health
Dept. of Health and Social Services
One West Wilson St.,
P. O. Box 309
Madison, WI 53701
(608) 267-3583

Wyoming

Administrator
Division of Health and Medical Services
Wyoming Dept. of Health
    and Social Services
Hathaway Bldg., 4th Floor
Cheyenne, WY 82002
(307) 777-7121

LOCAL RESOURCES
(By State)

Alabama

JEFFERSON COUNTY HEALTH
DEPARTMENT
STD Program
Box 2646
Birmingham, AL 35202
(205) 933-5419

Alaska

ALASKA DEPARTMENT
OF HEALTH
Communicable Disease Center Office
3601 C St., Suite 576
Box 240249
Anchorage, AK 99524
(907) 561-4233

Arkansas

ARKANSAS DEPARTMENT
OF HEALTH
AIDS Coordinator
4815 West Markham
Little Rock, AR 72205
(501) 661-2133

Arizona

PIMA COUNTY HEALTH
DEPARTMENT
150 W. Congress
Tucson, AZ 85701
(602) 792-8315

California

Los Angeles .
AID FOR AIDS
8235 Santa Monica Blvd. #311
West Hollywood, CA 90046
(213) 656-1107
Services:
    ...direct financial assistance
      for persons with AIDS
    ...education

AIDS POSITIVE ACTION LEAGUE
1154 North Lake Ave.
Pasadena, CA 91104
(213) 684-8411
Services:
    ...AIDS risk reduction information

AIDS PROJECT LOS ANGELES
7362 Santa Monica Blvd.
West Hollywood, CA 90046
(213) 876-AIDS (Hotline)
(800) 922-AIDS (Toll Free in
    S. California only)
Services:
    ...case management service
    ...counseling, support groups,
      people with AIDS,
      their families and lovers
    ...advocacy with community resources
    ...food vouchers, attendant care and
      emergency shelter programs
    ...limited temporary housing
    ...transportation
    ...legal, financial, insurance, and
      spiritual counseling
    ...dental clinic for AIDS patients
    ...volunteers will make house or
      hospital visits
    ...medical and mental health referrals
    ...educational programs for the public
      and health professionals
    ...educational materials, printed
      and audiovisual

AIDS RESPONSE PROGRAM
12832 Garden Grove Blvd., Suite E
Garden Grove, CA 92643
(714) 534-0862
Services:
...prevention
...education for people at risk
...support groups for HIV positives

AIDS SUPPORT GROUP
Wednesday Evenings at 7:00 PM
Plummer Park Hall A
7377 Santa Monica Blvd.
West Hollywood, CA
(213) 473-9253
Services:
...AIDS-related support group

ASIAN PACIFIC COUNSELING
AND TREATMENT CENTER
3407 West 6th St., Suite 510
Los Angeles, CA 90020
(213) 382-7311
Services:
...multilingual counseling

BEING ALIVE/PERSONS WITH
AIDS ACTION COALITION
4225 Santa Monica Blvd. #105
Los Angeles, CA 90029
Services:
...peer support for persons with AIDS
...monthly meetings
...newsletter

BEYOND FEAR
Monday Evenings, 7:30–9:30 pm
Crossroads of the World
6671 Sunset Blvd., #1500
Hollywood, CA
(213) 654-4117
Services:
...AIDS-related support group

CARES TEAM
8512 Santa Monica Blvd.
West Hollywood, CA 90069
(213) 659-4840
Services:
...education on safer sex
...condom distribution

EDMUND D. EDELMAN
HEALTH CENTER
Los Angeles Gay and Lesbian
  Community Services Center
1213 North Highland Ave.
Hollywood, CA 90038
(213) 464-7400
(213) 464-7276 appointments
Services:
...HIV Antibody testing alternative site
  — all testing is strictly confidential.
  An appointment must be made
  between 10:00 am and 12:00 pm,
  Tues–Sat. Results are given in person
  two weeks later during a follow-up
  appointment. No charge.

...AIDS prevention clinic — medical
  evaluation for any person who thinks
  he or she might have signs or symptoms
  of AIDS. Make appointments Mon–
  Thurs from 1:00–3:00 pm. No charge.

...Mobile Outreach — AIDS education
  and screening at various sites,
  including bath houses, throughout
  L.A. County.

EDWARD R. ROYBAL
COMPREHENSIVE
HEALTH CENTER
245 South Fetterly Ave.
Los Angeles, CA 90022
(213) 260-3033
Services:
...alternative testing site

EL CENTRO HEALTH AND
COUNSELING CENTER
972 Goodrich St.
Los Angeles, CA 90022
(213) 725-1337
Services:
...bilingual counseling

GAY AND LESBIAN
COMMUNITY SERVICES
CENTER
1213 N. Highland Ave.
P.O. Box 3877
Los Angeles, CA 90038
(213) 464-7400
Programs:
...Edmund D. Edelman Health Center
(see listing)
...CARES Team (see listing)
...Stop AIDS (see listing)

HARBOR/UCLA MEDICAL
CENTER
Dept. of Medicine, Immunology
& Allergy
1000 West Carson St
Torrance, CA 90509
(213) 533-2365
Services:
...AIDS medical evaluation
(by appointment only)

HEMOPHILIA FOUNDATION OF
SOUTHERN CALIFORNIA
33 South Catalina Ave.
Pasadena, CA 91106
(818) 793-6192

HOT, HORNY, AND HEALTHY
7985 Santa Monica Blvd.
Room 109-136
West Hollywood, CA 90069
(213) 664-4716
Services:
...sponsors safer sex parties

LONG BEACH DEPT. OF HEALTH
2655 Pine Ave.
Long Beach, CA 90806
(213) 427-7421 ext. 274
Services:
...alternative testing site

LOS ANGELES COUNTY
DEPARTMENT OF HEALTH
SERVICES
313 North Figueroa St.
Los Angeles, CA 90012
Programs:
...AIDS Program Office:
(213) 974-7803, coordination of
AIDS services in Los Angeles County
...AIDS Education Program:
(213) 730-3613, AIDS Health
Education
...AIDS Epidemiology Program, Acute
Communicable Disease Control:
(213) 974-8139, AIDS case reporting,
information and epidemiology

LOS ANGELES COUNTY/USC
MEDICAL CENTER
1200 North State St.
Los Angeles, CA 90033
(213) 226-5028
Services:
...AIDS medical evaluations
(by appointment only)

MIND AND BODY LIVING IN
HARMONY—HEALING
NETWORK
Friday and Sunday Evenings
Aerobics Unlimited
4370 Fountain Ave.
Silver Lake, CA 95666
(211) 622-6990
Services:
...AIDS-related support group

MINORITY AIDS PROJECT
5882 West Pico, #210
Los Angeles, CA 90019
(213) 936-4949
Services:
    ...AIDS buddies
    ...transportation
    ...housing
    ...financial help
      a) Social Security benefits
      b) food stamps

PROJECT AHEAD
2017 E. 4th St.
Long Beach, CA 90814
(213) 439-3948
Services:
    ...financial assistance
    ...food and shelter banks
    ...support groups
    ...education

RUTH TEMPLE HEALTH CENTER
3834 S. Western Ave.
Los Angeles, CA 90062
(213) 730-3838
Services:
    ...alternative testing site

SHANTI SHEP AIDS PROJECT
9060 Santa Monica Blvd., Suite 301
West Hollywood, CA 90069
(213) 273-7591
Services:
    ...AIDS-related support group
    ...seminars

SOUTH CA MOBILIZATION
AGAINST AIDS
1428 North McCadden Pl.
Los Angeles, CA 90028
(213) 463-3928
Services:
    ...political action

STOP AIDS LOS ANGELES
8512 Santa Monica Blvd.
West Hollywood, CA 90069
(213) 659-4778
Services:
    ...sponsors discussion groups for gay
      and bisexual men

THE CENTER—LONG BEACH
2017 Fourth St.
Long Beach, CA 90814
Services:
    ...alternative test site
    ...counseling

UCLA MEDICAL CENTER,
IMMUNOLOGY CLINIC
10833 Le Conte Ave.
Los Angeles, CA 90024
(213) 825-3718
Services:
    ...AIDS medical evaluations
      (by appointment only)

WATTS HEALTH FOUNDATION
AIDS Education Program
4116 East Compton
Compton, CA 90221
(213) 639-3068
Services:
    ...community education and
      awareness programs
    ...in-service training for churches
      and community groups
    ...speakers bureau

Sacramento .

SACRAMENTO AIDS
FOUNDATION
1900 K St., Suite 201
Sacramento, CA 95814
(916) 488-AIDS
Services:
    ...physician referral
    ...support groups for AIDS, ARC, and
      HIV antibody positive patients,
      family members, and significant
      others

San Bernardino   .

GAY AND LESBIAN COALITION
P.O. Box 2055
Pomona, CA 91769
(714) 623-1491

SAN BERNARDINO
GAY AND LESBIAN
COMMUNITY SERVICES CENTER
(714) 824-7618
Services:
...information
...referrals
...personal support
...arbitration commission
...peer counseling
...lending library

San Diego   .

MOTHERS OF AIDS PATIENTS
(MAP)
c/o Barbara Peabody
3403 E St.
San Diego, CA 92102
(619) 234-3432

OWEN CLINIC
University of CA, San Diego
Medical Center
225 Dickinson St.
San Diego, CA 92103
(619) 294-3995
Services:
...referrals
...medical evaluations and work ups

SAN DIEGO AIDS PROJECT
3777 4th Ave., P.O. Box 89409
San Diego, CA 92138
Services:
...community education
...buddies
...counseling
...support groups
   a) patients
   b) worried well
   c) health care workers
...housing
   a) temporary/emergency
   b) long-term
...transportation

San Francisco   .

AIDS INTERFAITH NETWORK
890 Hayes St.
San Francisco, CA 94117
(415) 558-HOPE
Services:
...spiritual support/counseling to
   persons with AIDS, their families

AIDS PROJECT OF THE
EAST BAY
400 40th St. #200
Oakland, CA 94609
(415) 420-8181
Services:
...community education
...buddies
...counseling for AIDS or ARC
...support groups
   a) patients
   b) others (lovers, family, friends,
      care partners)
   c) worried well
...transportation
...client advocacy

HAIGHT-ASHBURY FREE
MEDICAL CLINIC
IV Drug Users Program
San Francisco, CA 94117
(415) 621-2014
Services:
...community education
...professional education
...counseling
...funds research

MEN'S SEXUALLY
TRANSMITTED DISEASE
CLINIC
2339 Durant Ave.
Berkeley, CA 94704
(415) 644-0425
Services:
...testing & treatment of STD and AIDS
...education
...free drop-in clinic

NURSES COALITION ON AIDS
584 Castro St., Box 498
San Francisco, CA 94114
(415) 861-6182
Services:
...insure quality care in hospitals and
    homes
...work with other organizations
...support people though fear, grief, and
    lifestyle changes
...education
...disease prevention
...health promotion

OPERATION CONCERN
1853 Market St.
San Francisco, CA 94103
(415) 626-7000
Services:
...community education
...professional education
...counseling for AIDS patients and
    worried well
...support groups
    a) patients
    b) others (lovers, family, friends,
        care partners)

PACIFIC CENTER FOR HUMAN GROWTH
2712 Telegraph Ave.
Berkeley, CA 94705
(415) 841-6224
(415) 548-8283
Services:
...worried well group
...HIV positive support group

SAN FRANCISCO AIDS FOUNDATION WOMEN'S AIDS NETWORK
54 Tenth St.
San Francisco, CA 94103
(415) 864-4376
Services of the Foundation:
...community education
...professional education
...counseling
...support groups
    a) patients
    b) others (lovers, family, friends,
        care partners)
...transportation

Services of the Network:
...community education
...professional education
...support groups
    a) patients
    b) health care workers

SAN FRANCISCO AIDS FOUNDATION
333 Valencia St. 4th Floor
San Francisco, CA 94103
(415) 863-2437

SHANTI PROJECT
890 Hayes St.
San Francisco, CA 94117
(415) 558-9644
Services:
...provides emotional and practical
    support for persons with AIDS and
    significant others
...counseling
...long-term, low cost group housing for
    people with AIDS
...community education
...professional education
...legal aid

San Jose   .

AIDS FOUNDATION OF SANTA CLARA COUNTY
715 North First St., Suite 10
San Jose, CA 95112
(408) 298-AIDS

San Luis Obispo   .

SAN LUIS OBISPO AIDS TASK FORCE
2180 Johnson Ave.
San Luis Obispo, CA 93401
(805) 549-5540

Santa Barbara   .

QUADRI-COUNTIES AIDS TASK FORCE
300 San Antonio Rd.
Santa Barbara, CA 93110
(805) 967-2311 ext 455

WESTERN ADDICTION/GAY
RESOURCE CENTER
126 East Halley St., Suite A18
Santa Barbara, CA 93101
(805) 963-3636

Colorado

COLORADO AIDS PROJECT
Gay & Lesbian Community
   Center of Colorado
Drawer E
Denver, CO 80218
(303) 831-6268
Services:
   ...referrals
   ...support groups
   ...pamphlets

Connecticut

AIDS COORDINATOR
150 Washington St.
Connecticut Dept. of Health
Hartford, CT 06106
(203) 566-1157
Services:
   ...community education
   ...professional education
   ...counseling
   ...funds research

Delaware

DELAWARE DEPARTMENT OF
HEALTH AND SOCIAL SERVICES
AIDS Program Office
Emily Bissell Hospital
Building G
3000 Newport Gap Pike
Wilmington, DE 19808
(302) 995-8422

District of Columbia

DC AIDS TASK FORCE
Whitman-Walker Clinic
1407 S St., N.W.
Washington, DC 20009
(202) 332-5295
(202) 332-AIDS (Hotline)
(202) 332-EXAM (HIV testing line)
Services:
   ...community education
   ...professional education
   ...buddies
   ...counseling
   ...support groups
      a) patients
      b) others (lovers, family, friends,
         care partners)
      c) worried well
   ...financial assistance
   ...housing
      a) temporary/emergency
      b) long-term
   ...legal aid
   ...transportation
   ...home care
   ...referral services
   ...IV drug program
   ...HIV testing
   ...dental clinic

Florida

AIDS CENTER ONE
P.O. Box 8152
Ft. Lauderdale, FL 33312
(800) 325-5371 (Florida only)
(305) 561-0316
Services:
   ...buddies
   ...counseling
   ...support groups
      a) patients
   ...housing
      a) temporary/emergency
      b) long-term
   ...financial assistance
   ...community education
   ...professional education
   ...transportation
   ...housekeeping

HEALTH CRISIS NETWORK
P.O. Box 52-1546
Miami, FL 33152
(305) 326-8833
Services:
...community education
...professional education
...buddies
...counseling
...support groups
  a) patients
  b) others (lovers, family, friends,
    care partners)
  c) worried well
  d) health care workers
...housing
  a) temporary/emergency
  b) long-term
...funds research

Georgia

AIDS ATLANTA
1132 W. Peachtree St., N.W.
Atlanta, GA 30309
(404) 872-0600
Services:
...community education
...professional education
...counseling
...support groups
  a) patients
  b) others (lovers, family, friends,
    care partners)
  c) worried well
  d) health care workers
...financial assistance
...referrals
...housing

Hawaii

HAWAII DEPARTMENT OF HEALTH
P.O. Box 3378
1250 Punchbowl St.
Honolulu, HI 96813
(808) 548-5986
Services:
...counseling
...legal referrals
...medical referrals
...financial referrals
...education

Idaho

IDAHO DEPARTMENT OF HEALTH AND WELFARE
Division of Health Prevention
Medicine
Statehouse
450 West State St.
Boise, ID 83720
(208) 334-5930
Services:
...counseling
...testing

Illinois

AIDS SERVICES
Howard Brown Memorial Clinic
2676 North Halsted
Chicago, IL 60614
(800) 243-2437 (Hotline)
(312) 871-5777
Services:
...community education
...professional education
...counseling
...support groups
  a) patients
  b) others (lovers, family, friends,
    care partners)
  c) worried well
...funds research
...HIV testing
...buddies
...legal referrals
...speakers

SABLE-SHERER CLINIC
Fantus Health Center of Cook
County Hospital
1835 West Harrison, 2nd floor
Chicago, IL 60612
(312) 633-7810
Services:
...outpatient clinic
...community education
...professional education
...counseling
...HIV testing
...support groups
...buddies

Indiana

INDIANA STATE HEALTH
DEPARTMENT
Office of AIDS Activity
1330 West Michigan
Indianapolis, IN 46206
(317) 633-8406

Iowa

IOWA STATE DEPARTMENT OF
PUBLIC HEALTH
AIDS Education
Lucas State Office Building
Des Moines, IA 50319
(515) 281-4938
Services:
...education
...counseling
...referral to alternative testing sites

Kansas

STATE OF KANSAS
DEPARTMENT OF HEALTH
AND ENVIRONMENT
Department of Epidemiology
Forbes Field Bldg. 321, Room 13
Topeka, KS 66620

Kentucky

GAY AND LESBIAN SERVICE
ORGANIZATION
P.O. Box 11471
Lexington, KY 40575
(606) 231-0335
Services:
...referrals

Louisiana

LOUISIANA OFFICE OF
PREVENTIVE MEDICINE AND
PUBLIC HEALTH SERVICES
325 Loyola Ave., Room 615
New Orleans, LA 70012
(504) 568-5005

Maine

MAINE BUREAU OF HEALTH
Office on AIDS
Division of Disease Control
State House, Station 11
Augusta, ME 04333
(207) 289-3591

Maryland

BALTIMORE HEALTH
EDUCATION RESOURCE
ORGANIZATION (HERO)
Medical Arts Building
Read & Cathedral Sts.
Baltimore, MD 21201
(301) 945-AIDS
(800) 683-6252 (Maryland Hotline)
Services:
...community education
...professional education
...buddies
...support groups
  a) patients
  b) others (lovers, family, friends,
     care partners)
  c) worried well
  d) health care workers
...housing
  a) temporary/emergency
  b) long-term
...transportation
...funds research
...prison outreach
...IV drug program
...minority outreach
...referrals
...legal aid
...financial help

GAY COMMUNITY CENTER
OF BALTIMORE
HEALTH CLINIC
241 W. Chase St., 3rd floor
Baltimore, MD 21201
(301) 837-2050
Services:
...counseling
...medical examinations

Massachusetts

AIDS ACTION PROJECT
661 Boylston St.
Boston, MA 02111
(617) 437-6200
(800) 235-2331 (Massachusetts only)
(617) 536-7733 (Hotline)
Services:
...community education
...professional education
...buddies
...support groups
   a) patients
   b) others (lovers, family, friends,
      care partners)
   c) worried well
...housing
   a) temporary/emergency
   b) long-term
...legal aid
...transportation
...funds research
...IV drug task force
...newsletter
...referrals to mental health
   professionals
...holistic referrals
...meal delivery program
...religious counseling group
...financial counseling

Michigan

WELLNESS NETWORKS, INC.
P.O. Box 1046
Royal Oak, MI 48068
(313) 547-9040
(800) 872-2347 (in Michigan)

Minnesota

MINNESOTA DEPARTMENT
OF HEALTH
717 South East Delaware St.
Minneapolis, MN 55440
(612) 623-5414

Mississippi

MISSISSIPPI GAY ALLIANCE
P.O. Box 8342
Jackson, MI 39204
(601) 353-7611
Services:
...counseling
...medical referrals
...housing
...legal referrals

Missouri

MISSOURI DEPARTMENT
OF HEALTH
AIDS Program
P.O. Box 570
Jefferson City, MO 65102
(314) 751-6438

Montana

MONTANA DEPARTMENT
OF HEALTH AND
ENVIRONMENTAL SCIENCES
Cogswell Building
Helena, MT 59260
(406) 444-2457
Services:
...counseling
...education
...testing

Nebraska

NEBRASKA DEPARTMENT OF
HEALTH AIDS Prevention Program
P.O. Box 95007
Lincoln, NE 68509
(402) 541-2937

New Hampshire

NEW HAMPSHIRE DEPARTMENT
OF HEALTH AND WELFARE
6 Hazen Drive
Concord, NH 03301
(603) 271-4490

New Mexico

AIDS TASK FORCE
P.O. Box 968
124 Quincy, N.E.
Albuquerque, NM 87108
(505) 266-0911
Services:
...counseling
...support groups
...case management/advocacy
...legal aid
...transportation
...housekeeping

New Jersey

HYACINTH FOUNDATION
New Jersey AIDS Project
211 Livingston Ave.
New Brunswick, NJ 08901
(201) 246-0925
(800) 433-0254 (New Jersey only)
Services:
...community education
...professional education
...buddies
...counseling
...support groups
  a) patients
  b) others (lovers, family, friends,
     care partners)
  c) worried well
...transportation—limited
...advocacy
...legal aid
...financial referrals

New York

AIDS INSTITUTE
New York State Dept. of Health
Albany, NY 12237
(212) 340-3388
Services:
...community education
...professional education
...counseling
...legal aid
...housing
...pamphlets
...fund research
...HIV testing sites

AIDS RESOURCE CENTER
24 West 30th St., 10th floor
New York, NY 10001
(212) 481-1270
Services:
...housing
  a) temporary/emergency
  b) long-term

AIDS ROCHESTER
20 University Ave.
Rochester, NY 14605
(716) 232-3580
(716) 232-4430 (Hotline)
Services:
...counseling
...IV user/abuser program
...buddies
...financial assistance
...housing
  a) long-term
  b) temporary
...community education
...transportation
...legal aid

EAST END GAY ORGANIZATION
FOR HUMAN RIGHTS
P.O. Box 708
Bridgehampton, NY 11932
(516) 537-2480

GAY MEN'S HEALTH CRISIS, INC.
Box 274, 132 West 24th St.
New York, NY 10011
(212) 807-7035
(212) 807-6655 (Hotline)
Services:
...community education
...professional education
...buddies
...counseling
...support groups:
   a) patients
   b) others (lovers, family,
      friends, care workers)
   c) worried well
...financial assistance
...transportation
...legal aid

HISPANIC AIDS FORUM
c/o APRED
853 Broadway, Suite 2007
New York, NY 10003
(212) 870-1902
(212) 870-1864

LIAAC (LONG ISLAND
ASSOCIATION FOR AIDS CARE)
Box 2859
Huntington, NY 11746

MID-HUDSON VALLEY
AIDS TASK FORCE
Gay Men's Alliance
214 Central Ave.
White Plains, NY 10606
(914) 993-0606
(914) 993-0607 (Hotlines)
Services:
...community education
...professional education
...support groups
...referrals
...counseling
...legal referrals
...food pantry—limited
...housing referrals—limited

OFFICE OF GAY &
LESBIAN HEALTH
New York City Dept. of Health
Box 67
125 Worth St.,
New York, NY 10013
(212) 566-4995
Services:
...AIDS prevention programs
...community outreach and education
...forums

PWA (PEOPLE WITH AIDS)
COALITION
263A West 19th St., Room 125
New York, NY 10011
(212) 627-1810
Services:
...community education
...support groups
   a) AIDS and ARC patients
   b) women with AIDS
...publishes monthly newsletter
...handbook: *Striving and Thriving
   with AIDS*
...limited meal programs
...experimental treatment information

WESTERN NEW YORK
AIDS PROGRAM
220 Delaware Ave.
Buffalo, NY 14202
(716) 847-2437
Services:
...support group
...advocacy program
...limited financial aid
...community education and outreach

VISITING NURSE SERVICE
AIDS Task Force
350 Fifth Ave.
New York, NY 10118
(212) 560-5952

Nevada

AID FOR AIDS
2116 Paradise Rd., Suites C & D
Las Vegas, NV 89104
(702) 369-6162
Services:
...support groups
...buddies
...food bank
...printed material
...referrals
...financial information
...transportation
...volunteer training

North Carolina

STATE OF NORTH CAROLINA
HEALTH DEPARTMENT
P.O. Box 2091
Raleigh, NC 27602
(919) 733-3419

North Dakota

NORTH DAKOTA STATE
DEPARTMENT OF HEALTH
State Capitol Building
Bismark, ND 58505
(701) 224-2376/2378
Services:
...counseling
...referrals
...testing referrals
...professional education
...community education

Ohio

AMBROSE CLEMENT
HEALTH CLINIC
3101 Burnet Ave.
Cincinnati, OH 45229
312) 352-3102
(513) 421-AIDS (Hotline)
Services:
...support groups
...test site
...counseling
...referrals

CHOICES CLINIC
237 East 17th St.
Columbus, OH 43201
(614) 294-6337
Services:
...counseling
...medical referrals
...legal referrals

Oklahoma

OKLAHOMA FOR HUMAN
RIGHTS
2301 North Lincoln Blvd, Room 480
Oklahoma City, OK 73105
(405) 521-2360
Services:
...AIDS-related discrimination
  problems

Oregon

CASCADE AIDS PROJECT
408 Southwest 2nd, Suite 420
Portland, OR 97204
(503) 223-5907
Services:
...buddies
...support groups
  a) patients
  b) significant others
...crisis counseling
...housekeeping
...transportation
...emergency financial assistance
...emergency food assistance

PHOENIX RISING FOUNDATION
408 Southwest 2nd, Rm. 407
Portland, OR 97204
(503) 223-8299
Services:
...AIDS counseling

Pennsylvania

PHILADELPHIA AIDS
TASK FORCE
P.O. Box 53429
Philadelphia, PA 19105
(215) 732-AIDS (Hotline)
(215) 545-8686
Services:
...housing for PWAs
...HIV testing and counseling
...referrals: medical, dental, counseling
...education
...buddies

PHILADELPHIA DEPARTMENT
OF PUBLIC HEALTH
AIDS Control Program
500 South Broad St.
Philadelphia, PA 19146
(215) 875-5659

Rhode Island

RHODE ISLAND
DEPARTMENT OF HEALTH
AIDS Control Program
75 Davis, Room 105
Providence, RI 02908
(401) 277-2362

South Carolina

SOUTH CAROLINA
DEPARTMENT OF HEALTH
2600 Bull St.
Columbia, SC 29201
(803) 734-5010

South Dakota

SOUTH DAKOTA
DEPARTMENT OF HEALTH
523 East Capitol
Pierre, SD 57501
(605) 773-3357
Services:
...counseling
...testing referrals

Tennessee

TENNESSEE DEPARTMENT OF
HEALTH AND ENVIRONMENT
100 Ninth Ave., North
Nashville, TN 37219
(615) 741-7247

Texas

AIDS FOUNDATION OF
HOUSTON
3927 Essex Lane
Houston, TX 77027
(713) 524-2437 (Hotline 9am–9pm)
(713) 623-6796
Services:
...buddy program
...support groups
  a) patients
  b) health care workers
...legal referral
...transportation
...food and clothing bank
...rent assistance
...financial assistance
...temporary residence for people
  with AIDS
...physician referral

AIDS TASK FORCE
Dallas Gay Alliance
P.O. Box 190712
(214) 528-4233
(214) 559-AIDS (Hotline)
Services:
...community education
...food bank
...clothing bank
...limited financial assistance
...hospital/house visitation
...speakers bureau
...brochures
...newspaper

MONTROSE CLINIC
803 Hawthorne
Houston, TX 77006
(713) 528-5531
Services:
...HIV Testing
...counseling
...immune system screening
...medical referrals
...community education

OAK LAWN COUNSELING
CENTER AIDS PROJECT
6811 Nash St.
Dallas, TX 75235
(214) 351-1502
(214) 351-4335 (Hotline)
Services:
...counseling
...support groups
...holistic counseling
...buddies
...transportation
...housing referrals
...community education
...professional education

Utah

UTAH DEPARTMENT OF HEALTH
288 North 1460 West
P.O. Box 16660
Salt Lake City, UT 84116
(801) 538-6191
Services:
...literature
...referrals
...education
...counseling
...directory of references

Vermont

VERMONT DEPARTMENT
OF HEALTH
60 Main St.
P.O. Box 70
Burlington, VT 05402
(802) 863-7240

Virginia

VIRGINIA DEPARTMENT OF
HEALTH
James Madison Building, Room 719
109 Governor St.
Richmond, VA 23219

Washington

SEATTLE AIDS ACTION PROJECT
113 Summit Ave. East, #204
Seattle, WA 98102
(206) 323-1229
Services:
...phone referrals
...information

SEATTLE-KING COUNTY DEPT OF
PUBLIC HEALTH AIDS PROGRAM
1116 Summit Ave.
Seattle, WA 98101
(206) 587-4999
Services:
...testing
...counseling
...support groups
...direct services referrals

West Virginia

WEST VIRGINIA
DEPARTMENT OF HEALTH
151 11th Ave.
South Charleston, WV 25303
(304) 348-5358

Wisconsin

WISCONSIN DEPARTMENT
OF HEALTH
1 West Wilson St.
Madison, WI 53701
(608) 266-9853

Wyoming

WYOMING DEPARTMENT OF
HEALTH AND MEDICAL
SERVICES
Hathaway Building, 4th Floor
Cheyenne, WY 82002
(307) 777-7953

INTERNATIONAL RESOURCES

WORLD HEALTH
ORGANIZATION (WHO)
Special Programs on AIDS
20 Avenue Appia
1211 Geneva 27
Switzerland
Phone: 011 41 22 9126 73

WHO Regional Offices

Africa
WHO Regional Office
P.O. Box 6
Brazzaville, Congo
(011 91) 3860

The Americas
Pan American Health Organization
Coordinator, Epidemiology Program
525 23rd St., N.W.
Washington, DC 20037
(202) 861-4353

Eastern Mediterranean
WHO Regional Office
P.O. Box 1517
Alexandria, Egypt
(011-20) 3-30-090

Europe
WHO Regional Office
8 Schersigsvej
DK-2100
Copenhagen, Denmark
(011-45) 1-29-01-11

Southeast Asia
WHO Regional Office
World Health House
Indraprastha Estate
Ring Road
New Delhi 11002, India
(011-91) 11-27-01-81

Western Pacific
WHO Regional Office
P.O. Box 2932
12115 Manila, Philippines

Australia

AUSTRALIAN COUNCIL OF
TRADE UNIONS, OCCUPATIONAL
HEALTH AND SAFETY UNIT
Trades Hall, Box 93
Carlton South 3053
Victoria, Australia
(011 03) 662-3511
Services:
   ...publishers of "Information Paper on
   AIDS," 1985

Canada

AIDS COMMITTEE OF TORONTO
c/o Hassle Free Clinic
556 Church St., 2nd floor
Toronto, Ontario M4Y 2E3

AIDS VANCOUVER
c/o 19th Floor
355 Burrard St.
Vancouver, B.C. V6C 2J3

CENTRETOWN COMMUNITY
RESOURCES
100 Argyle Ave.
Ottawa, Ontario K2P 1B6

COLLECTIVE D'INTERVENTION
COMMUNAUTAIRE
AUPRES DES GAIS
C.P. 29 Succursale Victoria
Montreal, Quebec
(514) 484-2602

COMITE SOCIAL SERVICE
PROJECT
3757 rue Prud'homme
Montreal, Quebec H4A 3H8

GAY SOCIAL SERVICE
PROJECT
5 rue Weredale Park
Montreal, Quebec H3Z 1Y5

GAYS OF/GAIS DE OTTAWA
Box 2919
Stn. D
Ottawa, Ontario M5W 1X7

England

CAPITOL GAY
38 Mount Pleasant
London MC1XOAP

France

ASSOCIATION DES GAIS
MEDECINS
45 rue Sedaine
75011 Paris

The Netherlands

AIDS POLICY COORDINATOR
Jan K. van Wijngaarden, M.D.
Buro G.V.O.
Prins Hendriklaan 12
1075 BB Amsterdam

COC
Joop van der Linden
Rozenstraat 8
1016 NX Amsterdam

Puerto Rico

LATIN AMERICAN STD CENTER
Centro Medico
Rio Piedras 00922
(809) 754-8118

EDUCATIONAL MATERIALS

Computer Networks

CAIN—COMPUTERIZED AIDS
INFORMATION NETWORK
1213 North Highland Ave.
Hollywood, CA 90038
(213) 464-7400 ext 277
Services:
...nationally consolidated
computerized information on
AIDS or AIDS-related matters.
Available by subscription
by writing or calling.

Audiovisual

ADAIR FILMS
Public Television, KQED
San Francisco, CA
Titles:
..."The AIDS Show: Artists Involved
with Death and Survival"
An extremely moving film about the
pain, anguish and emotional turmoil
of AIDS patients and their loved
ones. It is presented with humor and
understanding.

ADVANCED IMAGING INC.
c/o Care Video Productions
P.O. Box 45132
Cleveland, OH 44145
(216) 835-5872
Titles:
...."AIDS and the Health Care Provider"
Health care professionals discuss
cause, transmission, and prevention
of AIDS. Deals with practical
control measures as well as the
innermost thoughts of the AIDS
patient. Produced in cooperation
with Yale–New Haven Hospital, CT.

AIDS PROJECT LOS ANGELES
7362 Santa Monica Blvd.
West Hollywood, CA 90046
(213) 876-9851
Titles:
..."AIDS: Questions and Answers"
..."Buying Time for a Cure"

ALFRED HIGGINS PRODUCTIONS
9100 Sunset Blvd.
Los Angeles, CA 90069
(213) 272-6580
Titles:
..."VD: More Bugs, More Problems"
20 minutes. An up-to-date review of
sexually transmitted diseases,
emphasizing AIDS and chlamydia.
Appropriate for junior high age and
up. Personal responsibility is
emphasized.

AMERICAN ASSOCIATION
OF BLOOD BANKS
Suite 600, 1117 N 19th St.
Arlington, VA 22209
Titles:
..."Blood Banks in the Age of AIDS"
A 10 minute videotape that helps
blood donor recruiters allay the fears
of potential donors with information
on how AIDS is transmitted.
Cost $99.

..."Fear of AIDS"
A public-service announcement that
stresses the message that blood
donors are not at risk. Cost $45.

AMERICAN COLLEGE
HEALTH ASSOCIATION
15879 Crabbs Branch Way
Rockville, MD 20855
(301) 963-1100
Titles:
..."The AIDS Dilemma: Higher
Education's Response"
90 minutes. Covers the history and
current development of the AIDS
dilemma, information on diagnosis,
treatment, prevention, implications
for institutions of higher education,
and recommendations on policy and
action appropriate for such
institutions.

AMERICAN HOSPITAL
ASSOCIATION
840 North Lakeshore Dr.
Chicago, IL
(312) 280-6000
Titles:
..."Fear of Caring"
20 minutes. Designed for hospital
workers, this docudrama covers the
fear of AIDS, duty to care,
epidemiology, transmission, and
infection control procedures.
Developed by the American Hospital
Association.

AMERICAN RED CROSS UNITS
(OR ANY LOCAL RED
CROSS UNIT)
2001 21st St.
Sacramento, CA 94131
(916) 452-6541
Titles:
..."Beyond Fear"
A series of three 20 minute
segments: The Virus; The Individual;

and The Community. Designed for the public and health professionals it addresses epidemiology, transmission, risk reduction, screening, the need for education, and discrimination issues. Interviews with a woman with AIDS, a woman with ARC, and a family with AIDS (mother, father, and 1-year old). Developed by the American Red Cross. Free.

AUDIO VIDEO DIGEST FOUNDATION
1577 Chevy Chase Dr.
Glendale, CA 91206
(800) 423-2308
(800) 232-2165 (California)
(213) 240-7500
Titles:
...."Epidemiology of AIDS"
   50 minutes. Examines the history of the Center for Disease Control's epidemiologic investigation, the risk groups, and the research that resulted in the isolation of the AIDS virus.
...."Immunology of AIDS"
   50 minutes. Presents an analysis of the immune system, its role in preventing infection, and the AIDS attack on it.
...."Kaposi's Sarcoma"
   50 minutes. Dr. Paul Volberding's discussion includes KS presentation, work-up and treatment, and the difficulties and precautions with an infectious agent.

CABISCO TELEPRODUCTIONS
Carolina Biological Supply Co.
2700 York Road
Burlington, NC 27215
(800) 334-5551
(800) 632-1231 (in North Carolina)
Titles:
...."AIDS Biology Video Programs"
   Series of on-location 28 minute videotape interviews with leading

AIDS researchers and clinicians: Dr. Robert Gallo on the search for the AIDS virus; Dr. Paul Volberding on the clinical story of AIDS; and Dr. Luc Montagnier on retroviruses and AIDS. Can be purchased as set starting at $348.85 (depending upon format) or starting at $149.95 individually.

CARLE MEDICAL COMMUNICATIONS
510 West Main
Urbana, IL 61081
(217) 384-4838
Titles:
...."An Institutional Response to AIDS"
   18 minutes. Dramatic film depicting a day in the life of a hospital after the admission of its first confirmed AIDS case. A candid portrayal of what can happen in a hospital that follows all the proper infection control procedures but is not prepared for the psychosocial impact of AIDS patients on its staff. Cost: $65 for 3-day rental of 16 mm or videotape, $365 for purchase of 16 mm film or videotape.

CHURCHILL EDUCATIONAL FILMS
662 N. Robertson Blvd.
Los Angeles, CA 90048
(213) 657-5110
Titles:
...."AIDS: What Everyone Needs to Know"
   18 minutes. Designed for schools and general audiences, the content includes the cause, transmission, prevention of transmission, symptoms, and diagnosis of AIDS. Produced in collaboration with CIRID at UCLA. Cost: Free previews for purchase consideration, $350 for 16 mm, $250 for videotape.

COMMUNITY TELEVISION
NETWORK
Video Services
11 East Hubbard St.
Chicago, IL 60611
Titles:
...."AIDS—Questions and Answers"
15 Minutes. For General audiences.
Culturally Sensitive. Cost $55.

CONTRA COSTA COUNTY
HOSPICE
2500 Alhambra Ave.
Martinez, CA 94553
(415) 674-0981
Titles:
...."AIDS: A Model for Care"

CREATIVE MEDIA
123 4th St., N.W.
Charlottesville, VA 22901
(804) 296-6138
Titles:
...."AIDS Alert"
17-minute cartoon videotape to
reduce anxiety about AIDS.
Cost: $125.

DOUBLE VISION
401 S St.
Sacramento, CA 95814
(916) 448-8220
Titles:
...."AIDS, A Nurses Responsibility"
Instructional program detailing
hospital care, discharge planning,
and home health needs of people
with AIDS. 30 minute videotape and
a Leader's Workbook written by
nurses. For health care providers.
Produced by California Nurses'
Association. Cost: $35 to preview,
$100 to purchase.

DURRIN FILMS, INC.
1748 Kalorama Rd., N.W.
Washington, DC 20009
(202) 387-6700
Titles:
...."The AIDS Movie"
29 minutes. A film on AIDS
prevention for teenagers and young
adults. Features a teacher talking to
a group of students who later ask
him questions most on their minds.
Three patients with AIDS also tell
their stories. Also distributed by
New Day Films, 22 Riverview Dr.,
Wayne, NJ 07470, (201) 633-0212.

EDUTECH COURSEWARE, INC.
7801 East Bush Lake Rd.
Suite 350
Minneapolis, MN 55435
(612) 831-0445
Titles:
...."AIDS Education Program"
45–60 minute interactive videodisk;
prerecorded format presenting AIDS
information, asking questions, and
providing answers in response to
user. Available for purchase of
videodisk only or disk plus player
and monitor, or rental of disk
only.

EDUCATIONAL DIMENSIONS
CORP.
Box 126
Stanford, CT 06904
(800) 243-9020
Titles:
...."The Truth About AIDS"
This program, available either as two
filmstrips with cassettes or on
videotape, includes a discussion of
diagnosis, treatment, transmission,
blood tests, vaccines, viruses, and
prevention. The presentation deals
with both patients and family.

FILMS FOR THE HUMANITIES, INC.
P.O. Box 2053
Princeton, NJ 08543
(800) 257-5126
(609) 452-1128 (in New Jersey)
Titles:
...."AIDS: Our Worst Fears"
57 minutes. This program purports to separate facts from hysteria and from wishful thinking. It explains what is known and not known about AIDS, who is most susceptible and most at risk, and what preventive actions and precautions can be taken.

HEALTH AND LIFE, INC.
25881 West 12 Mile Rd.
Southfield, MI 48034
(800) 624-8983
(800) 328-1240 (in Michigan)
Titles:
...."AIDS: What is it?"
26 minutes. Using documentary style interviews with medical experts, this tape explains AIDS, its transmission, prevention, and prospects for cure. Recommended for teens through adults.

HOSPITAL SATELLITE NETWORK
1901 Ave. of the Stars
Suite 1050
Los Angeles, CA 90067
(213) 277-6710
Titles:
...."Management of the AIDS Patient—San Francisco General Hospital's Approach"
Documentary on a clinically and economically successful multidisciplinary approach to the treatment of AIDS. Directed to hospital workers and administrators. Content includes medical facts about AIDS, infection control issues and practices, and guidance on establishing a dedicated AIDS unit involving all members of the health care team. Additional segments on outpatient care and psychosocial care are included. Developed by the California Medical Association, Hospital Satellite Network, and San Francisco General Hospital. (60 minutes).

INFOMEDIX
Educational Resources & Services
12800 Garden Grove Blvd.,
Suite F
Garden Grove, CA 92643
(714) 530-3454
Titles:
...."International Conference on AIDS"

INSERVICE VIDEO PRODUCTION
1191 Carey Dr.
Concord, CA 94520
(415) 827-2711
Titles:
...."AIDS and Grief"
...."AIDS and the Blood Supply"
...."AIDS and the Third World"
...."Immune System HTLV/III and Risk Reduction"
...."Infection Control"
...."Living with AIDS"
...."Putting the Puzzle Together"
A series of half-hour programs designed to assist health care workers to provide informed, compassionate care to people with AIDS. Includes: Introduction to AIDS, thanatology, infection control, discharge planning, nursing care, immunology, risk reduction, prevention of transmission, psychosocial issues, cultural and ethnic issues, and grief. Developed by the Santa Clara County Health Department AIDS Teaching Project and the Pacific Center for Human Growth. Cost: $50 per half-hour segment, $160 for four segments on a single videotape.

INTERNATIONAL BUREAU/
MODERN WORDS
P.O. Box 1093
Hermosa Beach, CA 90254
(213) 545-6278
Titles:
...."For Our Lives"

LAW VIDEO REVIEW
American Law Institute/
American Bar Association
4025 Chestnut St.
Philadelphia, PA 19104
(215) 243-1661
Titles:
...."AIDS and the Law"

MEDCOM PRODUCTS
12601 Industry St.
Garden Grove, CA 92641
(800) 223-2505
(714) 895-3882 (California)

MED-ED PRODUCTIONS
Division of MSI, Inc.
P.O. Box 1629
West Chester, PA 19380
(215) 436-8881
Titles:
...."AIDS: Medical Education for the
   Community"
   30 minute videotape and film
   designed for general viewing, refutes
   some of the common misconceptions
   about AIDS. Cost: $79.95 VHS/
   Beta, $225 3/4", or $425 16 mm film.

MERMAID PRODUCTIONS
118 King St.
San Francisco, CA 94107
(415) 777-3105
Titles:
...."Alternative Therapies I, II, & III"
...."Parasites and other Co-Factors in
   AIDS"
...."Politics of Drug Research and
   Treatment in AIDS"
...."Report on International Conference,
   Atlanta"

NATIONAL AUDIOVISUAL
CENTER
Order Section GA
8700 Edgeworth Dr.
Capital Heights, MD 20743
(800) 638-1300
Titles:
...."AIDS: Tracking the Mystery"
   20 minutes. Designed to provide the
   general public with information
   regarding the nature and extent of
   AIDS, populations at risk, risk
   reduction, and research in progress.
...."AIDS and Your Job"
   20 minutes. For people in
   occupations that do not require
   health science training, but that deal
   with patients and patient specimens.
   These may include hospital support
   personnel, security guards, police,
   firefighters, food service workers,
   and custodial personnel.
...."What if the Patient has AIDS?"
   22 minutes. The audience for this
   Public Health Service video includes
   nurses, physicians, dentists,
   ophthalmologists, laboratory
   technicians, and other health care
   personnel. Information is given on
   how to care for patients with AIDS
   or ARC and precautions to minimize
   infection. A written guide comes
   with the video. Order Section GA.
   Cost: $55.
...."AIDS: Fears and Facts"
   Videotape available for purchase at
   $55 from above address, or free on
   loan from Modern Talking Picture
   Service, 5000 Park St. North, St.
   Petersburg, FL 33709, Attn: Film
   Scheduling, or call (801) 541-5763.

NETWORK FOR CONTINUING
MEDICAL EDUCATION AIDS
1 Harmon Plaza
Secaucus, NY 07094
(800) 223-0772
Titles:
...."AIDS in the Hospital: Fears and
   Facts"

O.D.N. PRODUCTIONS, INC.
74 Varick St., Suite 304
New York, NY 10013
(212) 431-8923
Titles:
...."Sex, Drugs, and AIDS"
18 minutes. Factual information on
these important issues presented in
informal and direct style for use with
adolescents and adults. Emphasizes
the fact that the AIDS virus is
difficult to contract and risk
reduction behaviors. Cost: $75 to
preview, $385 to purchase.

PBS VIDEO
476 L'Enfant Plaza, S.W.
Washington, DC 20024
(800) 344-3337
Titles:
...."AIDS in the Workplace"
Discusses medical implications,
sociological implications, health and
human concerns, legal factors,
insurance aspects, public and
corporate responsibilities, and
methods of cost containment.
Available in 3/4″, VHS, and Beta
formats. Cost: $345 plus $15
shipping and handling.

SAN DIEGO AIDS PROJECT
4304 Third Ave.
P.O. Box 89049
San Diego, CA 92138
(619) 543-0300
Titles:
...."Psychosocial Aspects of Working
with People with AIDS"

SAN FRANCISCO AIDS
FOUNDATION
333 Valencia St., 4th Floor
San Francisco, CA 94103
(415) 864-4376
Titles:
...."HTLV-III Test Site"

...."Medical Treatment of AIDS"
...."AIDS Care Beyond the Hospital"
Videotape version of a slide
presentation designed as a teaching
tool for health care providers
working with people with AIDS in
the home. The 45 minute *Case
Management* version is directed to
visiting, public health, and hospice
nurses, social workers, discharge
planners, hospital nurses and
physicians. The 30 minute *Attendant
Care* version omits the case
management section and outlines
basic home hygiene techniques. The
content addresses the physical and
psychosocial needs of people with
AIDS and the continuum of illness.
NOT INTENDED FOR GENERAL
LAY AUDIENCES. Cost: $10 to
preview, $25 to rent for one week,
$15 for slide show, $75 to purchase
video, slide show not available for
purchase.
...."AIDS and the Women's
Community"
44 minutes. An analysis of the
impact of the AIDS epidemic on
women, especially lesbians. Includes
presentations by a physician, a
therapist, and an attorney. Topics
include risk factors, transmission,
safe sex, emotional issues, job
discrimination, and political aspects.
Cost: $45.

SHANTI PROJECT
890 Hayes St.
San Francisco, CA 94110
(415) 558-9644
Titles:
...."Volunteer Training Series:
Counseling, Medical, Psychosocial,
etc."
Series of videotapes ranging from
26–60 minutes, on range of topics,
reflecting the Project's training
session for counselors. Includes
discussions of death and dying,
grieving, psychosocial aspects,
sexuality of those with AIDS,
medical overview, etc. Cost: from
$14 for individual tape to $700
for set.

TACONIC CORRECTIONAL
FACILITY
Bedford Hills, NY
(914) 241-3010
Titles:
..."AIDS: A Bad Way to Die"
35 Minutes.

UCLA OFFICE OF
INSTRUCTIONAL DEVELOPMENT
46 Powell Library
10962 LeConte Ave.
Los Angeles, CA 90024
(213) 825-0755
Titles:
..."AIDS: Threats to the Individual and
Threats to the Public"

..."Update on AIDS: Therapy and
Research"

WITHOUT DEFENSES
811 Marigny
New Orleans, LA 70117
(504) 943-4209
Titles:
..."Without Defenses"
A dramatic presentation based on
actual experiences of people whose
lives have been touched by AIDS.
Describes the facts about AIDS
transmission and prevention of its
spread, and the effect AIDS has on a
family. Cost: $175 for VHS/Beta,
$195 for 3/4″, $150 for slide/film.

SELECTED BOOKS

AIDS
M.J. Fromer
New York: Pinnacle Books, 1983

AIDS
J.I. Galin
New York: Raven Press, 1985

AIDS
E.B. Helm
Munich: Zuckschwerdt, 1984

AIDS
H. Masur
Chicago: Year Book Medical Press,
1983

AIDS
I.J. Selikoff
New York: New York Academy of
Sciences, 1983

AIDS: A CATHOLIC CALL
FOR COMPASSION
Eileen Flynn
Kansas City: Sheed and Ward, 1986

AIDS: A MANAGER'S GUIDE
V. Schachter and S. Von Seeburg
New York: Executive Enterprises
Publications, 1986

AIDS: A STRATEGY FOR
NURSING CARE
Robert J. Pratt
Baltimore, Maryland:
Edward Arnold, 1986

AIDS: BASIC GUIDE FOR
CLINICIANS
P. Ebbesen
Copenhagen: Muksgaard, 1984

AIDS: CAUSATIVE AGENT &
EVOLVING PERSPECTIVE
P.J. Fishinger
Chicago: Year Book Medical
Publishers, 1985

AIDS: CLINICAL NURSING
CONFERENCE
B. Heller
Rockville, MD: Aspen Systems, 1984

AIDS: ETIOLOGY, DIAGNOSIS,
TREATMENT, & PREVENTION
V.T. DeVita, Jr.
Philadelphia: Lippincott, 1985

AIDS: EVERYTHING YOU MUST
KNOW ABOUT AIDS
J.Baker
Saratoga, CA: R & E Publishers,
1983

AIDS: FACTS AND ISSUES
Victor Gong and Norman Rudnick
New Brunswick, NJ: Rutgers
University Press, 1986

AIDS EPIDEMIC
K.M. Cahill
New York: St. Martin's Press, 1983

AIDS: MODERN CONCEPTS AND
THERAPEUTIC CHALLENGES
Samuel Broder, ed.
New York: Marcel Dekker Inc., 1987

AIDS & INFECTIONS OF
HOMOSEXUAL MEN
P. Ma and D. Armstrong
New York: Yorke Medical Books,
1984

AIDS: MEDICAL MYSTERY
F.P. Siegal
New York: Grove Press, 1983

AIDS: MYSTERY AND THE
SOLUTION
A. Cantwell, Jr.
Los Angeles: Aries Rising Press,
1983

AIDS: PRINICPALS, PRACTICES
AND POLITICS
Inge Corless & Mary Pitman-Lindeman
Washington DC: Hemisphere
Publishing Corporation, 1987

AIDS: THE FACTS
John Langone
Boston: Little, Brown, 1988

AIDS: THE SAFETY OF BLOOD
AND BLOOD PRODUCTS
J.C. Petricciani et al.
New York: John Wiley and Sons,
1987

AIDS: THE SPIRITUAL DILEMMA
John E. Fortunato
New York: Harper and Row, 1987

AIDS AND THE CHURCH
E.E. Shelp and R.H. Sunderland
Philadelphia: Westminster Press,
1987

AIDS AND PATIENT
MANAGEMENT: LEGAL,
ETHICAL, AND SOCIAL ISSUES
M.D. Witt, ed.
Owings Mills, MD:
Rynd Communications, 1986

AIDS AND THE LAW
William H.L. Dornette
New York: John Wiley and Sons,
1987

AIDS AND THE LAW: A GUIDE
FOR THE PUBLIC
H. Dalton and S. Burris
New Haven, CT: Yale University
Press, 1987

AN EPIDEMIC OF COURAGE:
FACING AIDS IN AMERICA
L.G. Nungesser
New York: St. Martin's Press, 1986

AND THE BAND PLAYED ON:
POLITICS, PEOPLE, AND THE
AIDS EPIDEMIC
R. Shilts
New York: St. Martin's Press, 1987

CONFRONTING AIDS
Institute of Medicine
Washington, DC: National Academy
Press, 1986

EUROPEAN STUDY GROUP ON
EPIDEMIC OF AIDS & KS
G. Giraldo
New York: Karger, 1984

FOCUS ON AIDS: A CLINICAL
APPRAISAL
Mirieux Institute
Miami: The Mirieux Institute, 1984

GAY MEN'S HEALTH: A GUIDE
TO AIDS AND STD
J. Kassler
New York: Harper & Row, 1983

HUMAN T-CELL
LEUKEMIA VIRUS
R.C. Gallo
Cold Springs Harbor, NY:
Cold Springs Harbor Laboratory,
1984

HUMAN T-CELL
LEUKEMIA VIRUS
P.K. Vogt
New York: Springer-Verlag, 1985

INFECTIOUS COMPLICATIONS
OF NEOPLASTIC DISEASE
A.E. Brown
New York: Yorke Medical Books,
1985

INTERNATIONAL CONFERENCE
ON AIDS
S. Gupta
New York: Plenum Press, 1985

INTERNATIONAL CONFERENCE
ON RNA TUMOR VIRUSES IN
HUMAN CANCER
P. Furmanski
New York: Kluwer Academic, 1985

MAXIMUM IMMUNITY
M.A. Weiner
New York: Pocket Books, 1987

MEDICAL ANSWERS ABOUT
AIDS
L. Mass
New York: Gay Men's Health Crisis,
1984

MOBILIZING AGAINST AIDS
Institute of Medicine
Washington DC: National Academy
Press, 1986

NURSING GUIDELINES ON THE MANAGEMENT OF PATIENTS IN THE HOSPITAL AND THE COMMUNITY SUFFERING FROM AIDS
Second Report of the RCN AIDS Working Party
London: Royal College of Nursing of the United Kingdom,
Ruislip Press, 1986

PSYCHIATRIC IMPLICATIONS OF AQUIRED IMMUNE DEFICIENCY SYNDROME
S.E. Nichols
Washington, D.C.: American Psychiatric Press, 1984

SAN FRANCISCO CANCER SYMPOSIUM: CANCER & AIDS
J.M. Vaeth
New York: Karger, 1985

STANDARDS OF ONCOLOGY NURSING PRACTICE
M.H. Brown et al.
New York: John Wiley and Sons, 1986

THE MANAGEMENT OF AIDS PATIENTS
D. Miller et al., Editors
New York: Macmillan, 1986

THE PERSON WITH AIDS: NURSING PERSPECTIVES
J.D. Durham and F.L. Cohen
New York: Springer Publishing, 1987

UNDERSTANDING AND PREVENTING AIDS
A book for everyone
Chris Jennings
Massachusetts: Health Alert Press, 1985

UNITED STATES CONGRESS/ RESPONSE TO AIDS
House Committee on Government Operations
Washington, D.C.: Government Printing Office, 1983

WHAT TO DO ABOUT AIDS: PHYSICIANS AND MENTAL HEALTH PROFESSIONALS DISCUSS THE ISSUES
L. McKusich
Berkeley: University of California Press, 1986

WHEN SOMEONE YOU LOVE HAS AIDS: A BOOK OF HOPE FOR FAMILY AND FRIENDS
B. Moffatt
New York: NAL/Plume, 1987

WOMEN AND AIDS
D. Richardson
New York: Methuen/Pandora, 1987

PAMPHLETS/TEACHING AND TRAINING MANUALS

AIDS AND THE HEALTH
  CARE WORKER
AIDS Education Committee of Service Employees International Union (SEIV)

Local 250, Hospital and Institutional Workers Union
240 Golden Gate Ave.
San Francisco, CA 94102
(415) 441-2500

AIDS AND HEALTH
   CARE WORKERS
AIDS AND IV DRUG USE
AIDS AND THE BLOOD SUPPLY
AIDS AND YOUR CHILDREN
AIDS AND YOUR JOB
AIDS, SEX, AND YOU
CARING FOR THE AIDS PATIENT
   AT HOME
GAY AND BISEXUAL MEN
IF YOUR ANTIBODY
   TEST IS POSITIVE
American Red Cross
U.S. Public Health Service
Rm. 725-H
200 Independence Ave., S.W.
Washington, DC 20201
All of the titles listed above are
leaflets about AIDS

AIDS AND THE PUBLIC
SCHOOLS
National School Boards Association
1680 Duke St.
Alexandria, VA 22314
This report hopes to dispel the myths
and misinformation surrounding
AIDS, allowing parents of school-age
children to make informed decisions.
Contains a review on the known
medical facts, information on the
legal implications of AIDS in schools
and an overview of possible school
board policy responses to AIDS. Cost
$15.

AIDS AND YOUR LEGAL RIGHTS
National Gay Rights Advocates
540 Castro St.
San Francisco, CA 94114
(415) 863-3624

AIDS: A MANAGER'S GUIDE
Schachter and von Seeburg
Executive Enterprises
   Publications Co., Inc.
22 West 21st St.
New York, NY 10010
This guide identifies key legal issues
and answers practical questions to
help managers lawfully respond to
AIDS issues in the workplace.

AIDS: A NURSE'S
RESPONSIBILITY
California Nurses' Association
1855 Folsom St.,
Suite 670
San Francisco, CA 94103
This 50 page booklet contains the
reprinted articles about AIDS which
were first published in the May 1986
issue of *California Nurse*. Cost: $4.20
including postage and handling.

AIDS HOME CARE AND
HOSPICE MANUAL
AIDS Home Care and Hospice
   Program
Visiting Nurses Association
San Francisco
225 30th St.
San Francisco, CA 94131
This comprehensive manual contains
excellent information about AIDS for
the home care worker as well as
guidelines for development of a home
care program for people with AIDS.
Cost: $50 for an individual, $95 for a
non-profit corporation, $195 for a for-
profit corporation.

AIDS IN THE BLACK
COMMUNITY: THE FACTS
National Coalition of Black Lesbians
and Gays
930 S St., N.W., Suite 514
Washington, DC 20004

AIDS: RECOMMENDATIONS
AND GUIDELINES
(NOV 1982–NOV 1986)
Centers for Disease Control
Atlanta, GA 30333

AIDS: REFERENCES AND
RESOURCES
School Nurse Organization of
Minnesota
41 Sherburne Ave.
St. Paul, MN 55103

AIDS: WHAT YOUNG ADULTS
SHOULD KNOW
American Alliance for Health
1900 Association Dr.
Reston, VA 22091

AIDS, YOUR CHILD AND
THE SCHOOL
R & E Research Associates
P.O. Box 2008
Saratoga, CA 95070
For parents and teachers. Includes
information on the virus, the CDC's
recommendations for determining
whether or not to admit an AIDS
sufferer to school , and advice for
day-to-day action, 1986. Cost $3.

AN UPDATED QUANTITATIVE
ANALYSIS OF AIDS IN
CALIFORNIA
Governer George Deukmejian
State of California
Sacramento, CA 95814

AUSTRALIAN COUNCIL OF
TRADE UNIONS INFORMATION
PAPER ON AIDS
Trades Hall
Box 93
Carlton South, 3053
Victoria, Australia
(03) 662-3511

CATALOGUE OF EDUCATION
AND PREVENTION PROJECTS
California Dept. of Health Services
Office of AIDS
Sacramento, CA 95814

CDC UPDATED SLIDES FOR
AIDS EDUCATION
Atlanta, GA 30333
(404) 639-1388

CDC—AIDS SURVEILLANCE
MONTHLY STATISTICS
Atlanta, GA 30333
(404) 639-3534

COPING WITH AIDS
U.S. Dept. of Health and Human
Services
Public Health Services
National Institute of Mental Health
Government Printing Office
DHHS Publication #(ADM)85-1432
Washington, DC
-or-
National Institute of Mental Health
Office of Scientific Information
5600 Fishers Lane
Rockville, MD 20857

FACTS ABOUT A.I.D.S.
American Red Cross
U.S. Public Health Service
Rm. 725-H
200 Independence Ave., S.W.
Washington, DC 20201

FAMILY'S GUIDE TO AIDS (1984)
San Francisco AIDS Foundation
333 Valencia St., 4th Floor
San Francisco, CA 94103
(415) 863-AIDS

GUIDELINES AND
RECOMMENDATIONS FOR
HEALTHFUL GAY SEXUAL
ACTIVITY
National Coalition of Gay Sexually
Transmitted Disease Services, 1981,
1982
P.O. Box 239
Milwaukee, WI 53201

GUIDE TO PUBLIC HEALTH
PRACTICE: HTLV-III ANTIBODY
TESTING AND COMMUNITY
APPROACHES
Publication #85, Oct. '85
ASTHO Foundation
Suite 207, 10400 Connecticut Ave.
Kensington, MD 20895

HEMOPHILIA AND AIDS:
INTIMACY AND SEXUAL
BEHAVIOR
National Hemophilia Foundation
19 West 34th St., Suite 1204
New York, NY 10001

KAPOSI'S SARCOMA
American Cancer Society
Service and Rehabilitation
90 Park Ave.
New York, NY 10013

LIVING WITH AIDS: AN
INFORMATION GUIDE FOR
ORANGE COUNTY
Gay and Lesbian Community
Services Center
12832 Garden Grove Blvd., Suite E
Garden Grove, CA 92634

LIVING WITH AIDS: A SELF-
CARE MANUAL
AIDS Project Los Angeles
7362 Santa Monica Blvd.
West Hollywood, CA 90046
This is a straightforward and very
complete manual written for people
with AIDS. It is a useful resource for
health care providers to have
available when working with people
with AIDS and ARC. Free of charge
to PWAs; 1–19 copies $5 each, 20–39
copies $4 each, 40–69 copies $3 each,
70+ copies $2 each; plus 6.5% sales
tax and .75 per book shipping and
handling.

MEDICAL EVALUATION
OF PERSONS AT RISK
FOR ACQUIRED
IMMUNODEFICIENCY
SYNDROME
San Francisco AIDS Foundation
333 Valencia St.,
4th Floor
San Francisco, CA 94103
Attn: Materials Dept.
This book covers diagnostic
information such as specific
symptoms of AIDS for physicians
and health care professionals. Cost:
$10.65.

PRESENTING AIDS: A RESOURCE
FOR INSERVICE EDUCATION ON
ACQUIRED IMMUNE
DEFICIENCY SYNDROME AND
EDUCATIONAL IMPLICATIONS
School Nurse Organization of
Minnesota
41 Sherburne Ave.
St. Paul, MN 55103

PREVENTING AIDS THROUGH
EDUCATION
Minnesota Curriculum Services
Center
3554 White Bear Ave.
White Bear Lake, MN 55110
(612) 770-3943

RECOMMENDATIONS FOR
PREVENTING THE
TRANSMISSION OF
HTLV-III/LAV
CDC, Office of Public Affairs
1600 Clifton Road, N.W.
Atlanta, GA 30333

SURGEON GENERAL'S REPORT
Acquired Immune Deficiency
Syndrome
U.S. Dept. of Health and
Human Services
National Institute of Mental Health
Office of Scientific Information
5600 Fishers Lane
Rockville, MD 20857

TEACHING ABOUT AIDS: A
TEACHER'S GUIDE
R & E Research Associates
P.O. Box 2008
Saratoga, CA 95070
A companion volume to "AIDS, Your
Child and the School" (see listing),
designed to help teachers educate
students on AIDS, 1987. Cost $6.50.

TEACHING AIDS: A RESOURCE
GUIDE ON ACQUIRED IMMUNE
DEFICIENCY SYNDROME
Network Publications
P.O. Box 1830
Santa Cruz, CA 95061

THE AIDS BOOK—
INFORMATION FOR WORKERS
Service Employees International
Union, AFL-CIO, CLC
Occupational Safety and Health Dept.
1313 L St., N.W.
Washington, DC 20005
(202) 898-3200
This manual provides general AIDS
information and guidelines for
specific groups of workers.

WHAT EVERYONE SHOULD
    KNOW ABOUT AIDS
WHAT GAY AND BISEXUAL MEN
    SHOULD KNOW ABOUT AIDS
U.S. Public Health Service
Rm. 725-H
200 Independence Ave. SW
Washington, DC 20201

WHAT EVERYONE SHOULD
    KNOW ABOUT AIDS
BE INFORMED ABOUT AIDS—
    INFORMATION FOR HEALTH
    CARE PROVIDERS
WHAT GAY AND BISEXUAL MEN
    SHOULD KNOW ABOUT AIDS
SHOOTING DRUGS AND AIDS
Channing L. Bete Co.
2000 State Rd.
South Deerfield, MA 01373
(413) 665-7611

WOMEN AND AIDS CLINICAL
RESOURCE GUIDE
Materials Distribution
San Francisco AIDS Foundation
333 Valencia St., 4th Floor
San Francisco, CA 94103
(415) 864-4376

DIRECTORIES

AIDS: A BIBLIOGRAPHY
R & E Publishers
A 1986 listing of AIDS information:
articles, reports, theses, dissertations,
books, and other bibliographies.

AIDS...A VIRUS THAT DOESN'T
DISCRIMINATE
AIDS Resource Guide
c/o FAPTP
P.O. Box 13372
Gainesville, FL 32604
An easy-to-use resource guide
cataloging all the major educational
materials on AIDS.

AIDS REFERENCE GUIDE FOR
MEDICAL PROFESSIONALS
CIRID at UCLA
c/o Dept. of Micro. and Immuno.
UCLA School of Medicine
Los Angeles, CA 90024-1747
Published by the Center for
Interdisciplinary Research in
Immunology and Diseases (CIRID) at
UCLA, and the UCLA AIDS Center.
Provides over 100 pages of
information including epidemiology,
case definitions, precautions for
various medical and non-medical
settings that come in contact with
HIV, national resources, educational
material, and medical referral centers.
Bound in a 3-ring notebook to
accommodate updated material.

ACQUIRED IMMUNE
DEFICIENCY SYNDROME:
REFERENCE LISTING:
Vol. 1, 1979–1982
AIDS Project Los Angeles

937 North Cole Ave. Suite 3
Los Angeles, CA 90038
This is a "cannot do without"
document which lists all the articles
known that describe research or
information in the area of AIDS or
ARC conditions. In addition, the
name and address of all of the
journals which are cited in the
document are included to obtain
further information. The 2nd volume
includes literature from Jan–June
1983, and a 3rd volume includes
literature from July–Dec 1983.
Additional volumes are planned.

MODEL PROGRAMS FOR
WOMEN'S AIDS EDUCATION
AND SERVICES
San Francisco AIDS Foundation
333 Valencia St., 4th Floor
San Francisco, CA 94103
Attn: Materials Dept.
A critical report on the transmission
and demographics of women with
AIDS. Includes a thorough overview
of networks, forum, research efforts,
and medical and support services
currently being offered in the San
Francisco Bay Area.

NATIONAL AND
INTERNATIONAL DIRECTORY
OF AIDS-RELATED SERVICES
Shanti Project
890 Hayes St.
San Francisco, CA 94117
-or
c/o FAPTP
P.O. Box 13372
Gainesville, FL 32604

NATIONAL DIRECTORY OF AIDS-
RELATED SERVICES
National Gay and Lesbian Task Force
of the US Conference of Mayors
666 Broadway
Suite 410
New York, NY 10012
(212) 741-5800

REPORTS ON AIDS
PUBLISHED IN THE MMWR,
June 1981–Feb 1986
National Technical Information
Service
Publication #PB86-182060/LAA
(703) 487-4650

SUPPORT SERVICES FOR
PEOPLE WITH AIDS
Federation of AIDS-Related
Organizations/AIDS Action Council
8630 Fenton St.
Silver Spring, MD 20910
(301) 588-5484

THE AIDS INFORMATION
SOURCEBOOK
2214 N. Central at Encanto
Phoenix, AZ 85504-1483
Lists resources for AIDS education.
Cost $35.

THE AIDS RECORD DIRECTORY
1518 K St., N.W.
Washington, DC 20005
(202) 783-0110

WOMEN AND AIDS CLINICAL
RESOURCE GUIDE
San Francisco AIDS Foundation
333 Valencia St., 4th Floor
San Francisco, CA 94103
(415) 864-4376
This 348 page Resource Guide was
prepared by the Women's Health
Outreach Project of the Women's
Program at the San Francisco AIDS
Foundation. It is designed to help
health, drug, and human service
providers educate their staffs about
AIDS and develop AIDS awareness
programs and policies.

NEWSLETTERS/PERIODICALS

AIDS '88 UPDATE
The Pacific Center
P.O. Box 908
Berkeley, CA 94701

AIDS ALERT: The Monthly
Update for Health Professionals
American Health Consultants, Inc.
67 Peachtree Park Drive, N.E.
Atlanta, GA 30309
(404) 351-4523

Published monthly. The AIDS
ALERT periodical presents the latest
news and expert advice on the full
spectrum of AIDS. Specific topics
include hazards, precautions,
screening, diagnosis, and treatment.
Management topics to be included
are: employment guidelines, school
policies, legal issues, reimbursement
for care, education, and prevention.
Cost: $79 for one year.

AIDS: AN INTERNATIONAL
BIMONTHLY JOURNAL
Gower Academic Journals
101 Fifth Ave.
New York, NY 10003
Original research papers on topics
ranging from epidemiology to
neuropsychiatry.

AIDS & PUBLIC POLICY
JOURNAL
University Publishing Group
107 East Church St.
Frederick, MD 21701
Published six times a year. This
publication covers issues such as
AIDS litigation, employment
practices, civil rights, and medical
decisions.

AIDS CENTER NEWS
World Hemophilia
AIDS Center
2400 South Flower St.
Los Angeles, CA 90007

AIDS FILE
San Francisco General Hospital
Medical Center Ward 84
99 S. Potrero Ave.
San Francisco, CA 94110
This is a free quarterly newsletter
designed to inform healthcare
providers of the latest treatment for
AIDS and ARC.

AIDS INFORMATION EXCHANGE
U.S. Conference of Mayors
1620 I St., N.W.
Washington, DC 20006

AIDS INSTITUTE NEWSLETTER
New York State Dept. of Health
Empire State Plaza
Tower Bldg., 14th floor
Albany, NY 12237

AIDS ISSUES IN METROPOLITAN
CHICAGO: A Guide for Hospital
Administration
Metropolitan Chicago Health
Care Council
840 North Lake Shore Drive
Chicago, IL 60611
This manual provides a synopsis of
information concerning the
administrative, operational, and legal
issues health care administrators
should understand to develop AIDS-
related policies.

AIDS LAW & LITIGATION
University Publishing Group
107 East Church St.
Frederick, MD 21701
Published six times a year with
monthly update supplements. Public
health and hospital law, medical
malpractice, and insurance law issues
are included.

AIDS MEDICAL UPDATE
UCLA AIDS Center/CIRID at UCLA
Division of Clinical Immunology
   & Allergy
UCLA School of Medicine
Los Angeles, CA 90024
Contains referenced abstracts of
10–12 medical journal articles on
AIDS in each monthly issue with
editorial opinion. Published by the
Center for Interdisciplinary Research
in Immunology and Diseases (CIRID)
at UCLA, and the UCLA AIDS
Center. One year subscription rate is
$24.00. For more information, call
(213) 825-3594.

AIDS NURSING UPDATE
UCLA AIDS Center/CIRID at UCLA
Division of Clinical Immunology
   & Allergy
UCLA School of Medicine
Los Angeles, CA 90024
Contains referenced AIDS abstracts
from current publications focusing on
AIDS issues of immediate importance
to the nursing profession.
Published quarterly by the Center for
Interdisciplinary Research in
Immunology and Diseases (CIRID) at
UCLA and the UCLA AIDS Center.
For more information, call
(213) 825-3594.

AIDS POLICY AND LAW
Buraff Publications, Inc.
1231 25th St., N.W.
Washington, DC 20037
Biweekly newsletter on legislation,
regulation, litigation concerning
AIDS, including policy statements
from various sources, economic
concerns, matters related to testing,
and AIDS education. Cost: $337.

AIDS REFERENCE & RESEARCH
COLLECTION
University Publishing Group
107 East Church St.
Frederick, MD 21701
Updated quarterly. This 1,200-page
collection includes articles on the
history of AIDS, an annotated
bibliography, federal and state
government reports, and a listing of
AIDS resources.

CALIFORNIA AIDS UPDATE
Senator David Roberti
State Capital, Rm. 205
Sacramento, CA 95814

CALIFORNIA MORBIDITY
SUPPLEMENT
Infectious Disease Section
2151 Berkeley Way
Berkeley, CA 94704

ECLIPSE
Shanti Project Newsletter
890 Hayes St.
San Francisco, CA 94117

FOCUS
AIDS Health Project
333 Valencia St., 4th Floor
San Francisco, CA 94103
This is a monthly publication of the
AIDS Health Project. It presents
AIDS research information relevant
to health care and service providers.
Cost: $24 for California residents,
$30 for other U.S. residents, $42 for
other countries, and free to residents
of the 94--- zip code.

HEART SPACE
Los Angeles Shanti Foundation
8568 Santa Monica Blvd.
West Hollywood, CA 90069

HEMOPHILIA INFORMATION
EXCHANGE
National Hemophilia Foundation
19 West 34th St., Suite 1204
New York, NY 10001

MORBIDITY AND MORTALITY
WEEKLY REPORT
Massachusetts Medical Society
C.S.P.O. Box 9120
Waltham, MA 02254

NATIONAL AIDS NETWORK
MONITOR
729 Eighth St., S.E.
Washington, DC 20003
A bimonthly publication. It contains a
digest of news and features
spotlighting the people, programs,
and opportunities which presently
make up the network.

NATIONAL COALITION OF GAY
STD SERVICES
P.O. Box 239
Milwaukee, WI 53201
Published 4–6 times a year. Provides
factual, up-to-date information to the
medical, scientific, and gay/lesbian
communities about sexually
transmitted diseases, AIDS, and
other health related issues.

NATIONAL GAY TASK FORCE
AIDS Update
80 Fifth Ave.
New York, NY 10011

OPTIMIST
AIDS Project Los Angeles
7362 Santa Monica Blvd.
West Hollywood, CA 90046

SAN FRANCISCO AIDS
FOUNDATION NEWS
333 Valencia St.,
4th Floor
San Francisco, CA 94103

THE AIDS RECORD
1518 K St., N.W.
Washington, DC 20005
(202) 783-0110

Appendix A

Abbreviations Used in the Text

AIDS—Acquired immunodeficiency syndrome

ANA—American Nurses' Association

ARC—AIDS-related complex

CDC—Centers for Disease Control

CIRID—Center for Interdisciplinary Research in Immunology and Diseases

CMV—Cytomegalovirus

CNS—Central nervous system

CSF—Cerebrospinal fluid

CT—Computed tomography

ELISA—Enzyme-linked immunosorbent assay

HCWs—Health care workers

HIV—Human immunodeficiency virus

HSV—Herpes simplex virus

IFA—Immunofluorescent assay

IPV—Inactivated polio virus

IV—Intravenous

KS—Kaposi's sarcoma

MMWR—*Morbidity and Mortality Weekly Report*

OI—Opportunistic infection

OPV—Oral polio virus

PAIDS—Pediatric AIDS

PCP—*Pneumocystis carinii* pneumonia

SNAs—State nurses associations

STDs—Sexually transmitted diseases

VZV—Varicella-zoster virus

WHO—World Health Organization

Appendix B

Vol. 36 / No. 1S   MMWR   3S

Revision of the CDC Surveillance Case Definition for Acquired Immunodeficiency Syndrome

Reported by
Council of State and Territorial Epidemiologists;
AIDS Program, Center for Infectious Diseases, CDC

INTRODUCTION

The following revised case definition for surveillance of acquired immunodeficiency syndrome (AIDS) was developed by CDC in collaboration with public health and clinical specialists. The Council of State and Territorial Epidemiologists (CSTE) has officially recommended adoption of the revised definition for national reporting of AIDS. The objectives of the revision are a) to track more effectively the severe disabling morbidity associated with infection with human immunodeficiency virus (HIV) (including HIV-1 and HIV-2); b) to simplify reporting of AIDS cases; c) to increase the sensitivity and specificity of the definition through greater diagnostic application of laboratory evidence for HIV infection; and d) to be consistent with current diagnostic practice, which in some cases includes presumptive, i.e., without confirmatory laboratory evidence, diagnosis of AIDS-indicative diseases (e.g., *Pneumocystis carinii* pneumonia, Kaposi's sarcoma).

The definition is organized into three sections that depend on the status of laboratory evidence of HIV infection (e.g., HIV antibody) (Figure 1). The major proposed changes apply to patients with laboratory evidence for HIV infection: a) inclusion of HIV encephalopathy, HIV wasting syndrome, and a broader range of specific AIDS-indicative diseases (Section II.A); b) inclusion of AIDS patients whose indicator diseases are diagnosed presumptively (Section II.B); and c) elimination of exclusions due to other causes of immunodeficiency (Section I.A).

Application of the definition for children differs from that for adults in two ways. First, multiple or recurrent serious bacterial infections and lymphoid interstitial pneumonia/pulmonary lymphoid hyperplasia are accepted as indicative of AIDS among children but not among adults. Second, for children<15 months of age whose mothers are thought to have had HIV infection during the child's perinatal period, the laboratory criteria for HIV infection are more stringent, since the presence of HIV antibody in the child is, by itself, insufficient evidence for HIV infection because of the persistence of passively acquired maternal antibodies < 15 months after birth.

The new definition is effective immediately. State and local health departments are requested to apply the new definition henceforth to patients reported to them. The initiation of the actual reporting of cases that meet the new definition is targeted for September 1, 1987, when modified computer software and report forms should be in place to accommodate the changes. CSTE has recommended retrospective application of the revised definition to patients already reported to health departments. The new definition follows:

1987 REVISION OF CASE DEFINITION FOR AIDS FOR SURVEILLANCE PURPOSES

For national reporting, a case of AIDS is defined as an illness characterized by one or more of the following "indicator" diseases, depending on the status of laboratory evidence of HIV infection, as shown below.

I. Without Laboratory Evidence Regarding HIV Infection

If laboratory tests for HIV were not performed or gave inconclusive results (*See* Appendix I) and the patient had no other cause of immunodeficiency listed in Section I.A below, then any disease listed in Section I.B indicates AIDS if it was diagnosed by a definitive method (*See* Appendix II).

  A. **Causes of immunodeficiency that disqualify diseases as indicators of AIDS in the absence of laboratory evidence for HIV infection**

    1. high-dose or long-term systemic corticosteroid therapy or other immuno-suppressive/cytotoxic therapy ≤3 months before the onset of the indicator disease

    2. any of the following diseases diagnosed ≤3 months after diagnosis of the indicator disease: Hodgkin's disease, non-Hodgkin's lymphoma (other than primary brain lymphoma), lymphocytic leukemia, multiple myeloma, any other cancer of lymphoreticular or histiocytic tissue, or angioimmu-noblastic lymphadenopathy

    3. a genetic (congenital) immunodeficiency syndrome or an acquired immu-nodeficiency syndrome atypical of HIV infection, such as one involving hypogammaglobulinemia

  B. **Indicator diseases diagnosed definitively (*See* Appendix II)**

    1. candidiasis of the esophagus, trachea, bronchi, or lungs

    2. cryptococcosis, extrapulmonary

    3. cryptosporidiosis with diarrhea persisting >1 month

    4. cytomegalovirus disease of an organ other than liver, spleen, or lymph nodes in a patient >1 month of age

    5. herpes simplex virus infection causing a mucocutaneous ulcer that persists longer than 1 month; or bronchitis, pneumonitis, or esophagitis for any duration affecting a patient >1 month of age

    6. Kaposi's sarcoma affecting a patient < 60 years of age

    7. lymphoma of the brain (primary) affecting a patient < 60 years of age

    8. lymphoid interstitial pneumonia and/or pulmonary lymphoid hyperplasia (LIP/PLH complex) affecting a child <13 years of age

    9. *Mycobacterium avium* complex or *M. kansasii* disease, disseminated (at a site other than or in addition to lungs, skin, or cervical or hilar lymph nodes)

    10. *Pneumocystis carinii* pneumonia

    11. progressive multifocal leukoencephalopathy

    12. toxoplasmosis of the brain affecting a patient >1 month of age

II. With Laboratory Evidence for HIV Infection

Regardless of the presence of other causes of immunodeficiency (I.A), in the presence of laboratory evidence for HIV infection (*See* Appendix I), any disease listed above (I.B) or below (II.A or II.B) indicates a diagnosis of AIDS.

A. **Indicator diseases diagnosed definitively (*See* Appendix II)**
    1. bacterial infections, multiple or recurrent (any combination of at least two within a 2-year period), of the following types affecting a child < 13 years of age:

    > septicemia, pneumonia, meningitis, bone or joint infection, or abscess of an internal organ or body cavity (excluding otitis media or superficial skin or mucosal abscesses), caused by *Haemophilus*, *Streptococcus* (including pneumococcus), or other pyogenic bacteria

    2. coccidioidomycosis, disseminated (at a site other than or in addition to lungs or cervical or hilar lymph nodes)
    3. HIV encephalopathy (also called "HIV dementia," "AIDS dementia," or "subacute encephalitis due to HIV") (*See* Appendix II for description)
    4. histoplasmosis, disseminated (at a site other than or in addition to lungs or cervical or hilar lymph nodes)
    5. isosporiasis with diarrhea persisting >1 month
    6. Kaposi's sarcoma at any age
    7. lymphoma of the brain (primary) at any age
    8. other non-Hodgkin's lymphoma of B-cell or unknown immunologic phenotype and the following histologic types:
        a. small noncleaved lymphoma (either Burkitt or non-Burkitt type) (*See* Appendix IV for equivalent terms and numeric codes used in the *International Classification of Diseases*, Ninth Revision, Clinical Modification)
        b. immunoblastic sarcoma (equivalent to any of the following, although not necessarily all in combination: immunoblastic lymphoma, large-cell lymphoma, diffuse histiocytic lymphoma, diffuse undifferentiated lymphoma, or high-grade lymphoma) (*See* Appendix IV for equivalent terms and numeric codes used in the *International Classification of Diseases*, Ninth Revision, Clinical Modification)

    Note: Lymphomas are not included here if they are of T-cell immunologic phenotype or their histologic type is not described or is described as "lymphocytic," "lymphoblastic," "small cleaved," or "plasmacytoid lymphocytic"

    9. any mycobacterial disease caused by mycobacteria other than *M. tuberculosis*, disseminated (at a site other than or in addition to lungs, skin, or cervical or hilar lymph nodes)
    10. disease caused by *M. tuberculosis*, extrapulmonary (involving at least one site outside the lungs, regardless of whether there is concurrent pulmonary involvement)
    11. *Salmonella* (nontyphoid) septicemia, recurrent
    12. HIV wasting syndrome (emaciation, "slim disease") (*See* Appendix II for description)

B. **Indicator diseases diagnosed presumptively (by a method other than those in Appendix II)**
    Note: Given the seriousness of diseases indicative of AIDS, it is generally important to diagnose them definitively, especially when therapy that would be used may have serious side effects or when definitive diagnosis is needed

for eligibility for antiretroviral therapy. Nonetheless, in some situations, a patient's condition will not permit the performance of definitive tests. In other situations, accepted clinical practice may be to diagnose presumptively based on the presence of characteristic clinical and laboratory abnormalities. Guidelines for presumptive diagnoses are suggested in Appendix III.

1. candidiasis of the esophagus
2. cytomegalovirus retinitis with loss of vision
3. Kaposi's sarcoma
4. lymphoid interstitial pneumonia and/or pulmonary lymphoid hyperplasia (LIP/PLH complex) affecting a child <13 years of age
5. mycobacterial disease (acid-fast bacilli with species not identified by culture), disseminated (involving at least one site other than or in addition to lungs, skin, or cervical or hilar lymph nodes)
6. *Pneumocystis carinii* pneumonia
7. toxoplasmosis of the brain affecting a patient >1 month of age

III. With Laboratory Evidence Against HIV Infection
With laboratory test results negative for HIV infection (*See* Appendix I), a diagnosis of AIDS for surveillance purposes is ruled out *unless*:
A. all the other causes of immunodeficiency listed above in Section I.A are excluded; **AND**
B. the patient has had either:
   1. *Pneumocystis carinii* pneumonia diagnosed by a definitive method (*See* Appendix II); **OR**
   2. a. any of the other diseases indicative of AIDS listed above in Section I.B diagnosed by a definitive method (*See* Appendix II); **AND**
      b. a T-helper/inducer (CD4) lymphocyte count <400/mm^3.

COMMENTARY
The surveillance of severe disease associated with HIV infection remains an essential, though not the only, indicator of the course of the HIV epidemic. The number of AIDS cases and the relative distribution of cases by demographic, geographic, and behavioral risk variables are the oldest indices of the epidemic, which began in 1981 and for which data are available retrospectively back to 1978. The original surveillance case definition, based on then-available knowledge, provided useful epidemiologic data on severe HIV disease (1). To ensure a reasonable predictive value for underlying immunodeficiency caused by what was then an unknown agent, the indicators of AIDS in the old case definition were restricted to particular opportunistic diseases diagnosed by reliable methods in patients without specific known causes of immunodeficiency. After HIV was discovered to be the cause of AIDS, however, and highly sensitive and specific HIV-antibody tests became available, the spectrum of manifestations of HIV infection became better defined, and classification systems for HIV infection were developed (2-5). It became apparent that some progressive, seriously disabling, and even fatal conditions (e.g., encephalopathy, wasting syndrome) affecting a substantial number of HIV-infected patients were not subject to epidemiologic surveillance, as they were not included in the AIDS

Vol. 36 / No. 1S   MMWR   7S

case definition. For reporting purposes, the revision adds to the definition most of those severe non-infectious, non-cancerous HIV-associated conditions that are categorized in the CDC clinical classification systems for HIV infection among adults and children (4,5).

Another limitation of the old definition was that AIDS-indicative diseases are diagnosed presumptively (i.e., without confirmation by methods required by the old definition) in 10%-15% of patients diagnosed with such diseases; thus, an appreciable proportion of AIDS cases were missed for reporting purposes (6,7). This proportion may be increasing, which would compromise the old case definition's usefulness as a tool for monitoring trends. The revised case definition permits the reporting of these clinically diagnosed cases as long as there is laboratory evidence of HIV infection.

The effectiveness of the revision will depend on how extensively HIV-antibody tests are used. Approximately one third of AIDS patients in the United States have been from New York City and San Francisco, where, since 1985, < 7% have been reported with HIV-antibody test results, compared with > 60% in other areas. The impact of the revision on the reported numbers of AIDS cases will also depend on the proportion of AIDS patients in whom indicator diseases are diagnosed presumptively rather than definitively. The use of presumptive diagnostic criteria varies geographically, being more common in certain rural areas and in urban areas with many indigent AIDS patients.

To avoid confusion about what should be reported to health departments, the term "AIDS" should refer only to conditions meeting the surveillance definition. This definition is intended only to provide consistent statistical data for public health purposes. Clinicians will not rely on this definition alone to diagnose serious disease caused by HIV infection in individual patients because there may be additional information that would lead to a more accurate diagnosis. For example, patients who are not reportable under the definition because they have either a negative HIV-antibody test or, in the presence of HIV antibody, an opportunistic disease not listed in the definition as an indicator of AIDS nonetheless may be diagnosed as having serious HIV disease on consideration of other clinical or laboratory characteristics of HIV infection or a history of exposure to HIV.

Conversely, the AIDS surveillance definition may rarely misclassify other patients as having serious HIV disease if they have no HIV-antibody test but have an AIDS-indicative disease with a background incidence unrelated to HIV infection, such as cryptococcal meningitis.

The diagnostic criteria accepted by the AIDS surveillance case definition should not be interpreted as the standard of good medical practice. Presumptive diagnoses are accepted in the definition because not to count them would be to ignore substantial morbidity resulting from HiV infection. Likewise, the definition accepts a reactive screening test for HIV antibody without confirmation by a supplemental test because a repeatedly reactive screening test result, in combination with an indicator disease, is highly indicative of true HIV disease. For national surveillance purposes, the tiny proportion of possibly false-positive screening tests in persons with AIDS-indicative diseases is of little consequence. For the individual patient, however, a correct diagnosis is critically important. The use of supplemental tests is, therefore, strongly endorsed. An increase in the diagnostic use of HIV-antibody tests could improve both the quality of medical care and the function of the new case definition, as well as assist in providing counselling to prevent transmission of HIV.

FIGURE I. Flow diagram for revised CDC case definition of AIDS, September 1, 1987

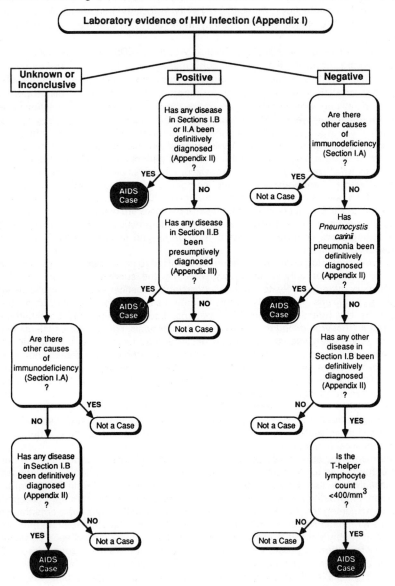

References
1. World Health Organization. Acquired immunodeficiency syndrome (AIDS): WHO/CDC case definition for AIDS. WHO Wkly Epidemiol Rec 1986;61:69-72.
2. Haverkos HW, Gottlieb MS, Killen JY, Edelman R. Classification of HTLV-III/LAV-related diseases [Letter]. J Infect Dis 1985;152:1095.
3. Redfield RR, Wright DC, Tramont EC. The Walter Reed staging classification of HTLV-III infection. N Engl J Med 1986;314:131-2.
4. CDC. Classification system for human T-lymphotropic virus type III/lymphadenopathy-associated virus infections. MMWR 1986;35:334-9.
5. CDC. Classification system for human immunodeficiency virus (HIV) infection in children under 13 years of age. MMWR 1987;36:225-30,235.
6. Hardy AM, Starcher ET, Morgan WM, et al. Review of death certificates to assess completeness of AIDS case reporting. Pub Hlth Rep 1987;102(4):386-91.
7. Starcher ET, Biel JK, Rivera-Castano R, Day JM, Hopkins SG, Miller JW. The impact of presumptively diagnosed opportunistic infections and cancers on national reporting of AIDS [Abstract]. Washington, DC : III International Conference on AIDS, June 1-5, 1987.

APPENDIX I

Laboratory Evidence For or Against HIV Infection

1. For Infection:
   When a patient has disease consistent with AIDS:
   a. a serum specimen from a patient ≥15 months of age, or from a child <15 months of age whose mother is not thought to have had HIV infection during the child's perinatal period, that is repeatedly reactive for HIV antibody by a screening test (e.g., enzyme-linked immunosorbent assay [ELISA]), as long as subsequent HIV-antibody tests (e.g., Western blot, immunofluorescence assay), if done, are positive; **OR**
   b. a serum specimen from a child < 15 months of age, whose mother is thought to have had HIV infection during the child's perinatal period, that is repeatedly reactive for HIV antibody by a screening test (e.g., ELISA), plus increased serum immunoglobulin levels and at least one of the following abnormal immunologic test results: reduced absolute lymphocyte count, depressed CD4 (T-helper) lymphocyte count, or decreased CD4/CD8 (helper/suppressor) ratio, as long as subsequent antibody tests (e.g., Western blot, immunofluorescence assay), if done, are positive; **OR**
   c. a positive test for HIV serum antigen; **OR**
   d. a positive HIV culture confirmed by both reverse transcriptase detection and a specific HIV-antigen test or in situ hybridization using a nucleic acid probe; **OR**
   e. a positive result on any other highly specific test for HIV (e.g., nucleic acid probe of peripheral blood lymphocytes).

2. Against Infection:
   A nonreactive screening test for serum antibody to HIV (e.g., ELISA) without a reactive or positive result on any other test for HIV infection (e.g., antibody, antigen, culture), if done.

3. Inconclusive (Neither For nor Against Infection):
   a. a repeatedly reactive screening test for serum antibody to HIV (e.g., ELISA) followed by a negative or inconclusive supplemental test (e.g., Western blot, immunofluorescence assay) without a positive HIV culture or serum antigen test, if done; **OR**
   b. a serum specimen from a child < 15 months of age, whose mother is thought to have had HIV infection during the child's perinatal period, that is repeatedly reactive for HIV antibody by a screening test, even if positive by a supplemental test, without additional evidence for immunodeficiency as described above (in 1.b) and without a positive HIV culture or serum antigen test, if done.

Vol. 36 / No. 1S   MMWR   11S

APPENDIX II

Definitive Diagnostic Methods for Diseases Indicative of AIDS

Diseases

Definitive Diagnostic Methods

cryptosporidiosis
cytomegalovirus
isosporiasis
Kaposi's sarcoma
lymphoma
lymphoid pneumonia
  or hyperplasia
Pneumocystis carinii
  pneumonia
progressive multifocal
  leukoencephalopathy
toxoplasmosis

microscopy (histology or cytology).

candidiasis

gross inspection by endoscopy or autopsy or by microscopy (histology or cytology) on a specimen obtained directly from the tissues affected (including scrapings from the mucosal surface), not from a culture.

coccidioidomycosis
cryptococcosis
herpes simplex virus
histoplasmosis

microscopy (histology or cytology), culture, or detection of antigen in a specimen obtained directly from the tissues affected or a fluid from those tissues.

tuberculosis
other mycobacteriosis
salmonellosis
other bacterial
  infection

culture.

HIV encephalopathy*   }   clinical findings of disabling cognitive and/or
(dementia)   motor dysfunction interfering with occupation or
                              activities of daily living, or loss of behavioral de-
                              velopmental milestones affecting a child,
                              progressing over weeks to months, in the
                              absence of a concurrent illness or condition other
                              than HIV infection that could explain the findings.
                              Methods to rule out such concurrent illnesses and
                              conditions must include cerebrospinal fluid exam-
                              ination and either brain imaging (computed to-
                              mography or magnetic resonance) or autopsy.

HIV wasting syndrome*   }   findings of profound involuntary weight loss
                              >10% of baseline body weight plus either chronic
                              diarrhea (at least two loose stools per day for
                              ≥ 30 days) or chronic weakness and documented
                              fever (for ≥ 30 days, intermittent or constant) in
                              the absence of a concurrent illness or condition
                              other than HIV infection that could explain the
                              findings (e.g., cancer, tuberculosis, cryptosporidi-
                              osis, or other specific enteritis).

*For HIV encephalopathy and HIV wasting syndrome, the methods of diagnosis described here
are not truly definitive, but are sufficiently rigorous for surveillance purposes.

APPENDIX III

Suggested Guidelines for Presumptive Diagnosis
of Diseases Indicative of AIDS

Diseases	Presumptive Diagnostic Criteria
candidiasis of esophagus	a. recent onset of retrosternal pain on swallowing; **AND** b. oral candidiasis diagnosed by the gross appearance of white patches or plaques on an erythematous base or by the microscopic appearance of fungal mycelial filaments in an uncultured specimen scraped from the oral mucosa.
cytomegalovirus retinitis	a characteristic appearance on serial ophthalmoscopic examinations (e.g., discrete patches of retinal whitening with distinct borders, spreading in a centrifugal manner, following blood vessels, progressing over several months, frequently associated with retinal vasculitis, hemorrhage, and necrosis). Resolution of active disease leaves retinal scarring and atrophy with retinal pigment epithelial mottling.
mycobacteriosis	microscopy of a specimen from stool or normally sterile body fluids or tissue from a site other than lungs, skin, or cervical or hilar lymph nodes, showing acid-fast bacilli of a species not identified by culture.
Kaposi's sarcoma	a characteristic gross appearance of an erythematous or violaceous plaque-like lesion on skin or mucous membrane. (**Note:** Presumptive diagnosis of Kaposi's sarcoma should not be made by clinicians who have seen few cases of it.)
lymphoid interstitial pneumonia	bilateral reticulonodular interstitial pulmonary infiltrates present on chest X ray for ≥ 2 months with no pathogen identified and no response to antibiotic treatment.
Pneumocystis carinii pneumonia	a. a history of dyspnea on exertion or nonproductive cough of recent onset (within the past 3 months); **AND** b. chest X-ray evidence of diffuse bilateral interstitial infiltrates or gallium scan evidence of diffuse bilateral pulmonary disease; **AND** c. arterial blood gas analysis showing an arterial pO_2 of <70 mm Hg or a low respiratory diffusing capacity (<80% of predicted values) or an increase in the alveolar-arterial oxygen tension gradient; **AND** d. no evidence of a bacterial pneumonia.

toxoplasmosis
of the brain

a. recent onset of a focal neurologic abnormality consistent with intracranial disease or a reduced level of consciousness; **AND**
b. brain imaging evidence of a lesion having a mass effect (on computed tomography or nuclear magnetic
resonance) or the radiographic appearance of which is
enhanced by injection of contrast medium; **AND**
c. serum antibody to toxoplasmosis or successful
response to therapy for toxoplasmosis.

APPENDIX IV

Equivalent Terms and International Classification
of Disease (ICD) Codes for AIDS-Indicative Lymphomas

The following terms and codes describe lymphomas indicative of AIDS in patients with antibody evidence for HIV infection (Section II.A.8 of the AIDS case definition). Many of these terms are obsolete or equivalent to one another.

ICD-9-CM (1978)

Codes	Terms
200.0	**Reticulosarcoma** lymphoma (malignant): histiocytic (diffuse) reticulum cell sarcoma: pleomorphic cell type or not otherwise specified
200.2	**Burkitt's tumor or lymphoma** malignant lymphoma, Burkitt's type

ICD-O (Oncologic Histologic Types 1976)

Codes	Terms
9600/3	**Malignant lymphoma, undifferentiated cell type** non-Burkitt's or not otherwise specified
9601/3	**Malignant lymphoma, stem cell type** stem cell lymphoma
9612/3	**Malignant lymphoma, immunoblastic type** immunoblastic sarcoma, immunoblastic lymphoma, or immunoblastic lymphosarcoma
9632/3	**Malignant lymphoma, centroblastic type** diffuse or not otherwise specified, or germinoblastic sarcoma: diffuse or not otherwise specified
9633/3	**Malignant lymphoma, follicular center cell, non-cleaved** diffuse or not otherwise specified
9640/3	**Reticulosarcoma, not otherwise specified** malignant lymphoma, histiocytic: diffuse or not otherwise specified reticulum cell sarcoma, not otherwise specified malignant lymphoma, reticulum cell type
9641/3	**Reticulosarcoma, pleomorphic cell type** malignant lymphoma, histiocytic, pleomorphic cell type reticulum cell sarcoma, pleomorphic cell type
9750/3	**Burkitt's lymphoma or Burkitt's tumor** malignant lymphoma, undifferentiated, Burkitt's type malignant lymphoma, lymphoblastic, Burkitt's type

Appendix C

Recommendations for Prevention of HIV Transmission in Health-Care Settings

Introduction

Human immunodeficiency virus (HIV), the virus that causes acquired immuno-deficiency syndrome (AIDS), is transmitted through sexual contact and exposure to infected blood or blood components and perinatally from mother to neonate. HIV has been isolated from blood, semen, vaginal secretions, saliva, tears, breast milk, cerebrospinal fluid, amniotic fluid, and urine and is likely to be isolated from other body fluids, secretions, and excretions. However, epidemiologic evidence has implicated only blood, semen, vaginal secretions, and possibly breast milk in transmission.

The increasing prevalence of HIV increases the risk that health-care workers will be exposed to blood from patients infected with HIV, especially when blood and body-fluid precautions are not followed for all patients. Thus, this document emphasizes the need for health-care workers to consider **all** patients as potentially infected with HIV and/or other blood-borne pathogens and to adhere rigorously to infection-control precautions for minimizing the risk of exposure to blood and body fluids of all patients.

The recommendations contained in this document consolidate and update CDC recommendations published earlier for preventing HIV transmission in health-care settings: precautions for clinical and laboratory staffs (1) and precautions for health-care workers and allied professionals (2); recommendations for preventing HIV transmission in the workplace (3) and during invasive procedures (4); recommendations for preventing possible transmission of HIV from tears (5); and recommendations for providing dialysis treatment for HIV-infected patients (6). These recommendations also update portions of the "Guideline for Isolation Precautions in Hospitals" (7) and reemphasize some of the recommendations contained in "Infection Control Practices for Dentistry" (8). The recommendations contained in this document have been developed for use in health-care settings and emphasize the need to treat blood and other body fluids from **all** patients as potentially infective. These same prudent precautions also should be taken in other settings in which persons may be exposed to blood or other body fluids.

Definition of Health-Care Workers

Health-care workers are defined as persons, including students and trainees, whose activities involve contact with patients or with blood or other body fluids from patients in a health-care setting.

Health-Care Workers with AIDS

As of July 10, 1987, a total of 1,875 (5.8%) of 32,395 adults with AIDS, who had been reported to the CDC national surveillance system and for whom occupational information was available, reported being employed in a health-care or clinical laboratory setting. In comparison, 6.8 million persons — representing 5.6% of the U.S. labor force — were employed in health services. Of the health-care workers with AIDS, 95% have been reported to exhibit high-risk behavior; for the remaining 5%, the means of HIV acquisition was undetermined. Health-care workers with AIDS were significantly more likely than other workers to have an undetermined risk (5% versus 3%, respectively). For both health-care workers and non-health-care workers with AIDS, the proportion with an undetermined risk has not increased since 1982.

AIDS patients initially reported as not belonging to recognized risk groups are investigated by state and local health departments to determine whether possible risk factors exist. Of all health-care workers with AIDS reported to CDC who were initially characterized as not having an identified risk and for whom follow-up information was available, 66% have been reclassified because risk factors were identified or because the patient was found not to meet the surveillance case definition for AIDS. Of the 87 health-care workers currently categorized as having no identifiable risk, information is incomplete on 16 (18%) because of death or refusal to be interviewed; 38 (44%) are still being investigated. The remaining 33 (38%) health-care workers were interviewed or had other follow-up information available. The occupations of these 33 were as follows: five physicians (15%), three of whom were surgeons; one dentist (3%); three nurses (9%); nine nursing assistants (27%); seven housekeeping or maintenance workers (21%); three clinical laboratory technicians (9%); one therapist (3%); and four others who did not have contact with patients (12%). Although 15 of these 33 health-care workers reported parenteral and/or other non-needlestick exposure to blood or body fluids from patients in the 10 years preceding their diagnosis of AIDS, none of these exposures involved a patient with AIDS or known HIV infection.

Risk to Health-Care Workers of Acquiring HIV in Health-Care Settings

Health-care workers with documented percutaneous or mucous-membrane exposures to blood or body fluids of HIV-infected patients have been prospectively evaluated to determine the risk of infection after such exposures. As of June 30, 1987, 883 health-care workers have been tested for antibody to HIV in an ongoing surveillance project conducted by CDC (*9*). Of these, 708 (80%) had percutaneous exposures to blood, and 175 (20%) had a mucous membrane or an open wound contaminated by blood or body fluid. Of 396 health-care workers, each of whom had only a convalescent-phase serum sample obtained and tested ≥90 days post-exposure, one — for whom heterosexual transmission could not be ruled out — was seropositive for HIV antibody. For 425 additional health-care workers, both acute- and convalescent-phase serum samples were obtained and tested; none of 74 health-care workers with nonpercutaneous exposures seroconverted, and three (0.9%) of 351 with percutaneous exposures seroconverted. None of these three health-care workers had other documented risk factors for infection.

Two other prospective studies to assess the risk of nosocomial acquisition of HIV infection for health-care workers are ongoing in the United States. As of April 30, 1987, 332 health-care workers with a total of 453 needlestick or mucous-membrane exposures to the blood or other body fluids of HIV-infected patients were tested for HIV antibody at the National Institutes of Health (10). These exposed workers included 103 with needlestick injuries and 229 with mucous-membrane exposures; none had seroconverted. A similar study at the University of California of 129 health-care workers with documented needlestick injuries or mucous-membrane exposures to blood or other body fluids from patients with HIV infection has not identified any seroconversions (11). Results of a prospective study in the United Kingdom identified no evidence of transmission among 150 health-care workers with parenteral or mucous-membrane exposures to blood or other body fluids, secretions, or excretions from patients with HIV infection (12).

In addition to health-care workers enrolled in prospective studies, eight persons who provided care to infected patients and denied other risk factors have been reported to have acquired HIV infection. Three of these health-care workers had needlestick exposures to blood from infected patients (13-15). Two were persons who provided nursing care to infected persons; although neither sustained a needlestick, both had extensive contact with blood or other body fluids, and neither observed recommended barrier precautions (16,17). The other three were health-care workers with non-needlestick exposures to blood from infected patients (18). Although the exact route of transmission for these last three infections is not known, all three persons had direct contact of their skin with blood from infected patients, all had skin lesions that may have been contaminated by blood, and one also had a mucous-membrane exposure.

A total of 1,231 dentists and hygienists, many of whom practiced in areas with many AIDS cases, participated in a study to determine the prevalence of antibody to HIV; one dentist (0.1%) had HIV antibody. Although no exposure to a known HIV-infected person could be documented, epidemiologic investigation did not identify any other risk factor for infection. The infected dentist, who also had a history of sustaining needlestick injuries and trauma to his hands, did not routinely wear gloves when providing dental care (19).

Precautions To Prevent Transmission of HIV

Universal Precautions

Since medical history and examination cannot reliably identify all patients infected with HIV or other blood-borne pathogens, blood and body-fluid precautions should be consistently used for **all** patients. This approach, previously recommended by CDC (3,4), and referred to as "universal blood and body-fluid precautions" or "universal precautions," should be used in the care of **all** patients, especially including those in emergency-care settings in which the risk of blood exposure is increased and the infection status of the patient is usually unknown (20).

1. All health-care workers should routinely use appropriate barrier precautions to prevent skin and mucous-membrane exposure when contact with blood or other body fluids of any patient is anticipated. Gloves should be worn for touching blood and body fluids, mucous membranes, or non-intact skin of all patients, for handling items or surfaces soiled with blood or body fluids, and for performing venipuncture and other vascular access procedures. Gloves should be changed after contact with each patient. Masks and protective eyewear or face shields should be worn during procedures that are likely to generate droplets of blood or other body fluids to prevent exposure of mucous membranes of the mouth, nose, and eyes. Gowns or aprons should be worn during procedures that are likely to generate splashes of blood or other body fluids.

2. Hands and other skin surfaces should be washed immediately and thoroughly if contaminated with blood or other body fluids. Hands should be washed immediately after gloves are removed.

3. All health-care workers should take precautions to prevent injuries caused by needles, scalpels, and other sharp instruments or devices during procedures; when cleaning used instruments; during disposal of used needles; and when handling sharp instruments after procedures. To prevent needlestick injuries, needles should not be recapped, purposely bent or broken by hand, removed from disposable syringes, or otherwise manipulated by hand. After they are used, disposable syringes and needles, scalpel blades, and other sharp items should be placed in puncture-resistant containers for disposal; the puncture-resistant containers should be located as close as practical to the use area. Large-bore reusable needles should be placed in a puncture-resistant container for transport to the reprocessing area.

4. Although saliva has not been implicated in HIV transmission, to minimize the need for emergency mouth-to-mouth resuscitation, mouthpieces, resuscitation bags, or other ventilation devices should be available for use in areas in which the need for resuscitation is predictable.

5. Health-care workers who have exudative lesions or weeping dermatitis should refrain from all direct patient care and from handling patient-care equipment until the condition resolves.

6. Pregnant health-care workers are not known to be at greater risk of contracting HIV infection than health-care workers who are not pregnant; however, if a health-care worker develops HIV infection during pregnancy, the infant is at risk of infection resulting from perinatal transmission. Because of this risk, pregnant health-care workers should be especially familiar with and strictly adhere to precautions to minimize the risk of HIV transmission.

Implementation of universal blood and body-fluid precautions for **all** patients eliminates the need for use of the isolation category of "Blood and Body Fluid Precautions" previously recommended by CDC (7) for patients known or suspected to be infected with blood-borne pathogens. Isolation precautions (e.g., enteric, "AFB" [7]) should be used as necessary if associated conditions, such as infectious diarrhea or tuberculosis, are diagnosed or suspected.

Precautions for Invasive Procedures

In this document, an invasive procedure is defined as surgical entry into tissues, cavities, or organs or repair of major traumatic injuries 1) in an operating or delivery

Vol. 36 / No. 2S   MMWR   7S

room, emergency department, or outpatient setting, including both physicians' and dentists' offices; 2) cardiac catheterization and angiographic procedures; 3) a vaginal or cesarean delivery or other invasive obstetric procedure during which bleeding may occur; or 4) the manipulation, cutting, or removal of any oral or perioral tissues, including tooth structure, during which bleeding occurs or the potential for bleeding exists. The universal blood and body-fluid precautions listed above, combined with the precautions listed below, should be the minimum precautions for **all** such invasive procedures.

1. All health-care workers who participate in invasive procedures must routinely use appropriate barrier precautions to prevent skin and mucous-membrane contact with blood and other body fluids of all patients. Gloves and surgical masks must be worn for all invasive procedures. Protective eyewear or face shields should be worn for procedures that commonly result in the generation of droplets, splashing of blood or other body fluids, or the generation of bone chips. Gowns or aprons made of materials that provide an effective barrier should be worn during invasive procedures that are likely to result in the splashing of blood or other body fluids. All health-care workers who perform or assist in vaginal or cesarean deliveries should wear gloves and gowns when handling the placenta or the infant until blood and amniotic fluid have been removed from the infant's skin and should wear gloves during post-delivery care of the umbilical cord.

2. If a glove is torn or a needlestick or other injury occurs, the glove should be removed and a new glove used as promptly as patient safety permits; the needle or instrument involved in the incident should also be removed from the sterile field.

Precautions for Dentistry*

Blood, saliva, and gingival fluid from **all** dental patients should be considered infective. Special emphasis should be placed on the following precautions for preventing transmission of blood-borne pathogens in dental practice in both institutional and non-institutional settings.

1. In addition to wearing gloves for contact with oral mucous membranes of all patients, all dental workers should wear surgical masks and protective eyewear or chin-length plastic face shields during dental procedures in which splashing or spattering of blood, saliva, or gingival fluids is likely. Rubber dams, high-speed evacuation, and proper patient positioning, when appropriate, should be utilized to minimize generation of droplets and spatter.

2. Handpieces should be sterilized after use with each patient, since blood, saliva, or gingival fluid of patients may be aspirated into the handpiece or waterline. Handpieces that cannot be sterilized should at least be flushed, the outside surface cleaned and wiped with a suitable chemical germicide, and then rinsed. Handpieces should be flushed at the beginning of the day and after use with each patient. Manufacturers' recommendations should be followed for use and maintenance of waterlines and check valves and for flushing of handpieces. The same precautions should be used for ultrasonic scalers and air/water syringes.

*General infection-control precautions are more specifically addressed in previous recommendations for infection-control practices for dentistry (*8*).

3. Blood and saliva should be thoroughly and carefully cleaned from material that has been used in the mouth (e.g., impression materials, bite registration), especially before polishing and grinding intra-oral devices. Contaminated materials, impressions, and intra-oral devices should also be cleaned and disinfected before being handled in the dental laboratory and before they are placed in the patient's mouth. Because of the increasing variety of dental materials used intra-orally, dental workers should consult with manufacturers as to the stability of specific materials when using disinfection procedures.
4. Dental equipment and surfaces that are difficult to disinfect (e.g., light handles or X-ray-unit heads) and that may become contaminated should be wrapped with impervious-backed paper, aluminum foil, or clear plastic wrap. The coverings should be removed and discarded, and clean coverings should be put in place after use with each patient.

Precautions for Autopsies or Morticians' Services

In addition to the universal blood and body-fluid precautions listed above, the following precautions should be used by persons performing postmortem procedures:
1. All persons performing or assisting in postmortem procedures should wear gloves, masks, protective eyewear, gowns, and waterproof aprons.
2. Instruments and surfaces contaminated during postmortem procedures should be decontaminated with an appropriate chemical germicide.

Precautions for Dialysis

Patients with end-stage renal disease who are undergoing maintenance dialysis and who have HIV infection can be dialyzed in hospital-based or free-standing dialysis units using conventional infection-control precautions (21). Universal blood and body-fluid precautions should be used when dialyzing **all** patients.

Strategies for disinfecting the dialysis fluid pathways of the hemodialysis machine are targeted to control bacterial contamination and generally consist of using 500-750 parts per million (ppm) of sodium hypochlorite (household bleach) for 30-40 minutes or 1.5%-2.0% formaldehyde overnight. In addition, several chemical germicides formulated to disinfect dialysis machines are commercially available. None of these protocols or procedures need to be changed for dialyzing patients infected with HIV.

Patients infected with HIV can be dialyzed by either hemodialysis or peritoneal dialysis and do not need to be isolated from other patients. The type of dialysis treatment (i.e., hemodialysis or peritoneal dialysis) should be based on the needs of the patient. The dialyzer may be discarded after each use. Alternatively, centers that reuse dialyzers—i.e., a specific single-use dialyzer is issued to a specific patient, removed, cleaned, disinfected, and reused several times on the same patient only— may include HIV-infected patients in the dialyzer-reuse program. An individual dialyzer must never be used on more than one patient.

Precautions for Laboratories[†]

Blood and other body fluids from **all** patients should be considered infective. To supplement the universal blood and body-fluid precautions listed above, the following precautions are recommended for health-care workers in clinical laboratories.

[†]Additional precautions for research and industrial laboratories are addressed elsewhere (22,23).

1. All specimens of blood and body fluids should be put in a well-constructed container with a secure lid to prevent leaking during transport. Care should be taken when collecting each specimen to avoid contaminating the outside of the container and of the laboratory form accompanying the specimen.
2. All persons processing blood and body-fluid specimens (e.g., removing tops from vacuum tubes) should wear gloves. Masks and protective eyewear should be worn if mucous-membrane contact with blood or body fluids is anticipated. Gloves should be changed and hands washed after completion of specimen processing.
3. For routine procedures, such as histologic and pathologic studies or microbiologic culturing, a biological safety cabinet is not necessary. However, biological safety cabinets (Class I or II) should be used whenever procedures are conducted that have a high potential for generating droplets. These include activities such as blending, sonicating, and vigorous mixing.
4. Mechanical pipetting devices should be used for manipulating all liquids in the laboratory. Mouth pipetting must not be done.
5. Use of needles and syringes should be limited to situations in which there is no alternative, and the recommendations for preventing injuries with needles outlined under universal precautions should be followed.
6. Laboratory work surfaces should be decontaminated with an appropriate chemical germicide after a spill of blood or other body fluids and when work activities are completed.
7. Contaminated materials used in laboratory tests should be decontaminated before reprocessing or be placed in bags and disposed of in accordance with institutional policies for disposal of infective waste (24).
8. Scientific equipment that has been contaminated with blood or other body fluids should be decontaminated and cleaned before being repaired in the laboratory or transported to the manufacturer.
9. All persons should wash their hands after completing laboratory activities and should remove protective clothing before leaving the laboratory.

Implementation of universal blood and body-fluid precautions for **all** patients eliminates the need for warning labels on specimens since blood and other body fluids from all patients should be considered infective.

Environmental Considerations for HIV Transmission

No environmentally mediated mode of HIV transmission has been documented. Nevertheless, the precautions described below should be taken routinely in the care of **all** patients.

Sterilization and Disinfection

Standard sterilization and disinfection procedures for patient-care equipment currently recommended for use (25,26) in a variety of health-care settings—including hospitals, medical and dental clinics and offices, hemodialysis centers, emergency-care facilities, and long-term nursing-care facilities—are adequate to sterilize or disinfect instruments, devices, or other items contaminated with blood or other body fluids from persons infected with blood-borne pathogens including HIV (21,23).

Instruments or devices that enter sterile tissue or the vascular system of any patient or through which blood flows should be sterilized before reuse. Devices or items that contact intact mucous membranes should be sterilized or receive high-level disinfection, a procedure that kills vegetative organisms and viruses but not necessarily large numbers of bacterial spores. Chemical germicides that are registered with the U.S. Environmental Protection Agency (EPA) as "sterilants" may be used either for sterilization or for high-level disinfection depending on contact time.

Contact lenses used in trial fittings should be disinfected after each fitting by using a hydrogen peroxide contact lens disinfecting system or, if compatible, with heat (78 C-80 C [172.4 F-176.0 F]) for 10 minutes.

Medical devices or instruments that require sterilization or disinfection should be thoroughly cleaned before being exposed to the germicide, and the manufacturer's instructions for the use of the germicide should be followed. Further, it is important that the manufacturer's specifications for compatibility of the medical device with chemical germicides be closely followed. Information on specific label claims of commercial germicides can be obtained by writing to the Disinfectants Branch, Office of Pesticides, Environmental Protection Agency, 401 M Street, SW, Washington, D.C. 20460.

Studies have shown that HIV is inactivated rapidly after being exposed to commonly used chemical germicides at concentrations that are much lower than used in practice (27-30). Embalming fluids are similar to the types of chemical germicides that have been tested and found to completely inactivate HIV. In addition to commercially available chemical germicides, a solution of sodium hypochlorite (household bleach) prepared daily is an inexpensive and effective germicide. Concentrations ranging from approximately 500 ppm (1:100 dilution of household bleach) sodium hypochlorite to 5,000 ppm (1:10 dilution of household bleach) are effective depending on the amount of organic material (e.g., blood, mucus) present on the surface to be cleaned and disinfected. Commercially available chemical germicides may be more compatible with certain medical devices that might be corroded by repeated exposure to sodium hypochlorite, especially to the 1:10 dilution.

Survival of HIV in the Environment

The most extensive study on the survival of HIV after drying involved greatly concentrated HIV samples, i.e., 10 million tissue-culture infectious doses per milliliter (31). This concentration is at least 100,000 times greater than that typically found in the blood or serum of patients with HIV infection. HIV was detectable by tissue-culture techniques 1-3 days after drying, but the rate of inactivation was rapid. Studies performed at CDC have also shown that drying HIV causes a rapid (within several hours) 1-2 log (90%-99%) reduction in HIV concentration. In tissue-culture fluid, cell-free HIV could be detected up to 15 days at room temperature, up to 11 days at 37 C (98.6 F), and up to 1 day if the HIV was cell-associated.

When considered in the context of environmental conditions in health-care facilities, these results do not require any changes in currently recommended sterilization, disinfection, or housekeeping strategies. When medical devices are contaminated with blood or other body fluids, existing recommendations include the cleaning of these instruments, followed by disinfection or sterilization, depending on the type of medical device. These protocols assume "worst-case" conditions of

Vol. 36 / No. 2S   MMWR   11S

extreme virologic and microbiologic contamination, and whether viruses have been inactivated after drying plays no role in formulating these strategies. Consequently, no changes in published procedures for cleaning, disinfecting, or sterilizing need to be made.

Housekeeping

Environmental surfaces such as walls, floors, and other surfaces are not associated with transmission of infections to patients or health-care workers. Therefore, extraordinary attempts to disinfect or sterilize these environmental surfaces are not necessary. However, cleaning and removal of soil should be done routinely.

Cleaning schedules and methods vary according to the area of the hospital or institution, type of surface to be cleaned, and the amount and type of soil present. Horizontal surfaces (e.g., bedside tables and hard-surfaced flooring) in patient-care areas are usually cleaned on a regular basis, when soiling or spills occur, and when a patient is discharged. Cleaning of walls, blinds, and curtains is recommended only if they are visibly soiled. Disinfectant fogging is an unsatisfactory method of decontaminating air and surfaces and is not recommended.

Disinfectant-detergent formulations registered by EPA can be used for cleaning environmental surfaces, but the actual physical removal of microorganisms by scrubbing is probably at least as important as any antimicrobial effect of the cleaning agent used. Therefore, cost, safety, and acceptability by housekeepers can be the main criteria for selecting any such registered agent. The manufacturers' instructions for appropriate use should be followed.

Cleaning and Decontaminating Spills of Blood or Other Body Fluids

Chemical germicides that are approved for use as "hospital disinfectants" and are tuberculocidal when used at recommended dilutions can be used to decontaminate spills of blood and other body fluids. Strategies for decontaminating spills of blood and other body fluids in a patient-care setting are different than for spills of cultures or other materials in clinical, public health, or research laboratories. In patient-care areas, visible material should first be removed and then the area should be decontaminated. With large spills of cultured or concentrated infectious agents in the laboratory, the contaminated area should be flooded with a liquid germicide before cleaning, then decontaminated with fresh germicidal chemical. In both settings, gloves should be worn during the cleaning and decontaminating procedures.

Laundry

Although soiled linen has been identified as a source of large numbers of certain pathogenic microorganisms, the risk of actual disease transmission is negligible. Rather than rigid procedures and specifications, hygienic and common-sense storage and processing of clean and soiled linen are recommended (26). Soiled linen should be handled as little as possible and with minimum agitation to prevent gross microbial contamination of the air and of persons handling the linen. All soiled linen should be bagged at the location where it was used; it should not be sorted or rinsed in patient-care areas. Linen soiled with blood or body fluids should be placed and transported in bags that prevent leakage. If hot water is used, linen should be washed with detergent in water at least 71 C (160 F) for 25 minutes. If low-temperature($\leqslant$70 C [158 F]) laundry cycles are used, chemicals suitable for low-temperature washing at proper use concentration should be used.

Infective Waste

There is no epidemiologic evidence to suggest that most hospital waste is any more infective than residential waste. Moreover, there is no epidemiologic evidence that hospital waste has caused disease in the community as a result of improper disposal. Therefore, identifying wastes for which special precautions are indicated is largely a matter of judgment about the relative risk of disease transmission. The most practical approach to the management of infective waste is to identify those wastes with the potential for causing infection during handling and disposal and for which some special precautions appear prudent. Hospital wastes for which special precautions appear prudent include microbiology laboratory waste, pathology waste, and blood specimens or blood products. While any item that has had contact with blood, exudates, or secretions may be potentially infective, it is not usually considered practical or necessary to treat all such waste as infective (23,26). Infective waste, in general, should either be incinerated or should be autoclaved before disposal in a sanitary landfill. Bulk blood, suctioned fluids, excretions, and secretions may be carefully poured down a drain connected to a sanitary sewer. Sanitary sewers may also be used to dispose of other infectious wastes capable of being ground and flushed into the sewer.

Implementation of Recommended Precautions

Employers of health-care workers should ensure that policies exist for:

1. Initial orientation and continuing education and training of all health-care workers—including students and trainees—on the epidemiology, modes of transmission, and prevention of HIV and other blood-borne infections and the need for routine use of universal blood and body-fluid precautions for **all** patients.

2. Provision of equipment and supplies necessary to minimize the risk of infection with HIV and other blood-borne pathogens.

3. Monitoring adherence to recommended protective measures. When monitoring reveals a failure to follow recommended precautions, counseling, education, and/or re-training should be provided, and, if necessary, appropriate disciplinary action should be considered.

Professional associations and labor organizations, through continuing education efforts, should emphasize the need for health-care workers to follow recommended precautions.

Serologic Testing for HIV Infection

Background

A person is identified as infected with HIV when a sequence of tests, starting with repeated enzyme immunoassays (EIA) and including a Western blot or similar, more specific assay, are repeatedly reactive. Persons infected with HIV usually develop antibody against the virus within 6-12 weeks after infection.

The sensitivity of the currently licensed EIA tests is at least 99% when they are performed under optimal laboratory conditions on serum specimens from persons infected for ≥12 weeks. Optimal laboratory conditions include the use of reliable reagents, provision of continuing education of personnel, quality control of procedures, and participation in performance-evaluation programs. Given this performance, the probability of a false-negative test is remote except during the first several weeks after infection, before detectable antibody is present. The proportion of infected persons with a false-negative test attributed to absence of antibody in the early stages of infection is dependent on both the incidence and prevalence of HIV infection in a population (Table 1).

The specificity of the currently licensed EIA tests is approximately 99% when repeatedly reactive tests are considered. Repeat testing of initially reactive specimens by EIA is required to reduce the likelihood of laboratory error. To increase further the specificity of serologic tests, laboratories must use a supplemental test, most often the Western blot, to validate repeatedly reactive EIA results. Under optimal laboratory conditions, the sensitivity of the Western blot test is comparable to or greater than that of a repeatedly reactive EIA, and the Western blot is highly specific when strict criteria are used to interpret the test results. The testing sequence of a repeatedly reactive EIA and a positive Western blot test is highly predictive of HIV infection, even in a population with a low prevalence of infection (Table 2). If the Western blot test result is indeterminant, the testing sequence is considered equivocal for HIV infection.

TABLE 1. Estimated annual number of patients infected with HIV not detected by HIV-antibody testing in a hypothetical hospital with 10,000 admissions/year*

Beginning prevalence of HIV infection	Annual incidence of HIV infection	Approximate number of HIV-infected patients	Approximate number of HIV-infected patients not detected
5.0%	1.0%	550	17-18
5.0%	0.5%	525	11-12
1.0%	0.2%	110	3-4
1.0%	0.1%	105	2-3
0.1%	0.02%	11	0-1
0.1%	0.01%	11	0-1

*The estimates are based on the following assumptions: 1) the sensitivity of the screening test is 99% (i.e., 99% of HIV-infected persons with antibody will be detected); 2) persons infected with HIV will not develop detectable antibody (seroconvert) until 6 weeks (1.5 months) after infection; 3) new infections occur at an equal rate throughout the year; 4) calculations of the number of HIV-infected persons in the patient population are based on the mid-year prevalence, which is the beginning prevalence plus half the annual incidence of infections.

14S   MMWR   August 21, 1987

When this occurs, the Western blot test should be repeated on the same serum sample, and, if still indeterminant, the testing sequence should be repeated on a sample collected 3-6 months later. Use of other supplemental tests may aid in interpreting of results on samples that are persistently indeterminant by Western blot.

Testing of Patients

Previous CDC recommendations have emphasized the value of HIV serologic testing of patients for: 1) management of parenteral or mucous-membrane exposures of health-care workers, 2) patient diagnosis and management, and 3) counseling and serologic testing to prevent and control HIV transmission in the community. In addition, more recent recommendations have stated that hospitals, in conjunction with state and local health departments, should periodically determine the prevalence of HIV infection among patients from age groups at highest risk of infection (32).

Adherence to universal blood and body-fluid precautions recommended for the care of all patients will minimize the risk of transmission of HIV and other blood-borne pathogens from patients to health-care workers. The utility of routine HIV serologic testing of patients as an adjunct to universal precautions is unknown. Results of such testing may not be available in emergency or outpatient settings. In addition, some recently infected patients will not have detectable antibody to HIV (Table 1).

Personnel in some hospitals have advocated serologic testing of patients in settings in which exposure of health-care workers to large amounts of patients' blood may be anticipated. Specific patients for whom serologic testing has been advocated include those undergoing major operative procedures and those undergoing treatment in critical-care units, especially if they have conditions involving uncontrolled bleeding. Decisions regarding the need to establish testing programs for patients should be made by physicians or individual institutions. In addition, when deemed appropriate, testing of individual patients may be performed on agreement between the patient and the physician providing care.

In addition to the universal precautions recommended for all patients, certain additional precautions for the care of HIV-infected patients undergoing major surgical operations have been proposed by personnel in some hospitals. For example, surgical procedures on an HIV-infected patient might be altered so that hand-to-hand passing of sharp instruments would be eliminated; stapling instruments rather than

TABLE 2. Predictive value of positive HIV-antibody tests in hypothetical populations with different prevalences of infection

	Prevalence of infection	Predictive value of positive test[*]
Repeatedly reactive enzyme immunoassay (EIA)[†]	0.2%	28.41%
	2.0%	80.16%
	20.0%	98.02%
Repeatedly reactive EIA followed by positive Western blot (WB)[§]	0.2%	99.75%
	2.0%	99.97%
	20.0%	99.99%

[*]Proportion of persons with positive test results who are actually infected with HIV.
[†]Assumes EIA sensitivity of 99.0% and specificity of 99.5%.
[§]Assumes WB sensitivity of 99.0% and specificity of 99.9%.

hand-suturing equipment might be used to perform tissue approximation; electro-cautery devices rather than scalpels might be used as cutting instruments; and, even though uncomfortable, gowns that totally prevent seepage of blood onto the skin of members of the operative team might be worn. While such modifications might further minimize the risk of HIV infection for members of the operative team, some of these techniques could result in prolongation of operative time and could potentially have an adverse effect on the patient.

Testing programs, if developed, should include the following principles:

- Obtaining consent for testing.
- Informing patients of test results, and providing counseling for seropositive patients by properly trained persons.
- Assuring that confidentiality safeguards are in place to limit knowledge of test results to those directly involved in the care of infected patients or as required by law.
- Assuring that identification of infected patients will not result in denial of needed care or provision of suboptimal care.
- Evaluating prospectively 1) the efficacy of the program in reducing the incidence of parenteral, mucous-membrane, or significant cutaneous exposures of health-care workers to the blood or other body fluids of HIV-infected patients and 2) the effect of modified procedures on patients.

Testing of Health-Care Workers

Although transmission of HIV from infected health-care workers to patients has not been reported, transmission during invasive procedures remains a possibility. Transmission of hepatitis B virus (HBV) — a blood-borne agent with a considerably greater potential for nosocomial spread — from health-care workers to patients has been documented. Such transmission has occurred in situations (e.g., oral and gynecologic surgery) in which health-care workers, when tested, had very high concentrations of HBV in their blood (at least 100 million infectious virus particles per milliliter, a concentration much higher than occurs with HIV infection), and the health-care workers sustained a puncture wound while performing invasive procedures or had exudative or weeping lesions or microlacerations that allowed virus to contaminate instruments or open wounds of patients (*33,34*).

The hepatitis B experience indicates that only those health-care workers who perform certain types of invasive procedures have transmitted HBV to patients. Adherence to recommendations in this document will minimize the risk of transmission of HIV and other blood-borne pathogens from health-care workers to patients during invasive procedures. Since transmission of HIV from infected health-care workers performing invasive procedures to their patients has not been reported and would be expected to occur only very rarely, if at all, the utility of routine testing of such health-care workers to prevent transmission of HIV cannot be assessed. If consideration is given to developing a serologic testing program for health-care workers who perform invasive procedures, the frequency of testing, as well as the issues of consent, confidentiality, and consequences of test results — as previously outlined for testing programs for patients — must be addressed.

16S   MMWR   August 21, 1987

Management of Infected Health-Care Workers

Health-care workers with impaired immune systems resulting from HIV infection or other causes are at increased risk of acquiring or experiencing serious complications of infectious disease. Of particular concern is the risk of severe infection following exposure to patients with infectious diseases that are easily transmitted if appropriate precautions are not taken (e.g., measles, varicella). Any health-care worker with an impaired immune system should be counseled about the potential risk associated with taking care of patients with any transmissible infection and should continue to follow existing recommendations for infection control to minimize risk of exposure to other infectious agents (7,35). Recommendations of the Immunization Practices Advisory Committee (ACIP) and institutional policies concerning requirements for vaccinating health-care workers with live-virus vaccines (e.g., measles, rubella) should also be considered.

The question of whether workers infected with HIV — especially those who perform invasive procedures — can adequately and safely be allowed to perform patient-care duties or whether their work assignments should be changed must be determined on an individual basis. These decisions should be made by the health-care worker's personal physician(s) in conjunction with the medical directors and personnel health service staff of the employing institution or hospital.

Management of Exposures

If a health-care worker has a parenteral (e.g., needlestick or cut) or mucous-membrane (e.g., splash to the eye or mouth) exposure to blood or other body fluids or has a cutaneous exposure involving large amounts of blood or prolonged contact with blood — especially when the exposed skin is chapped, abraded, or afflicted with dermatitis — the source patient should be informed of the incident and tested for serologic evidence of HIV infection after consent is obtained. Policies should be developed for testing source patients in situations in which consent cannot be obtained (e.g., an unconscious patient).

If the source patient has AIDS, is positive for HIV antibody, or refuses the test, the health-care worker should be counseled regarding the risk of infection and evaluated clinically and serologically for evidence of HIV infection as soon as possible after the exposure. The health-care worker should be advised to report and seek medical evaluation for any acute febrile illness that occurs within 12 weeks after the exposure. Such an illness — particularly one characterized by fever, rash, or lymphadenopathy — may be indicative of recent HIV infection. Seronegative health-care workers should be retested 6 weeks post-exposure and on a periodic basis thereafter (e.g., 12 weeks and 6 months after exposure) to determine whether transmission has occurred. During this follow-up period — especially the first 6-12 weeks after exposure, when most infected persons are expected to seroconvert — exposed health-care workers should follow U.S. Public Health Service (PHS) recommendations for preventing transmission of HIV (36,37).

No further follow-up of a health-care worker exposed to infection as described above is necessary if the source patient is seronegative unless the source patient is at high risk of HIV infection. In the latter case, a subsequent specimen (e.g., 12 weeks following exposure) may be obtained from the health-care worker for antibody testing. If the source patient cannot be identified, decisions regarding appropriate follow-up should be individualized. Serologic testing should be available to all health-care workers who are concerned that they may have been infected with HIV.

If a patient has a parenteral or mucous-membrane exposure to blood or other body fluid of a health-care worker, the patient should be informed of the incident, and the same procedure outlined above for management of exposures should be followed for both the source health-care worker and the exposed patient.

References
1. CDC. Acquired immunodeficiency syndrome (AIDS): Precautions for clinical and laboratory staffs. MMWR 1982;31:577-80.
2. CDC. Acquired immunodeficiency syndrome (AIDS): Precautions for health-care workers and allied professionals. MMWR 1983;32:450-1.
3. CDC. Recommendations for preventing transmission of infection with human T-lymphotropic virus type III/lymphadenopathy-associated virus in the workplace. MMWR 1985;34:681-6, 691-5.
4. CDC. Recommendations for preventing transmission of infection with human T-lymphotropic virus type III/lymphadenopathy-associated virus during invasive procedures. MMWR 1986;35:221-3.
5. CDC. Recommendations for preventing possible transmission of human T-lymphotropic virus type III/lymphadenopathy-associated virus from tears. MMWR 1985;34:533-4.
6. CDC. Recommendations for providing dialysis treatment to patients infected with human T-lymphotropic virus type III/lymphadenopathy-associated virus infection. MMWR 1986;35:376-8, 383.
7. Garner JS, Simmons BP. Guideline for isolation precautions in hospitals. Infect Control 1983;4 (suppl) :245-325.
8. CDC. Recommended infection control practices for dentistry. MMWR 1986;35:237-42.
9. McCray E, The Cooperative Needlestick Surveillance Group. Occupational risk of the acquired immunodeficiency syndrome among health care workers. N Engl J Med 1986;314:1127-32.
10. Henderson DK, Saah AJ, Zak BJ, et al. Risk of nosocomial infection with human T-cell lymphotropic virus type III/lymphadenopathy-associated virus in a large cohort of intensively exposed health care workers. Ann Intern Med 1986;104:644-7.
11. Gerberding JL, Bryant-LeBlanc CE, Nelson K, et al. Risk of transmitting the human immunodeficiency virus, cytomegalovirus, and hepatitis B virus to health care workers exposed to patients with AIDS and AIDS-related conditions. J Infect Dis 1987;156:1-8.
12. McEvoy M, Porter K, Mortimer P, Simmons N, Shanson D. Prospective study of clinical, laboratory, and ancillary staff with accidental exposures to blood or other body fluids from patients infected with HIV. Br Med J 1987;294:1595-7.
13. Anonymous. Needlestick transmission of HTLV-III from a patient infected in Africa. Lancet 1984;2:1376-7.
14. Oksenhendler E, Harzic M, Le Roux JM, Rabian C, Clauvel JP. HIV infection with seroconversion after a superficial needlestick injury to the finger. N Engl J Med 1986;315:582.
15. Neisson-Vernant C, Arfi S, Mathez D, Leibowitch J, Monplaisir N. Needlestick HIV seroconversion in a nurse. Lancet 1986;2:814.
16. Grint P, McEvoy M. Two associated cases of the acquired immune deficiency syndrome (AIDS). PHLS Commun Dis Rep 1985;42:4.
17. CDC. Apparent transmission of human T-lymphotropic virus type III/lymphadenopathy-associated virus from a child to a mother providing health care. MMWR 1986;35:76-9.
18. CDC. Update: Human immunodeficiency virus infections in health-care workers exposed to blood of infected patients. MMWR 1987;36:285-9.
19. Kline RS, Phelan J, Friedland GH, et al. Low occupational risk for HIV infection for dental professionals [Abstract]. In: Abstracts from the III International Conference on AIDS, 1-5 June 1985. Washington, DC: 155.
20. Baker JL, Kelen GD, Sivertson KT, Quinn TC. Unsuspected human immunodeficiency virus in critically ill emergency patients. JAMA 1987;257:2609-11.
21. Favero MS. Dialysis-associated diseases and their control. In: Bennett JV, Brachman PS, eds. Hospital infections. Boston: Little, Brown and Company, 1985:267-84.

22. Richardson JH, Barkley WE, eds. Biosafety in microbiological and biomedical laboratories, 1984. Washington, DC : US Department of Health and Human Services, Public Health Service. HHS publication no. (CDC) 84-8395.
23. CDC. Human T-lymphotropic virus type III/lymphadenopathy-associated virus: Agent summary statement. MMWR 1986;35:540-2, 547-9.
24. Environmental Protection Agency. EPA guide for infectious waste management. Washington, DC :U.S. Environmental Protection Agency, May 1986 (Publication no. EPA/530-SW-86-014).
25. Favero MS. Sterilization, disinfection, and antisepsis in the hospital. In: Manual of clinical microbiology. 4th ed. Washington, DC: American Society for Microbiology, 1985;129-37.
26. Garner JS, Favero MS. Guideline for handwashing and hospital environmental control, 1985. Atlanta: Public Health Service, Centers for Disease Control, 1985. HHS publication no. 99-1117.
27. Spire B, Montagnier L, Barré-Sinoussi F, Chermann JC. Inactivation of lymphadenopathy associated virus by chemical disinfectants. Lancet 1984;2:899-901.
28. Martin LS, McDougal JS, Loskoski SL. Disinfection and inactivation of the human T lymphotropic virus type III/lymphadenopathy-associated virus. J Infect Dis 1985; 152:400-3.
29. McDougal JS, Martin LS, Cort SP, et al. Thermal inactivation of the acquired immunodeficiency syndrome virus-III/lymphadenopathy-associated virus, with special reference to antihemophilic factor. J Clin Invest 1985;76:875-7.
30. Spire B, Barré-Sinoussi F, Dormont D, Montagnier L, Chermann JC. Inactivation of lymphadenopathy-associated virus by heat, gamma rays, and ultraviolet light. Lancet 1985;1:188-9.
31. Resnik L, Veren K, Salahuddin SZ, Tondreau S, Markham PD. Stability and inactivation of HTLV-III/LAV under clinical and laboratory environments. JAMA 1986;255:1887-91.
32. CDC. Public Health Service (PHS) guidelines for counseling and antibody testing to prevent HIV infection and AIDS. MMWR 1987;3:509-15..
33. Kane MA, Lettau LA. Transmission of HBV from dental personnel to patients. J Am Dent Assoc 1985;110:634-6.
34. Lettau LA, Smith JD, Williams D, et. al. Transmission of hepatitis B with resultant restriction of surgical practice. JAMA 1986;255:934-7.
35. Williams WW. Guideline for infection control in hospital personnel. Infect Control 1983;4 (suppl) :326-49.
36. CDC. Prevention of acquired immune deficiency syndrome (AIDS): Report of inter-agency recommendations. MMWR 1983;32:101-3.
37. CDC. Provisional Public Health Service inter-agency recommendations for screening donated blood and plasma for antibody to the virus causing acquired immunodeficiency syndrome. MMWR 1985;34:1-5.

Appendix D

MINI MENTAL STATE

I. ORIENTATION

Ask "What is today's date?" (Then ask specifically for parts omitted, e.g., "Can you also tell me what season it is?")

Ask "Can you tell me the name of this clinic (hospital)?" "What floor are we on?" "What city (town) are we in?" "What country are we in?" "What state are we in?"

II. REGISTRATION

Ask the subject if you may test his memory. Then say, "ball," "flag," and "tree" clearly and slowly, about one second for each. After you have said all 3 ask him to repeat them. This first repetition determines his score (0-3) but keep saying them until he can repeat all 3. If after 6 trials, he does not learn all 3, recall cannot be meaningfully tested.

III. ATTENTION AND CALCULATION

Ask the subject to begin with 100 and count backwards by 7. Stop after 5 subtractions (93, 86, 79, 72, 65). Score the total number of correct answers. If the subject cannot or will not perform this task, ask him to spell the word "world" backwards. The score is the number of letters in correct order. For example: dlrow=5, dlorw=3. Record how subject spelled "world" backwards.

Item 20 is scored only if items 15 thru 19 are blank.

	SCORE
I. ORIENTATION	
1. DATE	
2. YEAR	
3. MONTH	
4. DAY	
5. SEASON	
6. CLINIC (HOSPITAL)	
7. FLOOR	
8. CITY (TOWN)	
9. COUNTY	
10. STATE	
II. REGISTRATION	
11. "BALL"	
12. "FLAG"	
13. "TREE"	
14. # OF TRIALS _____	
III. ATTENTION AND CALCULATION	
15. "93"	
16. "86"	
17. "79"	
18. "72"	
19. "65"	
20. "WORLD" SPELLED BACKWARDS DLROW (SCORE 0-5)	

From Folstein, M.J., Folstein, F.E., & McHugh, P.R. (1975). Mini Mental State. *Journal of Psychological Research, 12,* 189–198. Used with permission.

MINI MENTAL STATE

IV. RECALL Ask the subject to recall the 3 words you previously asked him to remember. Score 0-3.	**IV. RECALL**	**SCORE**
	21. "BALL"	
	22. "FLAG"	
	23. "TREE"	
V. LANGUAGE Naming: Show the subject a wrist watch and ask him what it is. Repeat, using a pencil.	**V. LANGUAGE**	
	24. WATCH	
	25. PENCIL	
Repetition: Ask the subject to repeat, "No ifs, ands, or buts."	26. REPETITION	
3-Stage Command: Give the subject a piece of plain blank paper and say "Take the paper in your right hand, fold it in half, and put it on the floor."	27. TAKES PAPER IN RIGHT HAND	
	28. FOLDS PAPER IN HALF	
Reading: On a blank piece of paper, print the sentence "Close your eyes" in letters large enough for the subject to see clearly. Ask him to read it and do what it says. Score correct only if he actually closes his eyes.	29. PUTS PAPER ON FLOOR	
	30. CLOSES EYES	
	31. WRITES SENTENCE	
	32. DRAWS PENTAGONS	

Writing: Give the subject a blank piece of paper and ask him to write a sentence. It is to be written spontaneously. It must contain a subject and a verb and be sensible. Correct grammar and punctuation are not necessary.

Copying: On a clean piece of paper, draw intersecting pentagons, each side about 1 inch, and ask subject to copy it exactly as it is. All 10 angles must be present and two must intersect to score 1 point. Tremor and rotation are ignored.

TOTAL SCORE

ALL ITEMS EXCEPT No. 14 AND No. 20 ARE EACH SCORED 1 IF CORRECT AND 0 IF INCORRECT.

ITEM No. 20 IS SCORED 0-5

THE TOTAL SCORE IS THE SUM OF ITEMS 1 THROUGH 32 EXCLUDING No. 14.

TOTAL SCORE

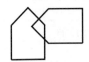

VI. LEVEL OF CONSCIOUSNESS
Rate the subject as to his level of consciousness.

VI. SUBJECT'S LEVEL OF CONSCIOUSNESS
CHECK ONE:

☐ COMA = 1   ☐ DROWSY = 3

☐ STUPOR = 2   ☐ ALERT = 4

Index

Note: Page numbers in *italics* refer to illustrations; page numbers followed by the letter t refer to tables.